Physical Evaluation and Treatment Planning in Dental Practice

Physical Evaluation and Treatment Planning in Dental Practice

Géza T. Terézhalmy, DDS, MA
Professor and Dean Emeritus, Case Western Reserve University School of Dental Medicine, Cleveland, Ohio, USA

Michaell A. Huber, DDS
Adjunct Professor, Department of Comprehensive Dentistry, UT Health San Antonio School of Dentistry, San Antonio, Texas, USA

Lily T. García, DDS, MS, FACP
Professor and Dean, University of Nevada, Las Vegas, School of Dental Medicine, Las Vegas, Nevada, USA

Ronald L. Occhionero, DDS
Professor and Associate Dean for Administration, Case Western Reserve School of Dental Medicine, Cleveland, Ohio, USA

Second Edition

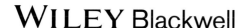

Registered Office
John Wiley & Sons, Inc., 111 River Street, Hoboken, NJ 07030, USA

Editorial Office
111 River Street, Hoboken, NJ 07030, USA

For details of our global editorial offices, customer services, and more information about Wiley products visit us at www.wiley.com.

Wiley also publishes its books in a variety of electronic formats and by print-on-demand. Some content that appears in standard print versions of this book may not be available in other formats.

Library of Congress Cataloging-in-Publication Data

Names: Terézhalmy, G. T. (Géza T.), author. | Huber, Michaell A., author. |
  García, Lily T., author. | Occhionero, Ronald L., author.
Title: Physical evaluation and treatment planning in dental practice /
  Géza T. Terézhalmy, Michaell A. Huber, Lily T. García, Ronald L.
  Occhionero.
Other titles: Physical evaluation in dental practice
Description: Second edition. | Hoboken, NJ : Wiley-Blackwell, 2021. |
  Preceded by Physical evaluation in dental practice / Géza T.
  Terézhalmy, Michaell A. Huber, and Anne Cale Jones with contributions
  by Vidya Sankar and Marcel Noujeim. 2009. | Includes bibliographical references and index.
Identifiers: LCCN 2021007898 (print) | LCCN 2021007899 (ebook) | ISBN 9781118646588 (paperback) |
  ISBN 9781118987513 (adobe pdf) | ISBN 9781118987506 (epub)
Subjects: MESH: Diagnosis, Oral–methods | Physical Examination–methods
Classification: LCC RK308 (print) | LCC RK308 (ebook) | NLM WU 141 | DDC 617.6/0754–dc23
LC record available at https://lccn.loc.gov/2021007898
LC ebook record available at https://lccn.loc.gov/2021007899

Cover Design: Wiley
Cover Image: © Gilitukha/iStock/Getty Images; © Courtesy of Lily T. Garcia; © David M. Bohnenkamp; © Guy Huynh-Ba

Set in 9.5/12.5pt STIXTwoText by Straive, Chennai, India

Printed in Singapore
M074168_110621

Contents

Preface to the Second Edition

It is an incredible honor to be asked to work on a second edition of a textbook. In effect, it is an opportunity to improve upon a concept that once in print, allows authors and contributors the ability to assess and review.

As we introduce the second edition of *Physical Evaluation and Treatment Planning in Dental Practice*, the authors acknowledge the true visionary force bringing this effort to fruition, our mentor and colleague Dr. Géza T. Terézhalmy. Dr. Terézhalmy has influenced many friends, colleagues, academicians, and professionals across dentistry and medicine. With his determination to improve on a solid concept, he invited a group of renowned, well-respected individuals to contribute to improving the content and expand the scope, all in an effort at building professional capabilities of those who directly care for patients. It is in the spirit of improving the quality of care that support for predictable, quality outcomes, improves the oral health and overall well-being of persons who seek expertise, compassion and care.

Géza's long and illustrious career has been underpinned by endless energy, academic discipline, and a passion to teach. He lives and teaches the motto of one of his favorite heroes, Sir William Ostler, to "never treat a stranger."

Learning physical evaluation of a patient from an overall health perspective, then adding the unique lens from dental specialists and discipline experts, provides fundamental information that focuses on the person seeking care. In a person-centered healthcare environment, this book is devoted to building capacity in oral healthcare.

Lily T. García

Preface to the First Edition

Learn to see, learn to hear, learn to feel, learn to smell, and know that by practice alone can you become an expert.

Sir William Osler

Diagnosis is the bridge between the study of disease and the treatment of illness. Making a distinction between disease and illness appears redundant because the words frequently are used interchangeably. However, diseases of the oral cavity and related structures may have profound physical and emotional effects on a patient, and a holistic approach to patient care makes this distinction significant. In oral pathology one studies disease; in clinical dentistry one treats illness. For example, necrotizing ulcerative gingivitis may be defined with special emphasis on the microbiological aspects of the disease, or one may speak of an inflammatory reaction featuring "punched-out" erosions of the interdental papillae. However, necrotizing ulcerative gingivitis is more complex. It is the totality of symptoms (subjective feelings) and signs (objective findings) that together characterize a single patient's reaction – not merely a tissue response – to infection by spirochetes. While disease is an abstraction, illness is a process.

Similarly, clinicians must recognize that systemic disease may affect the oral health of patients and to treat dental disease as an entity in itself is to practice a rigid pseudoscience that is more comforting to the clinician than to the patient. The diagnosis and treatment of advanced carious lesions afford little support to the patient if one overlooks obvious physical findings suggesting that the extensive restorative needs were precipitated by qualitative and quantitative changes in the flow of saliva secondary to an undiagnosed or uncontrolled systemic problem, or anti- cholinergic pharmacotherapy. The clinician with a balanced view of dentistry will recognize that caries is only a sign of disease and preventive and therapeutic strategies will have to be based on many patient-specific factors.

It is axiomatic that while dentists are the recognized experts on oral health, they must also learn of systemic diseases. Such an obligation is tempered only by the extent to which systemic diseases relate to the dental profession's anatomic field of responsibility, the extent to which illnesses require modification of dental therapy or alter prognoses, and the extent to which the presence of certain conditions (infectious diseases) may affect caregivers. Consequently, clinicians should not treat oral diseases as isolated entities. They should recall that physical signs and symptoms are produced by physical causes. Since physical problems are the determinants of physical signs and symptoms, these signs and symptoms must be recognized before the physical problems can be diagnosed and treated.

It is through the clinical process that clinical judgment is applied and, with experience, matures. Clinical judgment does not come early or easily to most clinicians. It is forged from long hours of clinical experience and a life-long commitment to the disciplined study of diseases and illnesses. Clinicians should study books to understand disease, study patients to learn of human nature and illness, and model mentors to develop clinical judgment. Ultimately, the experienced clinician will merge the science of understanding disease and the art of managing illness. These activities should be fostered by the clinician's sincere desire to minimize patient discomfort, both physical and emotional, and to maximize the opportunities to provide optimal care.

List of Contributors

David M. Bohnenkamp, DDS, MS, FACP
Prosthodontics
The University of Iowa College of Dentistry
Iowa City, Iowa, USA

Maria Cervantes Mendez, DDS, MS
Orthodontics
UT Health San Antonio, School of Dentistry
San Antonio, TX, USA

Joseph P. Connor, DDS
Restorative Dentistry
UT Health San Antonio, School of Dentistry
San Antonio, TX, USA

Anibal R. Diogenes, DDS, MS
Endodontics
UT Health San Antonio, School of Dentistry
San Antonio, TX, USA

Kevin M. Gureckis, DMD, ABGD, MAGD
Restorative Dentistry
UT Health San Antonio, School of Dentistry
San Antonio, TX, USA

Guy Huynh-Ba, DDS, MS
Periodontics
Private Practice
Bellevue, WA, USA

Theodoros Katsaros, DDS, MSD, FRCD(C)
Periodontics
Private Practice
Toronto, ON, Canada

Douglas E. Kendrick, DDS, FACS
Oral and Maxillofacial Surgery
The University of Iowa College of Dentistry
Iowa City, IA, USA

Fabricio B. Teixeira, DDS, MS, PhD
Endodontics
The University of Iowa College of Dentistry
Iowa City, IA, USA

Karen B. Troendle, DDS, MPH
Restorative Dentistry
UT Health San Antonio, School of Dentistry
San Antonio, TX, USA

Edward F. Wright, DDS, MS
Orofacial Pain
UT Health San Antonio, School of Dentistry
San Antonio, TX, USA

Zheng Xu, DMD, PhD
Pediatric Dentistry
University of Washington School of Dentistry
Seattle, WA, USA

About the Companion Website

This book also has a companion website:

www.wiley.com/go/terezhalmy/physical

This website includes:

- PowerPoints of figures

1

Introduction to the Clinical Process

Patients consult clinicians to obtain relief from symptoms and to return to full health. When cure is not possible, intervention to improve the quality of life is warranted. Consequently, oral healthcare providers' primary obligation is the timely delivery of quality care within the bounds of the clinical circumstances presented by patients. The provision of quality care will depend on timely execution of the clinical process.

1.1 Essential Elements of the Clinical Process

The clinical process represents a continuous interplay between science and art and may be conveniently divided into three phases.

Phase I

Phase I of the clinical process is physical evaluation and consists of eliciting a historical

Physical Evaluation and Treatment Planning in Dental Practice, Second Edition.
Géza T. Terézhalmy, Michaell A. Huber, Lily T. García and Ronald L. Occhionero.
© 2021 John Wiley & Sons, Inc. Published 2021 by John Wiley & Sons, Inc.
Companion Website: www.wiley.com/go/terezhalmy/physical

profile, performing an examination, obtaining appropriate radiographs, ordering laboratory tests, and, when indicated, initiating consultations with or referrals to other healthcare providers. The information obtained is systematically recorded. In order to optimize the yield, clinicians need to possess an inquiring mind, discipline, sensitivity, perseverance, and patience.

Phase II

Phase II of the clinical process involves an analysis of all data obtained during Phase I. Interpretation and correlation of these data, in the light of principles gained from basic biomedical and clinical sciences, will create the diagnostic fabric that will lead to a coherent, defendable, relevant, and timely diagnosis. This is an intellectual and, at times, intuitive activity. In making diagnoses, clinicians must recall their knowledge of disease.

Phase III

Phase III of the clinical process is centered around the timely development and implementation of necessary preventive and therapeutic strategies and communicating these strategies to the patient or guardian in order to obtain consent and to encourage compliance with and participation in the execution of the plan. In deciding on management strategies, clinicians must think in terms of illness and the total impact of a disease on a given patient and his or her immediate family.

1.2 Quality Management in the Clinical Process

A four-part control cycle (plan-do-check-act) introduced to industry in the 1930s is applicable to total quality management (TQM) in the clinical process and is reflected in the acronym CEAR (pronounced CARE):

Table 1.1 Activities intended to correct a problem identified by the control cycle.

- Reconsider the criteria (standard)
- Redesign the activities intended to achieve the criteria
- Review the assessment process
- Remediate without changing the criteria or the activities intended to achieve the criteria
- Reject the samples that do not meet the criteria
- Apply residual learning to the next control cycle

criteria-execution-assessment-response. Criteria are intended to maintain established standards. Ideally, standards should be based on knowledge derived from well-conducted trials or extensive, controlled observations. In the absence of such data, they should reflect the best-informed, most authoritative opinion available. Execution is the implementation of activities intended to meet stated standards. Assessment is comparing the impact of execution (outcome) against the stated standards. Response refers to the activities intended to reconcile differences between stated standards and observed outcome (Table 1.1).

TQM provides the fabric for a disciplined approach to work design, work practices, and constant reassessment of the clinical process. In TQM there is no minimum standard of "good enough"; there is only "better and better." Defects are signals that point to parts of a process that must be improved so that quality is the result.

Factors Affecting Quality

Amenities of Care

The amenities of care represent the desirable attributes of the setting within which the clinical process is implemented. They include convenience (access, availability of service), comfort, safety, and privacy. In private practice these are the responsibilities of the clinician. In institutional settings, the responsibility lies with the administrators of the institution.

Performance of the Clinician

The clinical process is a combination of intellectual and manipulative activities by which disease is identified and illness is treated. As we seek to define its quality, we must consider the performance of clinicians. There are two elements in the performance of clinicians that affect quality, one technical and the other interpersonal.

Technical performance depends on the knowledge and judgment used in arriving at appropriate diagnostic, therapeutic, and preventive strategies and on the skillful execution of those strategies. The quality of technical performance is judged in comparison with the best in practice. The best in practice, in turn, has earned that distinction because it is known or is believed to lead to the best outcome. The second element in the performance of the clinician that affects quality is interpersonal skills (see Section 1.3, Patient–Doctor Communication in the Clinical Process).

Performance of the Patient

In considering variables that affect the quality of the clinical process, contributions made by the patient, as well as by family members, must also be factored into the equation. In those situations in which the outcome of the clinical process is found to be inferior because of lack of optimal participation by the patient, the practitioner must be judged blameless.

Assessing Quality

Effective control over quality can best be achieved by designing and executing a clinical process that meets professional standards and also acknowledges patients' expectations. The information from which inferences can be drawn about quality may be classified under three headings: structure, process, and outcome.

Structure

In addition to the amenities of care discussed earlier, structure also denotes the attributes of material resources (e.g. facilities and equipment), human resources (e.g. the number and qualification of personnel), and organizational resources (e.g. convenience [access, availability of service], comfort, safety, privacy, methods of payment). Since structure affects the amenities of the oral healthcare setting, it can be inferred that good structure increases the likelihood of a good process.

Process

Process denotes what is actually done in the clinical process. It includes the clinician's activities in developing and recommending diagnostic, therapeutic, and preventive strategies; and the execution of those strategies, both by the clinician and the patient. Process also includes the values and virtues that the interpersonal patient–doctor relationship is expected to have (i.e. confidentiality, informed consent, empathy, congruence, honesty, tact, and sensitivity). In general, it can be assumed that a good process increases the likelihood of good outcome.

Outcome

Outcome denotes the effects of the clinical process on the identification and treatment of consequential problems, improvement in health, and changes in behavior. Because many factors influence outcome, it is not possible to determine the extent to which an observed outcome is attributable to an antecedent structure or process. However, outcome assessment does provide a mechanism to monitor performance to determine whether it continues to remain within acceptable bounds.

1.3 Patient–Doctor Communication in the Clinical Process

Poor skills in communicating with patients are associated with lower levels of patient satisfaction, higher rates of complaints, an increased risk of malpractice claims, and poorer health outcomes. Clearly, in the clinical process, the performance of clinicians as it relates to interpersonal skills is the very source of their vulnerability. The process of establishing a patient–doctor relationship, however, is not easy. To illustrate this point, let us consider the clinical process in dealing with a patient in pain, the most common complaint causing a person to seek the services of an oral healthcare provider.

Ideally, the clinician should initiate the clinical process in a quiet, comfortable, private setting and foster a warm, friendly, concerned, and supportive approach with the patient. However, this may be a challenging task since it is well-established that many patients experience anticipatory stress in the oral healthcare setting. Such stress may provoke patients to experience a state of disequilibrium or crisis characterized by anxiety, that is, an intense unpleasant subjective feeling and an inability to function normally. The sequence of events, which leads from equilibrium to a crisis situation (disequilibrium) and back to equilibrium, includes a hazardous event, a vulnerable state, a precipitating factor, an active crisis state, and a reintegration state.

Hazardous Event

A hazardous event is any stressful life event that challenges the patient's ability to cope. The experience can be either internal (the psychological stress of dental phobia) or external (such as a natural disaster, the death of a loved one, or the loss of employment). Clinicians may be unaware of such hazardous events and patients may not readily volunteer such information.

Vulnerable State

Depending on subjective interpretation, one person may see the hazardous event as a challenge, while another may see the same event as a threat. If one views the event as a threat, the increased physical and emotional tension may manifest itself as perceptions of helplessness, anxiety, anger, and depression.

Precipitating Factor

The precipitating factor (in our example, pain) is the actual event that moves the patient from the vulnerable state to the active crisis state. This event, especially when added onto other stressful life events (hazardous events), can cause a person to suffer a crisis. In susceptible patients, not only pain but even minor dental problems requiring a visit to the dentist can precipitate an active crisis state.

Active Crisis State

During the active crisis state, the patient is emotionally and psychologically aroused because of pain, negative self-critical thoughts about what brought him or her into the clinician's domain, unfamiliarity with the environment, and fear that the clinician will be judgmental or punitive. The model for crisis intervention has six characteristic phases and follows the acronym CRISIS: calm confidence, responsiveness, involvement, supportiveness, "I can" statements, and situation.

Calm Confidence

People who are in a crisis situation generally are not attuned to the words being spoken to them, but they are responsive to non-verbal communication. Behaviorally, calm confidence is displayed by establishing eye contact with the patient, by guiding the patient into the chair, or by touching the patient's shoulders. All of these measures reflect inner self-confidence and control over the situation. If the clinician is perceived as being calm and confident, the patient is more likely to calm down and give trust and control to the clinician.

Responsiveness

Responsiveness is conveyed through verbal communication. It requires a willingness to be directive and to give firm guidance while responding to both the emotional and oral healthcare needs of the patient. The clinician with empathy for the patient does not convey a negative value judgment and, therefore, builds rapport with the patient.

Involvement

A patient in crisis will exhibit behaviors suggesting helplessness or dependency, which might make the clinician feel all the more responsible. Clinicians must relinquish this sense of total responsibility and assist the patient to assume responsibility for his or her own health. The clinician can redirect responsibility by telling patients that their active involvement is needed for a successful long-term outcome. Positive encouragement increases the likelihood that patients will adopt the behaviors necessary to maintain their oral health.

Supportiveness

Listening to the patient relating his or her feelings, concerns, and experiences is a large part of being supportive. Expressing acceptance in a nonjudgmental style, such as sitting near the patient at eye level and nodding in an understanding manner, further conveys support. This does not imply that the clinician must agree with the ideas of the patient, but it does reflect a sense of support and concern for the patient.

"I Can" Statements

Individuals often aggravate a crisis situation by expressing negative thoughts such as "I can't handle this," "This is too much for me," or "I know this is going to be terrible." Here, the clinician's response may go a long way in determining a patient's success in developing coping skills. By saying nothing, the clinician tacitly agrees with and reinforces an unhealthy line of thinking. On the other hand, by teaching the patient to use positive self-statements, the clinician helps foster healthy coping skills.

Table 1.2 Primary goals of crisis intervention in the oral healthcare setting.

- Identify the problem
- Establish a working diagnosis
- Restore function (at least temporarily)
- Develop a plan for definitive treatment
- Help the patient to connect the current crisis with past ineffective behaviors
- Teach the patient new preventive healthcare skills

Examples of positive coping thoughts include "One step at a time," "I can handle this situation," or "I can handle this challenge." By positively confronting a crisis situation, the patient experiences less distress and is more responsive to intervention.

Situation

The situation is the crisis of the moment, and it reflects the physical and emotional state of the patient at that moment in time. It must be kept in mind that patients do not consult clinicians to obtain diagnoses, but to obtain relief from symptoms and to return to full health. When a cure is not possible, intervention to improve the quality of life is warranted. Successful resolution of the problem is often directly dependent on timely intervention. The situational component of the crisis mandates that the intervention produce both short-term and long-term results (Table 1.2).

Reintegration State

Reintegration refers to the transition back to equilibrium. Ideally, the patient feels that the clinician was responsive. The problem has been resolved in a timely fashion, function has been restored (at least temporarily), a plan for definitive treatment has been agreed upon, the current crisis has been successfully connected with past ineffective behaviors, and new preventive healthcare skills have been instituted.

1.4 Characteristics of the Patient–Doctor Relationship

Reflecting on the case of the patient in pain discussed above, it becomes clear that the characteristics that distinguish, promote, and maintain a healthy patient–doctor relationship are empathy, congruence, positive regard, and, as we shall see later, "due process."

Empathy

Empathy refers to the clinician's perception and awareness of the patient's feelings without participating in them. When the patient is sad, the clinician senses and acknowledges the sadness, but does not become sad. In contra-distinction, sympathy implies assumption of, or participation in, another person's feelings.

Congruence

Congruence relates to the matter of words and deeds conveying the same message. Patients will sense whether the clinician's words and deeds are congruent or convey divergent meanings. Similarly, if the patient says, "I am happy," but appears sad and dejected, the clinician should be alert to the discordant messages conveyed by what is heard and what is observed.

Positive Regard

Positive regard is the act of recognition and active demonstration to the patient that the clinician recognizes him or her as a worthy person. This means that the clinician makes a concentrated effort to get to know what the patient cares about; what makes the patient happy, sad, or angry; what makes the patient likable or unlikable; and identifies qualities that make the patient unique. In this process, the clinician transmits attitudes to the patient by the same unconscious word inflections, tones of voice, and body language by which the patient conveys underlying feelings to the clinician. The human qualities that the clinician and patient bring to the process of the patient–doctor interaction are crucial in either opening or closing the lines of communication (Figure 1.1).

1.5 Documentation of the Clinical Process

Attorneys, courts, and juries operate by the dictum "if it isn't written down, it didn't happen." Documentation of the clinical process should conform to state laws governing the practice of dentistry and the standards of care established by the American Dental Association and other relevant professional organizations.

Problem-Oriented Dental Record

Problem-oriented record keeping enjoys a significant degree of universality in both medical and dental settings. While there are many acceptable alternatives, the problem-oriented dental record facilitates the standardized

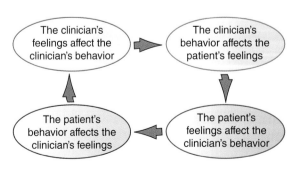

Figure 1.1 The patient–clinician interaction should be recognized and acknowledged in order to enhance the lines of communication.

Table 1.3 Essential elements of a progress note.

- Database
  - Subjective information
    - The reason for the visit, a statement of the problem (chief complaint), and a qualitative and quantitative description of the symptoms as described by the patient
  - Objective findings
    - "Measurements" (a record of actual clinical, radiographic and laboratory findings) taken by the clinician undistorted by bias
- Problem list
  - Assessment
    - Derived from the database, which leads to a provisional or definitive diagnosis, i.e. "needs" (existing conditions or pathoses
- Disposition
  - Plan
    - Proposed treatment plan and actual services (preventive, therapeutic) rendered to alleviate or resolve problems: include plans for consultation or referral to other healthcare providers, prescriptions written; and pre-and post-operative instructions

Table 1.4 The database.

Patient identification

Demographic data

A statement of the problem
   Chief complaint
      Qualitative and quantitative description of the symptoms provided by the patient
   Other reasons for the visit
     New patient
     Established patient
      Recall
      Emergency
      Follow-up
Historical profile
   Dental history
   Medical history
     Family history
     Social history
   Review of organ systems
Physical examination
   Vital signs, height, and weight
   Head and neck examination
   Examination of the oral cavity
   Radiographic studies
   Laboratory studies
Consultations
   Dental
   Medical
Risk stratification

sequencing of activities associated with the elicitation and documentation of demographic, diagnostic, preventive, and treatment planning, and treatment-related information.

Progress Notes

Logically structured progress notes provide the fabric to effectively document and promote continuing problem-oriented patient care. They facilitate the chronological recording of all patient encounters and are divided into three main components: the database (subjective and objective data), the problem list, and the disposition of the problem (Table 1.3).

The database is the product of those activities (e.g. history and physical examination) that are performed during Phase I of the clinical process (Table 1.4). These activities are effective to screen for significant disease, and the results are likely to be good reference points in the evaluation of future problems. Consequently,

screening measures should be validated and focused on identifying those problems that one cannot afford to miss.

A sample initial database that may be used to document the findings for the patient is shown in Tables 1.5 and 1.6. If using paper forms, the documentation must be legible, complete, and in ink. If corrections become necessary, they should be accomplished in a manner that does not obliterate the original entry, such as a single line drawn through the entry. In this regard, most electronic formats preserve or archive prior entries according to their unique time stamp. The use of symbols such as check marks and underlined or circled answers are best avoided. Responses to queries are to be recorded as "positive" (with appropriate elaboration), "negative," or "not applicable." The database is to be reviewed at all subsequent

Table 1.5 Documentation of initial historical profile.

NAME	ID NUMBER

Date of birth	Sex
Ethnic origin	Occupation
Address	City
State/Zip	Phone

Emergency contact   Name   Phone

                              Name   Phone

Insurance information

CHIEF COMPLAINT

DENTAL HISTORY

Frequency of visits to dentist?

Date of most recent radiographic examination?

Types of care received?

History of oro-facial injury (date, cause, type of injury)?

Difficulties with past treatment?

Adverse reactions (local anesthetics, latex products, and dental materials)?

MEDICAL HISTORY

Drug allergies or other adverse drug effects?

Medications (prescribed, OTC, vitamins, dietary supplements, special diets)?

Past and present illnesses?

Table 1.5 (Continued)

NAME	ID NUMBER

Last time examined by a physician (why)?

Females only (contraceptives, pregnancy, changes in menstrual pattern)?

Family history (DM, HTN, heart disease, seizures, cancer, bleeding problems, other)?

Social history (type, amount, frequency of tobacco, alcohol, and recreational drug use)?

REVIEW OF ORGAN SYSTEMS

Skin

  Itching

  Rash

  Ulcers

  Pigmentation

  Lack/loss of body hair

Extremities

  Varicose veins

  Swollen, painful joints

  Muscle weakness, pain

  Bone deformity, fractures

  Prosthetic joint

Eyes

  Conjunctivitis

  Blurred vision

  Double vision

  Drooping eyelids

  Glaucoma

Ear, nose, throat

  Earache

  Hearing loss

  Nosebleeds

  Sinusitis

  Sore throat

  Hoarseness

Gastrointestinal

  Eating disturbance

  GERD, abdominal pain, PUD

  Liver disease

  Jaundice, hepatitis

Genitourinary

  Difficulty urinating

  Excessive urination

  Blood in urine

  Kidney problem

  STDs

Endocrine

  Thyroid problem

  Weight change

  DM

  Excessive thirst

Hematopoietic

  Bruising/bleeding

  Anemia

  White blood cell problems

  HIV infection

  Spleen problem

Neurological

  Headaches

  Dizziness, fainting

Table 1.5 (Continued)

NAME	ID NUMBER
Respiratory	Seizures
Shortness of breath	Paresthesia/neuralgia
Coughing, blood in sputum	Paralysis
Bronchitis, emphysema	Psychiatric
Wheezing, asthma	Anxiety, phobia
TB, or exposure to	Depression
Cardiovascular	Other
Hypertension	Growth or tumor
Pain in chest, MI	Surgery
Congenital heart disease	Radiotherapy
Prosthetic valve/pacemaker	Chemotherapy

appointments and changes recorded in the progress notes of that day (Table 1.7).

A problem is anything that requires diagnosis or treatment or that interferes with the quality of life as perceived by the patient. It may be a firm diagnosis, a physical sign or symptom, or a psychological concern. Problems by their nature may fall into one of several categories (Table 1.8).

A complete database is so essential to the success of the clinical process that clinicians must consider an "incomplete database" as the number one problem until all required data have been obtained. An incomplete database may provide the basis for initial consultation with, and referral to, dental and medical specialists. Subsequently, the resolution of diagnostic problems may lead to further consultations with, or referrals to, colleagues, other healthcare professionals, and allied healthcare workers (see Chapter 16).

The clinical process culminates in the development of timely preventive and therapeutic strategies, along with the explanation of these strategies to the patient or guardian, in order to obtain consent and to encourage compliance with, and participation in implementing the treatment plan (see Chapter 16).

1.6 Designations and Abbreviations

The dental record is an important medico-legal document. Not only does it facilitates diagnosis, treatment planning, and practice management, it is also a valuable means of communication between the primary clinician and other providers, and it may be used in defense of allegations of malpractice and aid in the identification of a dead or missing person.

The record of the initial database shows missing teeth, existing restorations, and diseases and other abnormalities, while the chronological record of progress notes reflect treatment provided and diseases and other abnormalities that have occurred after the initial examination. The dental record is also a source of important information for the ongoing monitoring and evaluation of oral healthcare. Consequently, the charted record of the clinical process must be in conformity throughout the dental record.

Table 1.6 Documentation of initial physical examination.

NAME	ID NUMBER
VITAL SIGNS, HEIGHT, AND WEIGHT	
Blood pressure	Pulse
Respiration	Temperature
Weight	Height
HEAD AND NECK EXAMINATION	
Head	
Face	
Facial bones	
Ears	
Nose	
Eyes	
Hair	
Neck	
Lymph nodes	
TMJ	
Salivary glands	
Neurological findings	
INTRAORAL EXAMINATION	
Lips/commissures	
Mucosa	
Hard palate	
Soft palate/tonsillar area	
Tongue	
Floor of the mouth	
Gingivae	
Breath	

Table 1.6 (Continued)

Teeth/Occlusion/Periodontal status (PSR)	Remarks
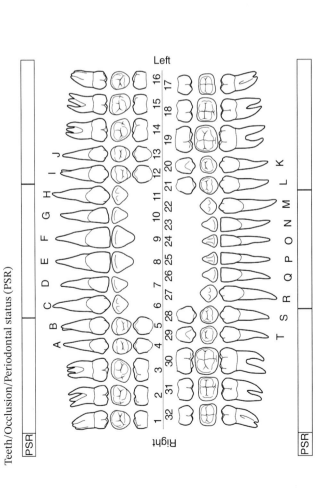	Example of an odontogram used to record missing teeth, existing restorations, and periodontal recordings (PSR).

Table 1.7 Progress notes.

PROGRESS NOTES	
Name:	ID number:

Date:

S	(subjective information): Reason for the visit; changes to the medical history
O	(objective findings): "Measurements" taken by the clinician (clinical, radiographic, and laboratory data; vital signs)
A	(assessment): diagnoses derived from subjective and objective data (reason for therapeutic intervention)
P	(plan): Treatment plan or actual treatment provided; prescriptions Written; post-operative instructions; disposition

Signature

Table 1.8 Problem categories with examples.

• Anatomic (developmental, acquired)	• Psychiatric (anxiety, depression)
• Physiological (pallor, jaundice)	• Abnormal diagnostic tests
• Symptomatic (pain, dyspnea)	• Risk factors (heart disease)
• Physical (paralysis)	• Socio-economic (uninsured)

Table 1.9 Alphabetical designation of primary teeth.

Tooth	Designation
Right maxillary primary second molar	A
Right maxillary primary first molar	B
Right maxillary primary canine	C
Right maxillary primary lateral incisor	D
Right maxillary primary central incisor	E
Left maxillary primary central incisor	F
Left maxillary primary lateral incisor	G
Left maxillary primary canine	H
Left maxillary primary first molar	I
Left maxillary primary second molar	J
Left mandibular primary second molar	K
Left mandibular primary first molar	L
Left mandibular primary canine	M
Left mandibular primary lateral incisor	N
Left mandibular primary central incisor	O
Right mandibular primary central incisor	P
Right mandibular primary lateral incisor	Q
Right mandibular primary canine	R
Right mandibular primary first molar	S
Right mandibular primary second molar	T

Table 1.10 Numerical designation of permanent teeth.

Tooth	Designation
Right maxillary third molar	1
Right maxillary second molar	2
Right maxillary first molar	3
Right maxillary second premolar	4
Right maxillary first premolar	5
Right maxillary canine	6
Right maxillary lateral incisor	7
Right maxillary central incisor	8
Left maxillary central incisor	9
Left maxillary lateral incisor	10
Left maxillary canine	11
Left maxillary first premolar	12
Left maxillary second premolar	13
Left maxillary first molar	14
Left maxillary second molar	15
Left maxillary third molar	16
Left mandibular third molar	17
Left mandibular second molar	18
Left mandibular first molar	19
Left mandibular second premolar	20
Left mandibular first premolar	21
Left mandibular canine	22
Left mandibular lateral incisor	23
Left mandibular central incisor	24
Right mandibular central incisor	25
Right mandibular lateral incisor	26
Right mandibular canine	27
Right mandibular first premolar	28
Right mandibular second premolar	29
Right mandibular first molar	30
Right mandibular second molar	31
Right mandibular third molar	32

Table 1.11 Standardized chart markings for missing teeth, existing restorations, and prostheses.

Missing teeth	Draw a large "X" on the root or roots of missing teeth.
Edentulous	Inscribe crossing lines, one extending from the maxillary right third molar area to the mandibular left third molar area and the other from the maxillary left third molar area to the mandibular right third molar area.
Edentulous arch	Inscribe crossing lines, each running from the uppermost aspect of the third molar area to the lowermost aspect of the third molar area on the opposite side.
Amalgam restoration	In the diagram of the tooth, draw an outline of the restoration showing size, location, and shape and block in solidly.
Nonmetallic permanent restoration	In the diagram of the tooth, draw an outline of the restoration showing size, location and shape.
Gold or other alloy restoration	In the diagram of the tooth, draw an outline of the restoration showing size, location, and shape and inscribe horizontal lines within the outline. If made of an alloy other than gold, indicate in the REMARKS section that the restoration is made of a metal other than gold (where possible, indicate type of alloy used).
Combination restoration	In the outline of the tooth, draw an outline of the restoration showing size, location, and shape; and partition at junction of materials used and indicate each as described in the amalgam restoration and nonmetallic permanent restoration above.
Porcelain or acrylic facings and pontic	In the diagram of the tooth, draw an outline of the restoration. Indicate in the REMARKS section that the facing or pontic is made of porcelain or acrylic.
Porcelain or acrylic post crown	In the diagram of the tooth, draw an outline of the restoration; outline approximate size and position of the post or posts. Indicate in the REMARKS section that the crown is made of porcelain or acrylic.
Porcelain or acrylic crown	In the diagram of the tooth, draw an outline of the restoration. Indicate in the REMARKS section that the crown is made of porcelain or acrylic.
Fixed partial denture	In the diagram of each tooth, draw an outline of the restoration; partition at junction of materials used. If made of gold, inscribe diagonal lines for both abutments and pontics. If made of an alloy other than gold, indicate in the REMARKS section that the restoration is made of a metal other than gold (where possible, indicate type of alloy used). Facing material should be indicated in the REMARKS section.
Removable prosthesis	Place a line over numbers of replaced teeth and describe briefly in REMARKS.
Root canal fillings	Outline each canal filled on the diagram of the root or roots of the tooth involved and block in solidly.
Apicoectomy	Draw a small triangle on the root of the tooth involved, apex away from the crown, the base line to show the approximate level of the root amputation.
Temporary restoration	In the diagram of the tooth, draw an outline of the restoration showing size, location and shape. If possible, describe the material in REMARKS.

Table 1.12 Standardized chart markings for diseases and abnormalities.

Caries	In the diagram of the tooth, draw an outline of the carious portion, showing size, location, and shape, and block in solidly.
Defective restorations	In the diagram of the tooth, outline the defective restoration and block in solidly.
Fractured tooth	Indicate approximate location of fracture with a zigzag line on outline of the tooth.
Partially erupted tooth	In the diagram of the tooth, draw an arcing line through the long axis.
Drifted teeth	Draw an arrow at the designating number of the tooth that has moved, with the point of the arrow indicating the direction of movement. Describe briefly in REMARKS.
Impacted tooth	Outline all aspects of each impacted tooth with a single oval. The long axis of the tooth should be indicated by an arrow pointing in the direction of the crown.
Radiolucency	Outline approximate size, form, and location.
Radiopacity	Outline approximate size, form, and location and block solidly.
Periodontal status	PSR scores (PSR periodontal probe with a 3.5 mm ball tip and a 3.5–5.5 mm color-coded band)
	0: Colored band of the probe remains completely visible in the deepest probing depth in the sextant. No calculus or defective margins are detected. Gingival tissues are healthy and no bleeding occurs after gentle probing.
	1: Colored band of the probe remains completely visible in the deepest probing depth in the sextant. No calculus or defective margins are detected. There is bleeding after gentle probing.
	2: Colored band of probe remains completely visible in the deepest probing depth in the sextant. Supra- or subgingival calculus or defective margins are detected.
	3: Colored band of probe is only partly visible in the deepest probing depth in the sextant.
	4: Colored band of probe completely disappears, indicating a probing depth of greater than 5.5 mm.

Table 1.13 Standard abbreviations and acronyms.

Acute necrotizing ulcerative gingivitis	ANUG	Oral health counseling	OHC
All caries not removed	ACNR	Oral surgery	OS
All caries removed	ACR	Panoramic radiograph	Pano.
Amalgam	Am.	Patient	Pt.
Anesthetic(thesia)	Anes.	Patient informed of examination findings and treatment plan	PTINF
Assessment	A	Periapical	PA
Camphorated paramonochlorophenol	CMCP	Pericoronitis	PCOR
Chief complaint	CC	Periodontal screening and recording	PSR
Complete denture	CD	Periodontics	Perio.
Copal varnish	Cop.	Plan	P
Crown	Cr.	Plaque control instructions	PCI
Curettage	Cur.	Porcelain	Porc.
Drain	Drn.	Post-operative treatment	POT
Electric pulp test	EPT	Preparation	Prep.
Endodontics	Endo.	Preventive dentistry	PD
Equilibrate(ation)	Equil.	Prophylaxis	Pro.
Eugenol	Eug.	Prosthodontics	Pros.
Examination	Exam.	Removable partial dentures	RPD
Extraction(ed)	Ext.	Restoration(s)	Rest.
Fixed partial denture	FPD	Return to clinic	RTC
Fluoride	Fl.	Root canal filling	RCF
Fracture	Fx.	Root canal therapy	RCT
Gutta percha	GP	Rubber dam	RD
Health questionnaire reviewed	HQR	Scaled(ing)	Scl.
History	Hx.	Subjective	S
Mandibular	Mand.	Surgical(ery)	Surg.
Maxillary	Max.	Suture(s)(d)	Su.
No significant findings	NSF	Temporary	Temp.
Objective	O	Topical	Top.
Operative	Oper.	Treatment(ed)	Tx.
Oral cancer screening exam	OCSE	Zinc oxide and eugenol	ZOE
Oral diagnosis	OD		

While there are acceptable alternatives, for purposes of brevity and exactness, the alphabetical designation of primary teeth (Table 1.9) and the numerical designation of permanent teeth are advocated (Table 1.10).

To record pathologic conditions and subsequent restorations of teeth, the following designations of tooth surfaces are used universally: facial (F), lingual (L), occlusal (O), mesial (M), distal (D), and incisal (I). Clinical circumstances may require the use of combinations of designations to identify and locate caries and to record treatment plans, operations, or restorations in the teeth involved. For example, 8-MID would refer to the mesial, incisal, and distal aspects of a right maxillary central incisor; 22-DF, the distal and facial aspects of a left mandibular cuspid; and 30-MODF, the mesial, occlusal, distal, and facial aspects of a right mandibular first molar.

When charting missing teeth, existing restorations, and prostheses as part of initial documentation of the database (Table 1.11); when charting diseases and abnormalities (Table 1.12); or when charting treatment completed (Table 1.11), standardized chart markings will further facilitate efficient continuity of care and may establish forensic identification.

Finally, when writing progress notes, the use of standard abbreviations and acronyms may be desirable for expediency (Table 1.13). In addition, the use of well-known medical and scientific signs and symbols, such as Rx, WNL, BP, H_2O, and others, is recommended.

1.7 Summary

It is axiomatic that in the clinical process the primary customer is the patient. However, the customer may also be a member of one's own organization (associates, staff) or individuals/organizations outside the institution (consultants, insurance companies, lawyers) who are "downstream" in the clinical process and must work with the product that is handed down to them. The licensed dental practitioner is solely responsible for all patient care-related activities including those legally provided by auxiliary personnel. This includes obtaining and documenting the patient's history, performing the physical examination, establishing diagnoses, developing and implementing preventive and therapeutic strategies, and properly documenting all services rendered and pertinent communications with patients.

Suggested Reading

American Dental Association. (2010). Council on Dental Practice Division of Legal Affairs. Dental Records. ADA: Chicago, IL. Available at: www.ada.org.

Chambers, D.W. (1998). TQM: the essential concepts. *J. Am. Coll. Dent.* 65: 6–13.

Deming, W.E. (1975). On probability as a basis for action. *Am. Stat.* 29: 146–152.

Donabedian, A. (1988). The quality of care. *JAMA* 260: 1743–1748.

Glassman, P. and Chambers, D.W. (1998). Developing competency systems: a never-ending story. *J. Dent. Educ.* 62: 173–182.

Low, S.B. (1998). Incorporating quality management into dental academics: a case report. *J. Am. Coll. Dent.* 65: 29–32.

Schleyer, T.K.L., Thyvalikakath, T.P., Malatack, P. et al. (2007). The feasibility of a three dimensional charting interface for general dentistry. *J. Am. Dent. Assoc.* 138 (8): 1072–1082.

Swenson, G.T., Kohler, K.A., and Lind, J.L. (1998). The integration of TQM at park dental. *J. Am. Coll. Dent.* 65: 19–22.

Tamblyn, R., Abramowitz, M., Dauphine, D. et al. (2007). Physician scores on a national clinical skills examination as predictors of complaints to medical regulatory authorities. *JAMA* 298 (9): 993–1001.

Waterman, B.D. (1998). Profile of TQM in a dental practice. *J. Am. Coll. Dent.* 65: 14–18.

2

The Historical Profile

"Never treat a stranger." Sir William Osler's statement is especially applicable to the practice of dentistry, in which the physical and emotional ability of the patient to undergo and respond to dental care is determined primarily by reviewing the medical/dental history. An initial historical profile (see Table 1.5) should identify the patient; determine the chief complaint; reflect the dental history; document drug allergies or other adverse drug effects; identify medications, vitamins, dietary supplements, or special diets; and provide a record of past and present illness, major hospitalizations, and a review of major organ systems. The historical profile shall be reviewed with the patient at each subsequent appointment

Physical Evaluation and Treatment Planning in Dental Practice, Second Edition.
Géza T. Terézhalmy, Michaell A. Huber, Lily T. García and Ronald L. Occhionero.
© 2021 John Wiley & Sons, Inc. Published 2021 by John Wiley & Sons, Inc.
Companion Website: www.wiley.com/go/terezhalmy/physical

and any new information obtained should be documented in the progress notes (see Table 1.7).

The current trend among dental practitioners is to use a combined printed and oral approach to establish the historical profile of a patient. A written questionnaire will elicit information that may be omitted by oral inquiry. Oral communication will provide important insight into a patient's feelings about past, present, and future illnesses and courses of treatment. This process is critical to the patient–doctor relationship and establishment of the rapport that precedes successful treatment.

Clinicians must be aware of the patient's overt and hidden concerns and develop a sense of the patient's reliability as an interpreter and reporter of events. Patients may suppress some information purposely or unknowingly. They may under-report other experiences or present them in a context that is less disconcerting than might be appropriate. Circumstances that may be of concern to clinicians might not be seen as unusual to patients.

Practitioners must be compulsive in compiling data, directing careful attention to the obvious and maintaining sensitivity to the less obvious "soft" clues that may be revealed in the history. An appreciation of the patient's perspective and an attitude of friendliness and respect will go a long way in assuring the patient's cooperation in gathering information.

Failure to obtain an initial historical profile, or to update it regularly, is not an excuse for being unaware of a patient's physical and emotional problems. Responses should be explored to determine whether the patient understands the question, is certain of the answer, and appreciates the importance of the question and the answer in the context of the care to be provided.

If the patient is confused, the dentist has an obligation to educate the patient to respond to questions, or the dentist may need to seek the necessary information from an additional informant. In all cases, the dentist should reduce those responses to writing. Failure to document and correctly interpret the historical profile of a patient may have devastating effects for the patient and the clinician.

2.1 Patient Identification

The basic biographical data should include the patient's name, age, sex, ethnic extraction, marital status, occupation, and place of residence. The date of the evaluation also must be recorded. Not only are these items essential for patient identification but also they may provide invaluable background information for the differential diagnosis of certain conditions, or identify patients in a high-risk category for a variety of diseases. For example, healthcare workers, military personnel, immigrants from developing countries, and people who work or live in institutions should be considered at higher risk for harboring certain infectious or communicable diseases.

2.2 Chief Complaint (Problem)

The clinician must record the patient's description of signs and symptoms associated with the current oral condition in a logical sequence. He/she should begin with the chief complaint, stated in the patient's own words. An attempt should be made to determine why the patient is consulting the dentist today and not yesterday or tomorrow. The answer may reveal an important clue to the severity of pain, underlying emotional problems, or other matters that are important in the overall understanding of the patient's illness.

Did acute symptoms prompt the visit, or was it the desire for a check-up because a neighbor, friend, or another family member was told they have oral cancer or have been diagnosed with HIV infection? The dentist should remember that a patient's expressed reason for seeking advice might mask underlying concerns. After an understandable statement of the chief complaint has been elicited, the chronology of the illness should be delineated.

Character of the Problem

The most common complaint causing a person to seek the services of a healthcare provider is pain. Determine its character. Is it sharp or dull? Is it pain or is it merely discomfort? Does it appear suddenly and disappear quickly, or does it gradually increase in intensity and subside slowly? A lesion should be inspected. Is it white, red, pigmented, ulcerative, vesicular, bullous, exophytic, or a combination of these various characteristics? Admittedly, this observation is part of the examination, not the history, but there are at least two good reasons for doing it at this point in time. First, it establishes the dentist's concern for the patient's problems, and second, it may suggest additional questions to be asked during the history-taking process.

Duration and Progression of the Problem

A number of questions should be considered. How long has the condition associated with the patient's chief complaint been present? Has the problem developed slowly or rapidly? Some conditions are characterized by a sudden onset, but others begin slowly and insidiously. Have the symptoms become worse or better? Are they better at times and worse at other times?

Domain of the Problem

One must determine whether the pain or discomfort remains localized or radiates to other anatomic locations. When dealing with a lesion, the clinician should determine if one specific area is affected or is it more wide-spread? This information is often helpful as certain diseases exhibit characteristic patterns of distribution.

Relationship Between Physiologic Function and the Problem

One should evaluate the effects of normal activities on the symptoms. What is the effect of the problem on mastication? Are the symptoms worse when the patient is chewing? In some instances, mastication relieves symptoms; in others, it aggravates them. Similar insights into the effects of swallowing, drinking, and speaking on the symptoms should be obtained.

2.3 Dental History

Important elements of a past dental history include frequency of visits to the dentist, history of radiographic examinations, type of care received in the past, history of oro-facial injuries, and difficulties with past treatment. A history of adverse reactions to local anesthetic agents, latex products (e.g. gloves, rubber dam), or other dental materials should also be investigated.

Note the attitude of the patient toward previous dentists and therapeutic interventions. Is this a patient who will never be satisfied no matter the skill of the clinician, or does the patient have significant undiagnosed problems that form the basis of the chief complaint? What is the patient's dental IQ and what priority is the patient likely to place on home care following periodontal surgery or extensive restorative care?

2.4 Medical History

The oral healthcare provider should document a history of allergic drug reactions and other adverse drug effects and investigate whether drugs or medications are being taken. Many patients habitually take drugs for minor complaints, a practice that should be documented carefully. Patients often do not recognize nonprescription medications as drugs and, therefore, do not mention the habitual use of aspirin, decongestants, antihistamines, vitamins, and many other over-the-counter medications. The clinician should inquire about dietary supplements or special diets the patient may be on. Immunosuppressant therapy may place a patient in the high-risk category for many viral, fungal, and bacterial infections and de novo malignancies.

The dentist should inquire about the patient's self-perceived general health and summarize past and present medical conditions. Significant hereditary or developmental abnormalities must be documented. Previous operations, injuries, accidents, and hospitalizations should be recorded, as well as comments about anesthesia, drug reactions, blood transfusions, or transmissible diseases. A history of repeated hospitalizations for the same condition, failure of an infection to resolve following therapy, recurrent infections with the same pathogen, and infection with unusual organisms, especially in the absence of "hard" signs of infection, may be suggestive of immunodeficiency (hereditary, acquired, or therapeutic).

2.5 Family History

Most diseases develop as a consequence of a multitude of internal or external contributing or causative factors. It is well established that some individuals exhibit a genetic predisposition or susceptibility to a given disease. Common examples which may run in families include cancer, diabetes mellitus (DM), cardiovascular diseases, mental health and asthma. Other diseases occur as a consequence of single genetic mutation, which predictably cause disease that may be passed down from generation to generation.

Commonly occurring examples of hereditary conditions include thalassemia, sickle cell anemia, hemophilia, cystic fibrosis, Fragile X syndrome and Huntington's disease. Finally, acquired infectious diseases may be transmitted from one family member to another, some requiring only casual contact, while others are transmitted only through repeated, intimate encounters (sometimes associated with child abuse).

Because of the frequency of facial and intraoral injuries and/or the presence of suspected sexually transmitted diseases associated with family violence (child abuse, elder abuse, spouse abuse), the oral healthcare provider is often the first professional to encounter the victim. While obtaining the history, careful attention must be paid to the explanation provided by the patient or other family members providing input. Look for any inconsistencies or behaviors suggestive of reluctance to provide information. Note nonverbal behaviors, which may not match verbal statements. Any suspicion of abuse should be reported to the appropriate local or state agency in accordance with local regulations.

2.6 Social History

The personal habits of patients may reveal important clues to diagnosis. Excessive use of tobacco and alcohol may produce symptoms whose significance is lost without knowledge of a patient's smoking and drinking habits. The daily use of tobacco products should be recorded in numbers of cigars, cigarettes (packs), or pipefuls smoked. Alcohol abuse is unequivocally associated with problems such as child abuse, fatal traffic accidents, homicides, rapes, and suicides.

Alcohol consumption should be recorded in terms of quantity and type over a specific period of time. Since patients with alcoholism are especially prone to certain diseases, it is important not to overlook this particular finding. The simple question "when was the last time you had more than X drinks in 1 day?" where X equals five for men and four for women should be asked as part of the interview. A response of "within the past 3 months" usually indicates the patient has a drinking problem and should undergo further assessment.

The patient's social history may also alert the clinician to the presence of environmental and cultural factors that may significantly influence the patient's general health and provide insight into the patient's personality and emotional state. A history of recreational drug use, frequent moves, sexual promiscuity (whether homosexual, bisexual, or heterosexual), frequent travels to developing countries, or recent immigration into the United States may signify a high risk for exposure to infectious diseases.

Information about educational, social, religious, and economic background and feelings of achievement or frustration can provide important insight into understanding the patient as a person. From this information, one can assess which factors might have a bearing on the current problem and whether they might be supportive or stressful influences.

2.7 Review of Organ Systems

The chief complaint and the medical, family, and social histories of the patient should guide the clinician to investigate areas of special concern. All signs and symptoms related to specific organ systems should be recorded. The status of organ systems may suggest the presence of concomitant systemic conditions, contribute to the diagnostic process, and influence projected treatment protocols and prognosis.

Skin

Itching, Rash, and Ulcers

An important cause of pruritus, especially associated with a bitter metallic taste and burning tongue, may be psychogenic (e.g. a reaction to stress and strain). Pruritus without a visible rash may be a reaction to drugs, such as aspirin, opiates and their derivatives, heroin, or amphetamines. Generalized pruritus is frequently the first sign of biliary cirrhosis and may occur many months before the onset

of jaundice. It may also be associated with carcinoma or a hematological disorder such as polycythemia, Hodgkin's lymphoma, or T-cell lymphoma (Sezary syndrome). Patients with pruritus in association with obvious skin lesions, such as papules, vesicles, bullae, or ulcerations, should be referred to a dermatologist. Many of these disorders require specialized dermatological approaches to establish the diagnosis.

Pigmentations

Vitiligo is an acquired disorder characterized by localized or generalized hypomelanosis of the skin and hair. Its etiopathogenesis is poorly understood but likely involves multiple overlapping pathogenic mechanisms. When localized, hypomelanosis of the skin and hair may be restricted to one region, such as the scalp. When generalized, the pattern of hypomelanosis is quite typical, with lesions evident on the face and neck coupled with loss of pigment in the hair.

Neurofibromatosis (von Recklinghausen disease) is inherited as an autosomal dominant trait. It is characterized by the appearance of numerous cutaneous café-au-lait spots. These lesions most commonly occur on the trunk and vary in diameter from less than 1 cm to more than 15 cm. The presence of six or more café-au-lait spots, each with a diameter greater than 1.5 cm (> 0.5 cm in children), is highly suggestive of neurofibromatosis even without a familial history of the disease.

Peutz–Jeghers syndrome is an autosomal dominant trait associated with intestinal polyposis and mucocutaneous pigmentation. The polyposis is most frequent in the ileum and jejunum and the mucocutaneous hypermelanosis is most noticeable in periorificial sites and the oral mucosa. It is now recognized that patients with Peutz–Jeghers syndrome are at increased risk for developing both gastrointestinal and nongastrointestinal malignancies.

Diffuse brown hypermelanosis is a striking feature of primary adrenocortical insufficiency

(Addison's disease). Most cases are caused by an autoimmune process or infiltration of the gland by an infectious agent (HIV, *Mycobacterium tuberculosis*). There is significant accentuation of pigmentation in certain mucocutaneous areas, namely along pressure points and oral mucous membranes. These patients are hypotensive and respond poorly to stress associated with infection, surgery, or trauma. An identical type of diffuse hyperpigmentation also has been reported as a sequela of adrenalectomy in patients with Cushing's disease (Nelson syndrome). A third example of an Addisonian type of hypermelanosis has been reported in patients with pancreatic and lung tumors. This phenomenon is known as a paraneoplastic syndrome.

In certain chronic nutritional deficiencies, splotches of dirty-brown hyperpigmentation may appear, especially on the trunk. Patients with protein deficiency may demonstrate a change in hair color, first to reddish brown and eventually to gray. In other selective deficiencies, such as sprue (faulty absorption of fats and carbohydrates), the hypermelanosis may be distributed over any area of the body, whereas in pellagra (niacin deficiency), it is limited to skin that is exposed to light or irritation. In vitamin B_{12} deficiency, the hair loses its original color and becomes gray and there is a diffuse cutaneous distribution of hypermelanosis.

Lack or Loss of Body Hair

Male-pattern baldness is inevitable in the presence of androgenic stimuli in patients with a genetic predisposition to baldness. The hypopituitary dwarf may completely lack hair, while patients with acquired hypopituitary states rapidly lose hair from the axillae, pubis, and, at times, the scalp. In congenital cretinism, lanugo hair may be retained, but the scalp hair is sparse and dry. In adults, hypothyroidism causes a decrease in secondary sexual or hormonal hair, in addition to the characteristic loss of the lateral third of the eyebrows. The loss of scalp hair in a male pattern along

with an increase in body and facial hair may be due to increased production of adrenal androgens (Cushing's syndrome) or exogenous adrenocorticotropic hormone administration.

In women, a temporary postpartum increase in hair loss is normal. The prolonged growth phase resulting from hormonal stimulation during pregnancy ends after delivery and a synchronized onset of the resting phase occurs in the scalp hair follicles. Prolonged febrile illnesses, systemic lupus erythematosus, dermatomyositis, severe cachexia, and lymphomas also may be associated with hair loss. Permanent hair loss on the extensor surfaces of the fingers is an early sign of systemic scleroderma.

Superficial ringworm infections of the scalp, deep pyogenic infections, and severe herpes zoster are associated with permanent hair loss in the affected area. Permanent alopecia may occur in lesions of discoid lupus erythematosus, localized scleroderma, and sarcoidosis, usually involving the scalp and eyebrows. Ionizing radiation in large doses causes permanent hair loss. Transient hair loss may be caused by certain medications such as antimetabolites, heparin, coumarin, and excessive doses of vitamin A.

Extremities

Swollen or Painful Joints

The causes of joint disorders are numerous and include traumatic, infectious, metabolic, immunologic, and neoplastic processes. Joint disorders may produce pain, stiffness, swelling, redness, increased warmth, or limitation of motion. Edema associated with heart failure tends to be most extensive in the ankles and accentuated in the evening, a feature determined largely by posture. Other evidence of heart disease usually indicates the pathogenesis of edema.

Muscle Weakness and Pain

Reduced strength of contraction, diminished power with single contractions, and repeated contractions are indubitable signs of muscle disease. In most of these diseases, some of the muscles are affected and others are spared. Each disease exhibits its own pattern. Ocular palsies are seen more or less exclusively as diplopia (double vision), ptosis (drooping eyelids), or strabismus (deviation of the eye that cannot be overcome by the patient).

Facial palsy is seen as an inability to close the eyes or smile and expose the teeth. Bulbar palsy is seen as dysphonia, dysarthria, and dysphasia, with or without a hanging jaw or facial weakness. Cervical palsy is often seen as the hanging-head syndrome, which is defined as an inability to lift the head from a pillow.

Bone Deformities or Fractures

Bone is a dynamic tissue that is remodeling itself throughout life. The response of bone to injuries, such as fracture, infection, interruption of blood supply, and the presence of expanding lesions, is relatively limited. Dead bone must be resorbed and new bone formed. Even in an architecturally disruptive disorder, remodeling appears to be dictated by mechanical forces. Disorders involving osseous tissues are associated with calcium, phosphorus, calcitonin, vitamin D, and parathyroid hormone interactions.

Prosthetic Joints

Of the many potential complications after total joint replacement, infection is by far one of the most catastrophic. The circumstantial association reported between certain invasive dental procedures and subsequent infectious seeding of artificial prostheses remains an area of professional debate and oral healthcare providers must be aware of current guidance.

Eyes

Conjunctivitis

Conjunctivitis associated with burning, itching, and runny eyes might be apparent in patients with allergies (e.g. pollens, dust mites, dander), viral infection (e.g. adenovirus, HSV, EBV, VZV, influenza), and bacterial infection (*Staphylococcus aureus*, *Neisseria gonorrhea*, *Chlamydia trachomatis*). Other potential causes include Sjögren's syndrome and chemical burn.

Blurred Vision

The dentist should record whether the patient wears glasses or contact lenses. The appearance of black spots moving in front of the eyes, followed by nausea, is often the first symptom of pending migraine headache. Blurred vision may also result from cataracts (often aggravated by DM), Stevens–Johnson syndrome, or benign mucous membrane pemphigoid.

Double Vision

Diplopia occurs when the disparate points (visual receptors) are too far apart. The images formed are separate and do not fuse. Diplopia may occur when the area in the cerebrum responsible for visual acuity is compromised by trauma, stroke, or vascular abnormalities. It is also the predominant symptom of dysfunction of the optic nerve.

Drooping Eyelids

Paresis of the third cranial nerve (oculomotor) will result in ptosis (drooping of the upper eyelid). Ptosis and/or diplopia are the most frequently observed initial sign of myasthenia gravis, occurring in 85% of patients. Ptosis is an essential finding in Horner's syndrome (paralysis of the cervical sympathetic nerves characterized by ptosis, miosis, anhydrosis, and flushing on the affected side of the face).

Glaucoma

Glaucoma is characterized by increased intraocular pressure associated with progressive irreversible damage to the optic nerve, resulting in defects in the visual field. It is the second most common cause of blindness in the United States. The most common type is chronic primary open-angle glaucoma, in which the ocular pressure builds up painlessly and gradually over time. In contrast, the acute primary open-angle type of glaucoma is a medical emergency characterized by a sudden increase in intraocular pressure, ocular immobility, dilated pupils, and severe pain.

Ears, Nose, and Throat

Seasonal/Environmental Allergies

Patients with a history of seasonal or environmental allergies are often prescribed antihistamines and/or corticosteroid sprays to manage their condition. These medications may contribute to oral dryness and increase the risk of epistaxis. The most common cause of epistaxis is probably nose picking, which results in tearing of the rich network of veins (Kiesselbach plexus) in the anterior naris. Other conditions associated with epistaxis are upper respiratory tract infection, atheromas of the nasal vessels, hypertension, bleeding diatheses (e.g. thrombocytopenia, coagulopathies), polycythemia, rhinoliths, acute sinusitis (especially involving the ethmoid sinus), tumors of the nose or paranasal sinuses, nasal angiomas, hereditary hemorrhagic telangiectasia, and Wegener granulomatosis. The number of bleeding episodes along with the severity of epistaxis is frequently increased in patients taking antithrombotic agents or anticoagulants.

Earache and Tinnitus

Patients with a history of recurrent ear infections may exhibit pain referred to the dentition or temporomandibular joint, while pain of odontogenic or myofacial origin may mimic otitis media. Tinnitus, or ringing of the ears, is a purely subjective phenomenon affecting about 10% of adults, but often of no clinical significance. Potential causes include noise-induced hearing loss, presbycusis, wax in the external auditory canal, otitis media, or an adverse medication reaction. Commonly implicated medications are NSAIDs, loop diuretics, aminoglycosides, and chemotherapy agents.

Hearing Loss

The most common causes of middle ear deafness are otitis media, rupture of the eardrum, and osteosclerosis. Nerve deafness has many causes, including damage from rubella or syphilis. The auditory nerve may be affected by tumors of the cerebellopontine angle. Deafness also may result from a demyelinating plaque in the brain stem. Fullness, vertigo, tinnitus, and fluctuating hearing loss may be due to Ménière's disease, a rare nonsuppurative disease of the labyrinth.

Sinusitis

The most common predisposing factor for acute purulent sinusitis is a viral infection of the upper respiratory tract. This may lead to obstruction of the paranasal sinuses along with the development of localized pain, tenderness, and low-grade fever. Frontal sinusitis is characterized by pain over the forehead. Pain, swelling, and tenderness in the anterior portions of the maxilla characterize maxillary sinusitis. Ethmoid sinusitis is characterized by pain in the upper lateral areas of the nose, frontal headache, redness of the skin, and tenderness to pressure over the nasal bones adjacent to the inner canthus of the eye.

Sphenoid sinusitis is characterized by tenderness and pain over the vertex of the skull, mastoid bones, and occipital portion of the head. These manifestations usually clear as the viral disease subsides. In a number of instances, however, invasion by pyogenic bacteria supervenes and causes a purulent sinusitis to develop. The cause of chronic sinusitis may be the same as that for the acute form, but more than one pathogen may be present. A neoplastic lesion should be ruled out in patients who experience repeated episodes of acute sinusitis or who have chronic symptoms.

Sore Throat

A sore throat, regardless of the cause, is the outstanding symptom of acute pharyngitis. Approximately two-thirds of all acute illnesses are viral infections (e.g. coronavirus, rhinovirus, influenza) of the upper respiratory tract that demonstrate varying degrees of pharyngeal discomfort. Fifteen to 30% of pharyngitis cases are caused by Group A streptococci and less common bacterial causes include *N. gonorrhea, Corynebacterium diphtheria, Treponema pallidum*. Potential serious complications of acute pharyngitis are peritonsillar cellulitis and abscess. The persistence of pain in an enlarged firm tonsil, in the absence of an infectious process, warrants a biopsy. The presence of fever does not rule out a neoplastic lesion because the temperature may be elevated in lymphomas.

Hoarseness

Laryngitis is the most common symptom of a disorder involving the larynx and it often interferes with normal phonation. Although hoarseness is usually of short duration and associated with an upper respiratory infection, it may persist as a chronic complication of gastroesophageal reflux disease (GERD), allergies, or smoking. When hoarseness persists for more than two to three weeks, further medical assessment is indicated to rule out laryngeal cancer or a thyroid problem.

Respiratory Tract

Shortness of Breath

Dyspnea, difficult or labored breathing, is associated with abnormalities resulting in hypoxia, or even more commonly with disorders associated with excess carbon dioxide retention. It is a cardinal manifestation of diseases involving the respiratory and cardiovascular systems. Dyspnea that is present at rest or when performing a menial task is an early manifestation of left ventricular heart failure. Orthopnea and acute paroxysmal nocturnal dyspnea may also be present. The dyspnea of chronic obstructive pulmonary disease tends (COPD) to develop more gradually than that of heart disease.

Coughing

Cough is a defensive mechanism triggered by stimulation of a complex reflex arc consisting of inflammatory, mechanical, chemical, and thermal cough receptors. It is an explosive expiration that helps clear the tracheobronchial tree of secretions and foreign bodies. Acute cough (<3 weeks in duration) is usually caused by an upper respiratory tract viral infection. Subacute cough (three to eight weeks duration) is usually postinfectious and typically resolves without treatment. Chronic cough (>8 weeks duration) is usually caused by postnasal drip syndrome, asthma, or gastroesophageal reflux (GERD), alone or in combination. An estimated 5–20% of patients using angiotensin-converting enzyme (ACE) inhibitors develop a dry hacking cough. Finally, coughing is so common in cigarette smokers that it is often ignored or minimized. Any change in the nature and character of a chronic cough by a cigarette smoker should prompt an immediate diagnostic evaluation, with particular attention directed to the detection of pulmonary tuberculosis and bronchogenic carcinoma.

Hemoptysis

Hemoptysis, or blood in the sputum, may be evidence of a respiratory tract infection or a pulmonary neoplasm. A productive cough in the morning characterized by hemoptysis is highly suggestive of tuberculosis, especially if associated with fever or night sweats, chest pain, and weight loss. Although hemoptysis may occur during the course of a viral or bacterial pneumonia, its occurrence always should raise the question of a more serious underlying process.

Bronchitis and Emphysema

Chronic bronchitis and emphysema represent the two main clinical manifestations of COPD. Chronic bronchitis is defined by the presence of excessive bronchial secretions that persist for at least three months per year for at least two consecutive years. The patient has been classically described as being overweight, blue or red-blue around the face, and having distended neck veins and ankle edema.

Emphysema is defined by the permanent destructive enlargement of the airspaces distal to the terminal bronchioles. The patient with emphysema has been classically described as being thin, pinkish in color, and using their intercostal muscles to breathe. In reality, the patient with COPD may manifest features of both chronic bronchitis and emphysema. Significant risk factors for COPD are smoking, environmental pollutants, and α_1-antitrypsin deficiency. Oxygen must be used with care in patients with COPD because the respiratory center in the brain readjusts so that the basic stimulus to respiration becomes oxygen instead of carbon dioxide.

Wheezing and Asthma

Wheezing is a whistling sound made during expiration and usually occurs in association with asthma. Bronchial asthma is a respiratory disease characterized by inflammation of alveolar epithelium, hypersecretion of mucus, and bronchial smooth muscle spasm presenting as the triad of coughing, wheezing, and labored breathing (dyspnea). In its most common form, asthma is an episodic disease. Allergens, upper respiratory tract infections, exercise, NSAIDs, and emotional stress may provoke an asthmatic attack.

The association of aspirin-induced asthma, aspirin sensitivity, and nasal polyps is known as Samter triad. Dental treatment may also trigger a reaction in the hyperactive airways. A clinically significant decrease in lung function has been reported in up to 15% of children with asthma. Wheezing is regarded as the sine qua non of asthma.

Tuberculosis and Latent Tuberculosis

The lung is the most common target for infections with *Mycobacterium tuberculosis* (MBT) and two distinct forms of the tuberculosis are recognized. Active tuberculosis is characterized by a productive, chronic cough (more than three weeks in duration); fever, chills, and night sweats; loss of appetite, weight loss, easy fatigability; and hemoptysis. Ten to 42% of active tuberculosis patients have extrapulmonary disease. Patients co-infected with HIV often experience active tuberculosis which is more severe and atypical. The patient with active tuberculosis is infectious and thus managed by initial isolation and prolonged multidrug therapy.

Latent tuberculosis occurs far more commonly than active tuberculosis. In this scenario, the patient is able to immunologically contain the disease as an asymptomatic infection. The diagnosis of latent tuberculosis is established either by a tuberculin skin test or an interferon-gamma release assay. Unfortunately, an estimated 5% of the patients develop active tuberculosis within 18 months of their initial exposure and another 5% of patients with latent TB develop active disease throughout life. Immunosuppression, acquired or therapeutic, increases the risk of developing active tuberculosis. Patients at high-risk are prescribed preventive treatment to reduce the risk of reactivation, typically a 9–12 month course of isoniazid.

Cardiovascular System

Hypertension and Hypotension

Arterial blood pressure (BP) must be maintained at levels sufficient to permit adequate perfusion of the extensive capillary networks in the systemic vascular bed. Hypertension (HTN) is a sustained elevation of arterial pressure and is the number one risk factor for death throughout the world. HTN is typically asymptomatic but invariably causes secondary organ damage (i.e. cardiac, renal, and cerebrovascular). The goal in the management of HTN is to reduce morbidity and mortality by lifestyle modification and pharmacotherapy. This may be accomplished by achieving and maintaining systolic BP below 130 mmHg and diastolic BP below 80 mmHg, while also controlling other modifiable risk factors for cardiovascular disease. For every 20 mmHg systolic or 10 mmHg diastolic increase in BP, the risk of death from ischemic heart disease and stroke doubles.

Hypotension is generally defined as a systolic BP reading of 90 mmHg or less or diastolic reading of 60 mmHg or less. Hypotensive patients are at increased risk for syncope and severe hypotension can be life-threatening. Causes of hypotension include cardiovascular disease, endocrinopathies, pregnancy, septicemia, blood loss and dehydration. Several medications can lower the BP including diuretics, adrenergic blockers, tricyclic antidepressants, and erectile dysfunction drugs such as sildenafil.

Chest Pain and Myocardial Infarction

Chest pain is a common presenting complaint in healthcare, representing about 1% of initial presenting complaints. The three most common causes of chest pain are chest wall pain, costochondritis, and reflux esophagitis. Other causes include anxiety, pneumonia, pulmonary embolism, heart failure, and acute coronary syndrome (ACS). ACS is an umbrella term covering both unstable angina and myocardial infarction (MI). ACS occurs when there is inadequate oxygen supply to the myocardium, often due to organic narrowing of the coronary arteries secondary to atherosclerosis.

Angina pectoris is defined as chest pain that is described as being aching, heavy or squeezing and may affect the arms, jaw, neck, back or stomach. Angina pectoris may be either stable or unstable. Stable angina pectoris is usually precipitated by heavy exercise. Unstable angina pectoris may be spontaneous or precipitated mild exercise. The symptoms of MI are similar to angina pectoris but persist and often include additional symptoms such as dyspnea, diaphoresis, dizziness, and nausea. About 25% of MIs produce no pain and are "silent." Both unstable angina and MI within the last 60 days are major predictors for a cardiac event occurring in the future.

Congenital Heart Disease, Endocarditis, Prosthetic Heart Valve, and Heart Transplant

Certain cardiac conditions appear to be associated with a higher risk of infective endocarditis and there is concern that manipulation of the gingival tissue or the periapical region of teeth or perforation of the oral mucosa may further contribute to this risk. In an effort to address these concerns, the American Heart Association (AHA) periodically publishes consensus guidelines intended to prevent infective endocarditis. Oral healthcare providers must be aware of current recommendations.

Pacemakers

Cardiac pacemakers (intravascular or epicardial) or implanted cardiac defibrillators (ICD) are often placed in patients to override potentially life-threatening cardiac conduction abnormalities that may develop as a consequence of atherosclerotic heart disease, MI, or heart block. For these patients, antibacterial prophylaxis is not recommended because the risk of developing IE is negligible. However, patients with ICDs may be susceptible to electromagnetic interference generated by dental devices. Inhibition of pacing has been noted with electrosurgery units, ultrasonic scalers, and ultrasonic cleaners. The rate and rhythm of pacing appear not to be affected by dental handpieces, amalgamators, dental units and lights, endodontic ultrasonic instruments, sonic scalers, and radiographic units.

Gastrointestinal Tract

Eating Disturbances

Difficulty swallowing or dysphagia is estimated to affect about 15% of patients over the age of 65 years. Contributing conditions include neurologic diseases (e.g. stroke, dementia, myasthenia gravis, and cerebral palsy), rheumatologic diseases (e.g. progressive systemic sclerosis, Sjögren's disease), tumors, medications, irradiation and chemotherapy.

Patients with dysphagia are at increased risk of malnutrition and pneumonia.

Bulimia nervosa and anorexia nervosa are eating disorders that are 10 times more common in women than men. The bulimic patient can regurgitate at will, and as a consequence experience frequent episodes of acid reflux into the oral cavity. This in turn might result in chemical erosion of teeth in a peculiar pattern. Dramatic weight change is not an essential characteristic of bulimia. In contrast, the anorexic patient refuses to maintain body weight at or above the 85th percentile of expected weight. Any patient with a suspected eating disorder should be referred for medical evaluation.

Reflux and Gastroesophageal Reflux Disease

Virtually everyone experiences reflux at some time or another, such as after an overindulgent meal. This frequently occurring phenomena serves to help relief stomach distention, is short-lived, and not pathologic. However, excessive or extensive reflux can damage to the esophageal tissues resulting in GERD. The etiopathogenesis of reflux involves a complex interplay of esophageal sphincter function and esophageal epithelial tissue sensitivity to the digestive action of gastric juice.

The primary determinant of GERD appears to be a transient relaxation of the lower esophageal sphincter not induced by swallowing. Episodes of transient relaxation are more common after meals, in association with slow gastric emptying, and in the presence of increased intra-abdominal pressure. Transient relaxation of the lower esophageal sphincter is more likely to be followed by an episode of reflux when there is a hiatal pouch (hernia) containing retained gastric acid. GERD is further exacerbated by obesity and smoking (nicotine relaxes the lower esophageal sphincter).

Complications of GERD include peptic strictures due to scarring and esophageal hemorrhage. Additionally, persistent reflux disease may lead to metaplastic transformation of the esophageal squamous epithelium (Barrett's esophagus) and an increased risk of esophageal carcinoma. Oral manifestations of GERD may include a burning or itching sensation affecting the oral mucosa, mouth ulcers, erosion of tooth structure, altered salivary flow, halitosis, and bad taste.

Abdominal Pain and Peptic Ulcer Disease

Patients with abdominal pain relate classic patterns of pain distribution. Pain in the right upper quadrant may be a sign of liver disease, such as hepatitis; gall bladder dysfunction (cholecystitis); or carcinoma at the head of the pancreas. Pain in the right lower quadrant may result from acute appendicitis (McBurney point) or pneumonia in the superior aspect of the lower right lung lobe.

Pain in the left upper quadrant may result from an enlarged spleen or pancreatic involvement (carcinoma or inflammation of the tail of the pancreas). Pain in the left lower quadrant may be a sign of diverticulitis. In a diabetic patient, vague, diffuse abdominal pain associated with hyperventilation is a possible sign of a diabetic coma.

Peptic ulcer disease (PUD) typically affects the lining of the stomach and proximal small intestine (duodenum). The pain of a duodenal ulcer is localized to the right side of the abdomen, with a focal spot of tenderness, and a characteristic cycle of pain-food-pain relief-pain. Gastric ulcers produce a diffuse pain on the left side. The two most common causes of PUD are *Helicobacter pylori* infection and chronic exposure to NSAIDs.

Major complications of PUD are hemorrhage, gut perforation, or gastric outlet obstruction. Therapy for PUD is focused on eradicating *H. pylori* in the gut, prescribing a proton pump inhibitor or H_2 blocker, and reducing exposure to thrombolytic medications. All patients with abdominal pain require early and thorough evaluation because proper therapy often requires urgent action.

Liver Disease

The liver, the largest organ in the body, is involved in a myriad of essential metabolic processes to include the formation of bile, urea, plasma albumin, coagulation factors glycogen, and ketones. In addition, the detoxification of drugs and toxins, deamination of proteins, storage of glycogen, and excretion of drugs also occurs in the liver. Hepatic structural and functional abnormalities occur in chronic cirrhosis, hepatitis, and a variety of pathophysiologic states, including congestive heart failure and metabolic, inflammatory, toxic, infectious, and neoplastic diseases. Disease-induced morphologic and functional changes of the liver can adversely affect hemostasis, alter drug metabolism, and impair the immune response to infections.

Jaundice

Jaundice refers to the yellow discoloration of the skin, mucous membranes, and sclera resulting from increased concentrations of bilirubin in the blood. Bilirubin is a by-product of hemoglobin catabolism and clinical jaundice typically becomes evident once the bilirubin level exceeds 2.5 to 3.0 mg/dl. This water-insoluble molecule is attached to albumin and is conjugated with glucuronic acid in the liver, rendering it water-soluble.

The conjugated bilirubin becomes a constituent of the bile and is transported to the duodenum, where it gives the fecal matter its characteristic color. The predominance of conjugated or unconjugated bilirubin can pinpoint the metabolic problem as prehepatic (excess destruction of red blood cells), hepatic (hepatitis, cirrhosis, infectious mononucleosis, liver carcinoma), or posthepatic (cholelithiasis, carcinoma of the head of the pancreas).

Hepatitis

The major causes of hepatitis are alcohol, drugs, and viruses. Approximately 80% of viral hepatitis infections are caused by the hepatotropic viruses A (HAV), B (HBV), C (HCV), D (HDV), or E (HEV). Other viral agents that can cause hepatitis include the Epstein–Barr virus, cytomegalovirus, and human herpesvirus types 1, 2, and 6. Liver disease may also occur following infections with rubella, rubeola, coxsackie, varicella-zoster, and adenoviruses.

Because of their parenteral mode of transmission and ability to establish chronic infection, HBV and HCV are of particular concern for oral healthcare personnel. Hepatitis lasting for six months or more is generally defined as chronic and is classified according to the etiology and modified by the histologic status of the liver. Chronic HBV and HCV infection is estimated to cause 57% of cirrhosis cases and 78% of liver cancer cases.

Genitourinary Tract

Difficulty or Pain Urinating

Difficulty with urination (dysuria), with or without pain, may result from a wide variety of pathologic conditions. Common causes include cystitis, prostatitis, urethritis, post-streptococcal glomerulonephritis, and sexually transmitted diseases (e.g. gonorrhea). Dysuria may also be caused by trauma and prostatic enlargement (e.g. hypertrophy or carcinoma).

Blood in Urine (Hematuria)

Bleeding from the urinary tract, whether microscopic or gross, is a serious sign, and must be regarded with the same gravity as abnormal bleeding from any other body orifice. The most common cause of hematuria is acute cystitis, but it may also be caused by hypertension with secondary renal damage, acute glomerulonephritis, trauma, a toxic response to drugs such as acetylsalicylic acid or acetaminophen, bladder carcinoma, and gonorrhea.

Excessive Urination (Polyuria)

Polyuria is generally defined as the output of more than 3 L of urine per day. There are four important disorders, which may be associated with polyuria: DM, diabetes insipidus, acquired renal lesions, and psychogenic polydipsia.

Kidney Disease

Bacterial infections of the urinary tract are extremely common and most frequently affect women. Many of these infections resist treatment and are likely to recur. Lower urinary tract infections are known as cystitis and urethritis, and the most common causative organisms are colonic flora and gonococci. Upper urinary tract infections are known as pyelitis and pyelonephritis.

Chronic renal insufficiency, chronic renal failure, and end-stage renal disease represent a continuum and are most frequently associated with DM and hypertension. Impaired renal function affects both pharmacodynamic and pharmacokinetic mechanisms and may lead to significant drug toxicity.

Sexually Transmitted Diseases

Many sexually transmitted diseases have reached epidemic proportions. Syphilis, gonorrhea, chlamydia, herpes, condyloma acuminata (HPV), and HIV infection may present significant oral manifestations. Diagnosis requires a thorough review of the patient's medical and social histories, as well as an appreciation of potential oral manifestations.

Endocrine System

Thyroid Abnormalities

Thyroid hormone influences cellular growth, maturation, and energy expenditure. An obese patient who demonstrates symptoms of fatigue, drowsiness, cold intolerance, and poor memory and has physical signs that include dry, coarse skin and hair, a decreased heart rate, and slow reflexes may have hypothyroidism. Conversely, a patient who relates symptoms of headache, increased appetite, weight loss, and heat intolerance and has physical signs that include exophthalmia, increased heart rate, and agitation may have hyperthyroidism.

Weight Change

Causes of weight gain may include overeating, hypothyroidism, edema with congestive heart failure, hepatic and renal failure, and Cushing's disease or Cushing's syndrome. Weight loss may be associated with diet, gastrointestinal dysfunction (e.g. peptic ulcer, gallbladder disease, enteritis, and colitis), hyperthyroidism, malignancy, affective disorders (e.g. anxiety, depression, and hysteria), adrenal insufficiency (Addison's disease), and infection (e.g. HIV, tuberculosis, and syphilis).

Diabetes Mellitus

The hallmark of DM is hyperglycemia. Patients with Type I DM are usually younger, thinner, and ketosis prone; whereas patients with Type II DM tend to be older, obese, and generally ketosis resistant. Long-term complications of hyperglycemia include diabetic retinopathy, ulcers on the legs and feet, increased cardiovascular disease, renal failure, stroke, and oral complications. Hypoglycemia is the immediate life-threatening adverse effect of treatment with insulin and some oral hypoglycemic agents.

Polydipsia

Excessive thirst usually suggests the possibility of DM or diabetes insipidus. This complaint may also occur as a result of severe hypokalemia (e.g. primary hyperaldosteronism, Cushing's syndrome, and excessive diuretic therapy).

Hematopoietic Abnormalities

Easy Bruising and Excessive Bleeding

Easy bruising is observed more often in women and tends to increase with advancing age. Antithrombotic and anticoagulant medications, corticosteroids, and some over-the counter (OTC) dietary supplements increase bruising risk. It is important to determine if the bruising is provoked or unprovoked and a change in the frequency and severity of bruising may indicate the presence of a serious underlying condition such as thrombocytopenia.

Excessive bleeding is one of the most serious and cardinal manifestations of disease. It may occur in an isolated area or be more generalized in distribution. Bleeding associated with a localized lesion may be superimposed on a normal or defective hemostatic mechanism. In contrast, generalized bleeding usually is associated with a bleeding diathesis. Excessive bleeding may be induced pharmacologically by antithrombotic agents, warfarin sodium, and heparin; or it may result from a defect in the hemostatic system.

Anemia

Anemia should never be thought of as a diagnosis in and of itself, but rather as a manifestation of an underlying disease or physiologic process. Typical signs and symptoms include fatigue, lack of energy, weakness, lightheadedness, shortness of breath, and pallor. In severe anemia, cardiac output increases and the patient may be aware of this increased cardiac activity and complain of palpitations.

On examination, tachycardia and an increased pulse pressure may be noted. The adequacy of the cardiovascular adjustments to anemia depends on the degree of the anemia, the rapidity with which it has developed, and the pre-existing status of the cardiovascular system. A patient with anemia may develop cardiac disease (e.g. angina pectoris, MI, heart failure).

Abnormal White Blood Cell Count and Problems with the Immune System

Alterations in leukocyte count and function occur in a wide variety of hematological, infectious, inflammatory, metabolic, and neoplastic diseases. Infections are a major cause of morbidity and mortality during periods of granulocytopenia. These infections are often associated with cancer chemotherapy, acute leukemia, aplastic anemia, and immunosuppression. The risk of infection is greatest when the polymorphonuclear leukocyte count falls below $500/mm^3$. When the granulocyte count is less than $100/mm^3$ for more than a few days, bacteremia and severe infection are inevitable.

Spleen Dysfunction

The spleen is an integral component of the body's reticuloendothelial system and supports numerous body functions. It filters the blood to remove old erythrocytes, serves as a reservoir of platelets and white blood cells, and helps fight certain forms of bacteria that cause pneumonia and meningitis. Spleen dysfunction, either through disease or trauma, may necessitate its removal.

Removal of the spleen predisposes the patient to post-splenectomy sepsis (PSS), a condition characterized by the onset of bacteremia without a primary site of infection. Characteristically, the bacteremia is followed by the sudden onset of nausea and vomiting, meningitis, disseminated intravascular coagulation, acute respiratory distress syndrome, shock, and death in less than 72 hours.

Neurologic System

Headaches

The significance of headache is often obscure; however, it may be a symptomatic expression of tension and fatigue. The degree of incapacity, location, duration, and time-intensity curve of headaches, in the attack itself and its historical pattern, are most useful in establishing a diagnosis. The two most frequently observed headache types are migraine and tension. Other notable forms include cluster headache and sinus headache.

Dizziness and Fainting

Loss of consciousness secondary to transient ischemia to the brain and a generalized weakness of muscles characterize syncope. In contrast, the term faintness refers to a lack of strength with a sensation of impending loss of consciousness. Two-thirds of syncope episodes are autonomic reflex responses to a specific trigger such as emotional or orthostatic stress.

These conditions rarely appear when the patient is recumbent. Pallor is an early and invariable finding. The onset is deliberate. Injury from falling is rare and the return to consciousness is usually prompt.

Seizures

Seizures occur as a consequence of uncontrolled electrical discharge in the brain. Most seizures can be classified as either generalized or partial. A seizure may occur any time regardless of the position of the patient. The attack is sudden, and if an aura is present (characterized by seeing intermittent lights or hearing a continuous buzzing sound), it rarely lasts longer than a few seconds before unconsciousness. Injury from falling is frequent because protective reflexes are abolished. The classic tonic–clonic (grand mal) seizure starts with a stiffening of the limbs (the tonic phase), followed by jerking of the limbs and face (the clonic phase). Unconsciousness, mental confusion, headache, and drowsiness are commonly observed after the seizure.

Paresthesia and Neuralgia

Paresthesia refers to a burning or prickling sensation usually affecting the hands, arms, legs, or feet and may be of short duration (e.g. crossed legs) or chronic (e.g. nerve damage). Patient often use terms such as tingling, numbness, skin crawling, or itching to describe it. Potential causes include an underlying nutritional, toxic, or metabolic abnormality.

The two most common types of neuralgia are postherpetic neuralgia and trigeminal neuralgia. Trigeminal neuralgia, also known as tic douloureux, is a striking form of neuralgia that affects the head and neck area. It typically occurs in middle-aged and elderly individuals and causes excruciating paroxysms of pain involving the lips, gums, cheek, or chin, and rarely, the distribution of the ophthalmic division of the fifth cranial nerve.

Glossopharyngeal neuralgia is a syndrome that resembles trigeminal neuralgia in many respects. The pain is intense and paroxysmal; it originates in the throat, approximately in the tonsillar fossa. In some cases the pain is localized to the ear or may radiate from the throat to the ear. Spasms may be initiated by swallowing.

Postherpetic neuralgia occurs when the nerves are damaged during a recurrence of varicella virus infection (shingles). Patients over the age 60 who experience shingles are at highest risk for postherpetic neuralgia and the pain can be debilitating.

Paralysis

The two most common causes of paralysis are cerebrovascular accidents (CVAs) and spinal cord injury. Paralysis resulting from a stroke may involve the mouth, arms, and hands, thereby making it difficult to wear prostheses and maintain good oral hygiene. Patients with a history of CVA are likely to be taking oral anticoagulants. Since CVAs are almost always associated with evidence of cardiovascular disease.

There are numerous paralytic conditions specific to the head and neck. Bell's palsy is the most common disease affecting the facial nerve and is thought to result from an inflammatory reaction in or around the facial nerve near the stylomastoid foramen. The onset is acute and the paralysis may evolve over a period of several hours.

Bulbar palsy results from weakness or paralysis of the muscles supplied by the medulla oblongata. A syndrome of dysphasia and dysphonia secondary to complete interruption of the intracranial portion of the vagus nerve results in a characteristic paralysis. In this situation, the soft palate droops and does not rise in phonation. There is loss of the gag reflex on the affected side, the voice is hoarse and slightly nasal, and the vocal cord lies immobile in a cadaveric position.

Psychiatric Problems

Anxiety

The stress associated with contemporary society, along with the prospect of a real or imaginary illness, is thought to induce anxiety. When this occurs in a clear relationship to a stressful event or situation, it can be accepted as normal. Only when it is excessively intense and uncontrollable or accompanied by derangement of visceral function does it become the basis for medical intervention.

The anxiety state is characterized by a subjective feeling of fear and uneasy anticipation with the physiologic accompaniments of strong emotion. Behavioral clues include fidgeting and hyperactivity or rigidity, facial expressions of panic and stammering, or speech blocks. In adults, behavioral displays are frequently masked because they are perceived as socially inappropriate or embarrassing. Despite the potential limitations of patient self-report, behavioral clues remain an important component of anxiety assessment.

Asking patients how they feel, in a manner that avoids the appearance of being evaluative or judgmental, often facilitates disclosure of anxiety. A phobia is a persistent, irrational fear of and compelling desire to avoid an object or a situation. Affected patients often exhibit a single phobia that involves a fear of animals, illness, heights, or closed spaces.

The most common simple phobia seen in dentistry is dental phobia and affects an estimated 9–15% of the population. It is a persistent and recurrent fear of dentistry. The patient recognizes it as unreasonable, tries to resist avoidance behavior, yet the fear is not under voluntary control. Factors associated with dental phobia include unfavorable attitudes toward dentists, infrequent visits to the dentist, and dissatisfaction with appearance.

Depression

Most individuals experience periodic episodes of discouragement and despair throughout life. As with anxiety, depression is appropriate in a given life situation and is a natural, healthy reaction that is seldom the basis for medical consultation. According to the DSM-IV diagnostic criteria for affective disorders, a major depressive episode is a cluster of depressive symptoms characterized by the presence of low mood and/or loss of interest or pleasure

for at least two weeks and at least five of the following: (i) depressed mood most of the day; (ii); diminished interest or pleasure in all or most activities; (iii) significant unintentional weight loss or gain; (iv) insomnia or sleeping too much; (v) agitation or psychomotor retardation noticed by others; (vi) fatigue or loss of energy; (vii) feelings of worthlessness or excessive guilt; (viii) diminished ability to think or concentrate, or indecisiveness; and (ix) recurrent thoughts of death. It is the presence of these accompanying symptoms that helps to differentiate a significant depressive condition from the low mood or depressed feelings that most individuals experience from time to time, often in the context of an environmental stress.

Growths and Tumors

Radiotherapy and Chemotherapy

Optimal oral health is important for patients who are undergoing or who have undergone cancer therapy. Good oral hygiene and elimination of existing or potential sources of infection or irritation help to minimize mucositis, infection, hemorrhage, xerostomia, neurologic disorders, and nutritional problems and improve the patient's quality of life.

2.8 Summary

In eliciting and interpreting the historical profile, the clinician must exercise a degree of skill, care, and judgment ordinarily possessed by other members of the profession in similar circumstances. A breach of this duty constitutes negligence, for which the dentist may be held liable. Although consultation with a patient's physician(s) is desirable in many cases, it is the dentist, not the physician, who is responsible for the physical and emotional well-being of the patient undergoing dental treatment.

In addition to gathering, documenting, and interpreting data about the patient's health, the dentist also is charged with maintaining confidentiality. The need to maintain confidentiality extends to the office staff as well. A breach of that duty may lead to the possibility of a damage claim in tort law. Patients must give consent before any information can be disclosed to a third party unless allowed or required by law.

Suggested Reading

Alcaide, M.L. and Bisno, A.L. (2007). Pharyngitis and epiglottitis. *Infect. Dis. Clin. North Am.* 21 (2): 449–469.

Alter, H. and Messner, A.H. (2013). Patient information: Nosebleeds (Epistaxis). UpToDate. Available at: http://www.uptodate .com/contents/nosebleeds-epistaxis-beyond- the-basics?detectedLaguage=en& source=search_result&search=nosebleed& selectedTitle=7percent7E150& provider=noProvider (accessed 16 December 2020).

American Diabetes Association. Eye complications. Available at: http://www .diabetes.org/living-with-diabetes/ complications/eye-complications (accessed 16 December 2020).

American Speech-Language-Hearing Association. Causes of hearing loss in adults. Available at: www.asha.org/public/hearing/ disorders/causes_adults.htm (accessed on 16 December 2020).

Aring, A.M. and Chan, M.M. (2011). Acute rhinosinusitis in adults. *Am. Fam. Physician* 83 (9): 1057–1063.

Armstrong, C. (2012). ACP updates guideline on diagnosis and management of stable COPD. *Am. Fam. Physician* 85 (2): 204–205.

Baddour, L.M., Bettmann, M.A., Bolger, A.F. et al. (2003). Nonvalvular cardiovascular device-related infections. *Circulation* 108 (16): 2015–2031.

Baumgarten, M. and Gehr, T. (2011). Chronic kidney disease: detection and evaluation. *Am. Fam. Physician* 84 (10): 1138–1148.

Benich, I.I.I.J.J. and Carek, P.J. (2011). Evaluation of the patient with chronic cough. *Am. Fam. Physician* 84 (8): 887–892.

Cartwright, S.L. (2008). Evaluation of acute abdominal pain in adults. *Am. Fam. Physician* 77 (7): 971–978.

Center for Substance Abuse Treatment. Managing depressive symptoms in substance abuse clients during early recovery. Rockville (MD): Substance Abuse and Mental Health Services Administration (US); 2008. (Treatment Improvement Protocol (TIP) Series, No. 48.) Appendix D: DSM-IV-TR Mood Disorders. Available from: www.ncbi .nlm.nih.gov/books/NBK64063 (accessed 16 December 2020).

Chan, Y. (2009). Tinnitus: etiology, classification, characteristics, and treatment. *Discov. Med.* 8 (42): 133–136.

Cronau, H., Kankanala, R.R., and Mauger, T. (2010). Diagnosis and management of red eye in primary care. *Am. Fam. Physician* 81 (2): 137–144.

Dietlein, T.S., Hermann, M.M., and Jordan, J.F. (2009). The medical and surgical treatment of glaucoma. *Dtsch. Arztebl. Int.* 106 (37): 597–605; quiz 606.

Fan, B.J. and Wiggs, J.L. (2010). Glaucoma: genes, phenotypes, and new directions for therapy. *J. Clin. Invest.* 120 (9): 3064–3072.

Feierabend, R.H. and Shahram, M.N. (2009). Hoarseness in adults. *Am. Fam. Physician* 80 (4): 363–370.

Friedman, B.W. and Grosberg, B.M. (2009). Diagnosis and management of the primary headache disorders in the emergency department setting. *Emerg. Med. Clin. North Am.* 27 (1): 71–87.

Gawkrodger, D.J., Ormerod, A.D., Shaw, L. et al. (2010). Vitiligo: concise evidence based guidelines on diagnosis and management. *J. Postgrad. Med.* 86 (1018): 466–471.

Gwaltney, J.M. (2002). Clinical significance and pathogenesis of viral respiratory infections. *Am. J. Med.* 112 (Suppl 6A): 13S–18S.

Hauck, F.R., Neese, B.H., Panchal, A.S., and El-Amin, W. (2009). Identification and management of latent tuberculosis infection. *Am. Fam. Physician* 79 (10): 879–886.

Mayo Clinic. Low blood pressure (hypotension). Available at: www.mayoclinic.com/health/low-blood-pressure/DS00590 (accessed 16 December 2020).

McConaghy, J.R. and Oza, R.S. (2013). Outpatient diagnosis of acute chest pain in adults. *Am. Fam. Physician* 87 (3): 177–182.

Meriggioli, M.N. and Sanders, D.B. (2009). Autoimmune myasthenia gravis: emerging clinical and biological heterogeneity. *Lancet Neurol.* 8 (5): 475–490.

Mintz, M. (2004). Asthma update: part I. Diagnosis, monitoring, and prevention of disease progression. *Am. Fam. Physician* 70 (5): 893–898.

Miravitlles, M., Calle, M., and Soler-Cataluña, J.J. (2012). Clinical phenotypes of COPD: identification, definition and implications for guidelines. *Arch Bronconeumol.* 48 (3): 86–98.

Mishra, N. and Hall, J. (2012). Identification of patients at risk for hereditary colorectal cancer. *Clin. Colon Rectal Surg.* 25 (2): 67–82.

Mounsey, A.L. and Reed, S.W. (2009). Diagnosing and treating hair loss. *Am. Fam. Physician* 80 (4): 356–362.

National Cancer Institute. Pruritus. Available at: www.cancer.gov/cancertopics/pdq/supportivecare/pruritus/HealthProfessional/page1/AllPages (accessed 16 December 2020).

National Institute on Alcohol Abuse and Alcoholism. Alcohol Alert. Screening for alcohol use and alcohol-related problems. Available at: http://pubs.niaaa.nih.gov/publications/aa65/AA65.pdf (accessed 16 December 2020).

Oh, R.C. and Hustead, T.R. (2011). Causes and evaluation of mildly elevated liver transaminase levels. *Am. Fam. Physician* 84 (4): 1003–1008.

Ohar, J., Fromer, L., and Donohue, J.F. (2011). Reconsidering sex-based stereotypes of COPD. *Prim. Care Respir. J.* 20 (4): 370–378.

O'Neill, S.M., Rubinstein, W.S., Wang, C. et al. (2009). Familial risk for common diseases in primary care: the Family Healthware Impact Trial. 4th; Family Healthware Impact Trial group. *Am. J. Prev. Med.* 36 (6): 506–514.

Pfaar, O. and Klimek, L. (2006). Aspirin desensitization in aspirin intolerance: update on current standards and recent improvements. *Curr. Opin. Allergy Clin. Immunol.* 6 (3): 161–166.

Pollart, S.M. and Elward, K.S. (2009). Overview of changes to asthma guidelines: diagnosis and screening. *Am. Fam. Physician* 79 (9): 761–767.

Pritts, S.D. and Susman, J. (2003). Diagnosis of eating disorders in primary care. *Am. Fam. Physician* 67 (2): 297–304.

Ramakrishnan, K. (2007). Peptic ulcer disease. *Am. Fam. Physician* 76 (7): 1005–1012.

Roche, S.P. and Kobos, R. (2004). Jaundice in the adult patient. *Am. Fam. Physician* 69 (2): 299–304.

Sollecito, T.P., Abt, E., Lockhart, P.B. et al. (2015). The use of prophylactic antibiotics prior to dental procedures in patients with prosthetic joints: Evidence-based clinical practice guideline for dental practitioners–a report of the American Dental Association Council on Scientific Affairs. *J. Am. Dent. Assoc.* 146 (1): 11–16.

Springer, K., Brown, M., and Stulberg, D.L. (2003). Common hair loss disorders. *Am. Fam. Physician* 68 (1): 93–102.

Sura, L., Madhavan, A., Carnaby, G., and Crary, M.A. (2012). Dysphagia in the elderly: management and nutritional considerations. *Clin. Interv. Aging* 7: 287–298.

Taj, N., Devera-Sales, A., and Vinson, D.C. (1998). Screening for problem drinking: does a single question work? *J. Fam. Practice* 46 (4): 328–335.

Tuder, R.M. and Petrache, I. (2012). Pathogenesis of chronic obstructive pulmonary disease. *J. Clin. Invest.* 122 (8): 2749–2755.

Viegi, G., Pistelli, F., Sherrill, D.L. et al. (2007). Definition, epidemiology and natural history of COPD. *Eur. Respir. J.* 30 (5): 993–1013.

Viehweg, T.L., Roberson, J.B., and Hudson, J.W. (2006). Epistaxis: diagnosis and treatment. *J. Oral Maxillofac. Surg.* 64 (3): 511.

Wahls, S.A. (2012). Causes and evaluation of chronic Dyspnea. *Am. Fam. Physician* 86 (2): 173–180.

Wald, E.R. (2011). Acute otitis media and acute bacterial sinusitis. *Clin. Infect. Dis.* 52 (Suppl 4): S277–S283.

Whelton, P.K., Carey, R.M., Aronow, W.S. et al. (2018). 2017 ACC/AHA/AAPA/ABC/ACPM/ AGS/APhA/ASH/ASPC/NMA/PCNA Guideline for the Prevention, Detection, Evaluation, and Management of High Blood Pressure in Adults: Executive Summary: A Report of the American College of Cardiology/American Heart Association Task Force on Clinical Practice Guidelines. *Hypertension* 71 (6): 1269–1324.

Wilkins, T., Khan, N., Nabh, A., and Schade, R.R. (2012). Diagnosis and management of upper gastrointestinal bleeding. *Am. Fam. Physician* 85 (5): 469–476.

Wilson, W., Taubert, K.A., Gewitz, M. et al. (2007). Prevention of infective endocarditis: guidelines from the American Heart Association: a guideline from the American Heart Association Rheumatic Fever, Endocarditis, and Kawasaki Disease Committee, Council on Cardiovascular Disease in the Young, and the Council on Clinical Cardiology, Council on Cardiovascular Surgery and Anesthesia, and the Quality of Care and Outcomes Research Interdisciplinary Working Group. *Circulation* 116 (15): 1736–1754.

Workowski, K.A. and Berman, S.M. (2011). Centers for Disease Control and Prevention sexually transmitted diseases treatment guidelines. *Clin. Infect. Dis.* 53 (Suppl 3): S59–S63.

World Health Oragnization. Genes and human disease. Available at: www.who.int/genomics/ public/geneticdiseases/en/index2.html# (accessed 16 December 2020).

Zumla, A., Raviglione, M., Hafner, R., and von Reyn, C.F. (2013). Tuberculosis. *N. Engl. J. Med.* 368 (8): 745–755.

3

Basic Procedures in Physical Examination

Time-tested basic procedures in physical examination include inspection, palpation, percussion, auscultation, olfaction, and evaluation of function. The process begins the moment the patient presents for care. Note the patient's general appearance, body language, and mannerisms, as these are reliable indicators of their physical and mental state. When shaking the patient's hand, does the patient respond in kind? A patient who shuns a handshake may be doing so for cultural reasons, or the handshake may be painful, as for a patient suffering from arthritis. Does the patient maintain or avoid eye contact when spoken to? Reticence to maintain eye contact and poor personal hygiene may indicate depression or some other psychological disorder.

Determine the patient's level of consciousness, cognitive function, and language comprehension during the initial contact with the patient. When the patient speaks, note voice quality. Abnormalities in volume may indicate hearing loss, while hoarseness may be due to laryngeal pathoses. Peculiarities of speech such as an unusual accent or pattern of communication, slurring, dysphasia, aphasia, garbled speech, or lapses of speech may be consequential observations.

3.1   Inspection

Inspection is defined as the process of examination that relies on the sense of vision. It is not only the most common but often the most successful examination technique.

Note the patient's physical characteristics such as anatomical architecture, mobility, gait, color, and respiratory function. Alterations in

Physical Evaluation and Treatment Planning in Dental Practice, Second Edition.
Géza T. Terézhalmy, Michaell A. Huber, Lily T. García and Ronald L. Occhionero.
© 2021 John Wiley & Sons, Inc. Published 2021 by John Wiley & Sons, Inc.
Companion Website: www.wiley.com/go/terezhalmy/physical

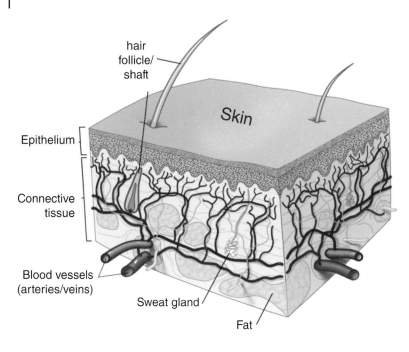

Figure 3.1 Normal skin.

body size, shape, and symmetry may suggest developmental or acquired abnormalities. Mobility, gait, and postural abnormalities may indicate skeletal or neuromuscular defects. Pallor may be an indicator of anemia, while cyanosis may indicate problems associated with the respiratory and/or cardiovascular system. Jaundice may be a sign of hemolytic anemia, liver disease, or a pancreatic

abnormality. Evidence of respiratory difficulty may be associated with allergic, pulmonary, or cardiac disorders.

Once the global inspection of the patient is accomplished, the clinician should proceed to the more focused inspection of specific tissues such as visible skin and the oral mucosa. The skin (Figure 3.1) and oral mucosa (Figure 3.2) are metabolically active tissues. Both serve a

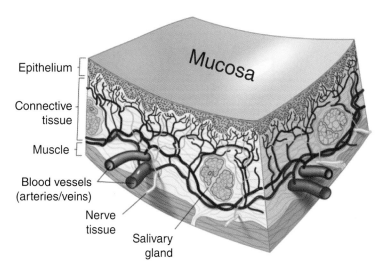

Figure 3.2 Normal mucosa.

primary protective function for the body, and through their rich innervation and vascularity mediate sensory contact with the environment and help regulate temperature.

To the uninitiated, many skin and mucosal lesions may look alike, but most have characteristic presentations. Lesions are dynamic and typically evolve as a consequence of such factors as normal maturation, trauma, secondary infection, or therapy. For example, an initial vesicle on the lip may quickly break down, become eroded or ulcerate and eventually crust as healing progresses.

Careful inspection of the skin and oral mucosa may reveal the first signs of internal or systemic disease and, on occasion, skin lesions may provide the first clues essential for the diagnosis of certain oral conditions. Changes in color (pigmentation, vascularity); the presence of edema, swelling, and bulging; surface characteristics such as moistness, dryness, or oiliness; and other unusual findings should be noted.

The terminology used to describe mucocutaneous lesions is not only descriptive but may at times be suggestive of the underlying cause. The pattern of distribution of the various lesions is also important and may be described with terms such as linear, annular (in a ring), or serpiginous (in a curvilinear pattern, serpent-like).

Lesions of the Skin and Oral Mucosa

Macule

A macule (Figure 3.3a and b) is a circumscribed, flat lesion less than 1 cm in size, varied in shape and color, and may represent hyperpigmented, hypopigmented, or vascular abnormalities. Figure 3.3b is an example of multiple macules on the lower lip due to physiologic pigmentation.

Patch

A patch (Figure 3.4a and b) is a circumscribed, flat lesion larger than 1 cm in size, varied in shape and color, and may represent hyperpigmented, hypopigmented, or vascular abnormalities. Figure 3.4b is an example of a patch on the dorsum of the tongue due to physiologic pigmentation.

Papule

A papule (Figure 3.5a and b) is a circumscribed, elevated, superficial, solid lesion less than 1 cm in size, varied in shape and color, and may reflect hyperplasia of cellular structures or represent cellular infiltrates. Figure 3.5b is an example of a dermal papule in a patient with lichen planus.

Plaque

A plaque (Figure 3.6a and b) is a circumscribed, elevated, superficial, solid lesion larger than

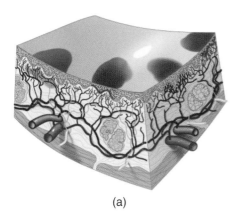
(a)

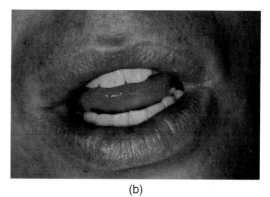
(b)

Figure 3.3 (a) and (b) Macule.

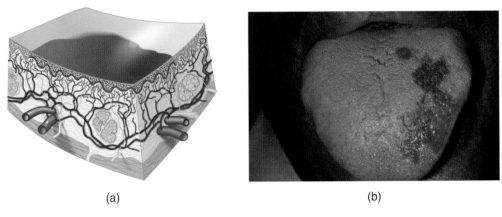

(a)   (b)

Figure 3.4 (a) and (b) Patch.

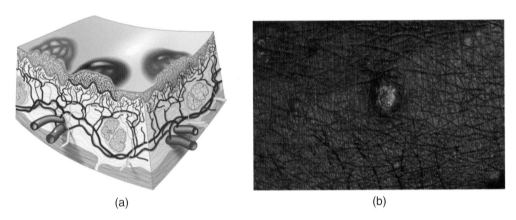

(a)   (b)

Figure 3.5 (a) and (b) Papule.

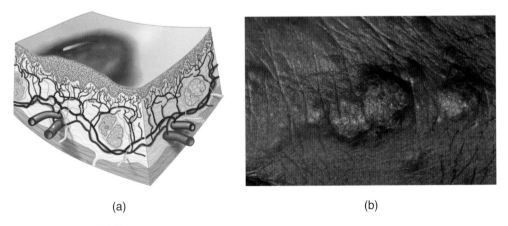

(a)   (b)

Figure 3.6 (a) and (b) Plaque.

1 cm in size, varied in shape and color, and may reflect hyperplasia of cellular structures, represent cellular infiltrates, or may be formed by a confluence of papules. Figure 3.6b is an example of a dermal plaque in a patient with lichen planus.

Nodule

A nodule (Figure 3.7a and b) is a solid palpable lesion less than 1 cm in size. Its depth may be above, level with, or beneath the skin or mucosal surface. Nodules may be the result of inflammatory, neoplastic, or metabolic processes. Descriptors such as soft, firm, hard (bony), fixed, movable, pedunculated (has a stem-like connecting part, a stalk by which a nodule or a tumor is attached to normal tissue), or sessile (attached by a base; not pedunculated or stalked) are helpful when describing these lesions. Figure 3.7b is an

example of a pedunculated nodule on the right lateral surface of the tongue.

Tumor

A tumor (Figure 3.8a and b) is a solid palpable lesion larger than 1 cm in size. Its depth may be above, level with, or beneath the skin or mucosa. Tumors may be the result

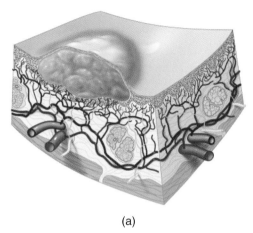

(a)

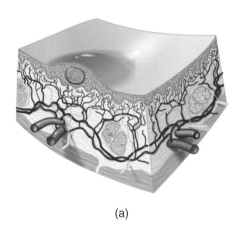

(a)

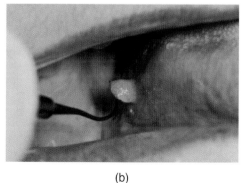

(b)

Figure 3.7 (a) and (b) Nodule.

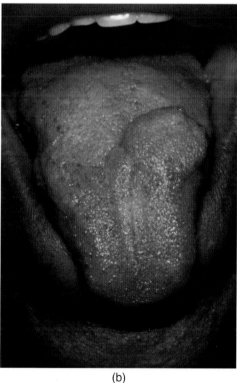

(b)

Figure 3.8 (a) and (b) Tumor.

of inflammatory, metabolic, and neoplastic processes. Descriptors such as soft, firm, hard (bony), fixed, movable, pedunculated, or sessile are helpful when describing these lesions. Figure 3.8b is an example of a tumor affecting the dorsum of the tongue.

Wheal

A wheal (Figure 3.9a and b) is an edematous, rounded or oval transitory papule of variable size, usually the result of an allergic reaction. Figure 3.9b is an example of wheals on the face of a patient with an allergy to latex.

Vesicle

A vesicle (Figure 3.10a and b) is a circumscribed elevated intraepithelial or subepithelial lesion less than 1 cm in size, which contains a serous fluid. Figure 3.10b is an example of a vesicle associated with recurrent herpes labialis.

Bulla

A bulla (Figure 3.11a and b) is a circumscribed elevated intraepithelial or subepithelial lesion larger than 1 cm in size, which contains a serous fluid. Figure 3.11b is an example of multiple bullae occurring on the inner aspect of the lower lip in a patient with pemphigus vulgaris.

Cyst

A cyst (Figure 3.12a and b) is an encapsulated lesion of variable size in subcutaneous or submucosal tissue filled with liquid or semisolid material. Figure 3.12b is an example of a dermoid cyst; the lesion is located about 2 cm lateral to the commissure of the mouth.

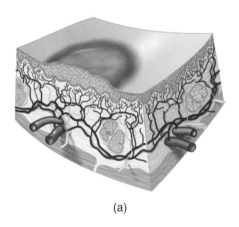
(a)

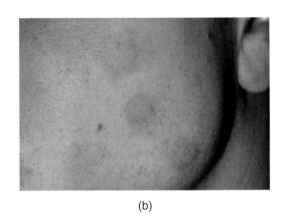
(b)

Figure 3.9 (a) and (b) Wheal.

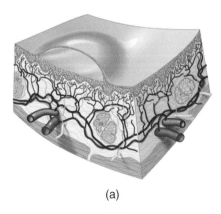
(a)

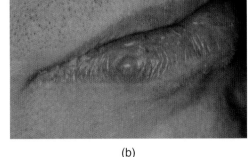
(b)

Figure 3.10 (a) and (b) Vesicle.

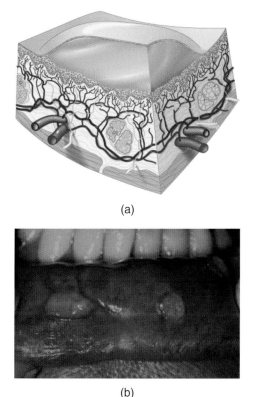

(a)

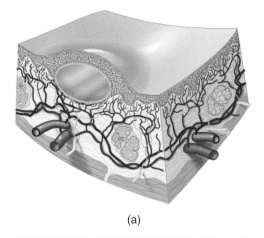

(a)

(b)

Figure 3.11 (a) and (b) Bulla.

Pustule

A pustule (Figure 3.13a and b) is a circumscribed elevation of variable size and shape containing a purulent exudate. Depending on the color of the purulent exudates, it may appear white, yellow, or greenish-yellow. Figure 3.13b is an example of a dermal pustule.

Hemangioma A hemangioma (Figure 3.14a and b) is a red irregular macule or patch of variable size and shape caused by dilation of dermal or mucosal capillaries. Figure 3.14b is an example of capillary hemangioma located on the patient's lower lip.

Telangiectasia Telangiectases (Figure 3.15a and b) are serpiginous lesions caused by permanent dilation of superficial capillaries. Figure 3.15b is an example of multiple telangiectases on the face of a patient with alcoholic cirrhosis of the liver.

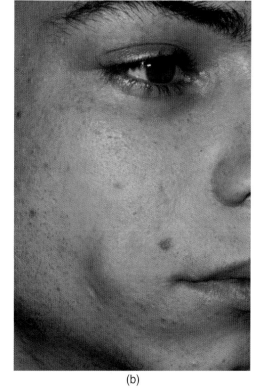

(b)

Figure 3.12 (a) and (b) Cyst.

Petechia

A petechia (Figure 3.16a and b) is a circumscribed deposit of extravasated blood or blood pigments less than 2 mm in size. Figure 3.16b is an example of multiple petechiae occurring on the soft palate in a patient taking clopidogrel, an antithrombotic agent.

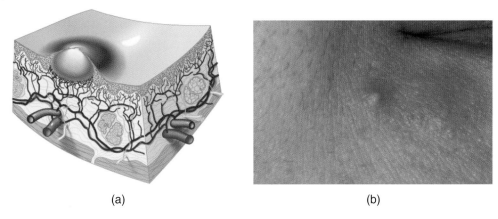

(a)   (b)

Figure 3.13 (a) and (b) Pustule.

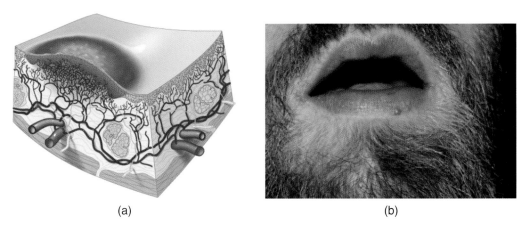

(a)   (b)

Figure 3.14 (a) and (b) Hemangioma.

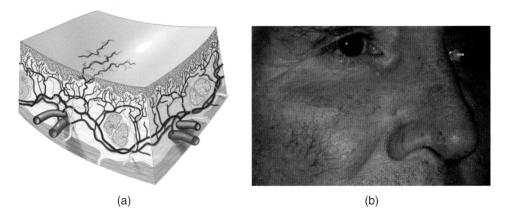

(a)   (b)

Figure 3.15 (a) and (b) Telangiectasia.

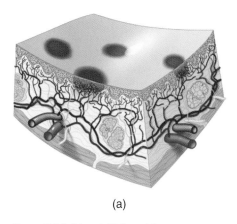

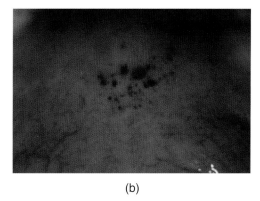

(a)   (b)

Figure 3.16 (a) and (b) Petechiae.

Purpura

A purpura (Figure 3.17a and b) is a circumscribed deposit of extravasated blood or blood pigments between 2 and 10 mm in size. Figure 3.17b is an example of a purpura on the left buccal mucosa secondary to trauma in a patient taking warfarin, an oral anticoagulant.

Ecchymosis

An ecchymosis (Figure 3.18a and b) is a circumscribed deposit of extravasated blood or blood pigments larger than 1 cm in size. Figure 3.18b is an example of a large ecchymotic lesion secondary to trauma associated with a minor salivary gland biopsy.

Hematoma A hematoma (Figure 3.19a and b) is an accumulated mass of extravasated blood that usually clots to form a solid swelling of variable size and shape within a tissue. Figure 3.19b is an example of a hematoma affecting the lateral border of the tongue in a patient who was taking heparin, a parenteral anticoagulant.

Scale

Scales (Figure 3.20a and b) are characterized by abnormal shedding (desquamating), usually of dry and flaky, dead epithelial cells. Figure 3.20b is an example of scaly lesions occurring on the forearm of a patient with psoriasis.

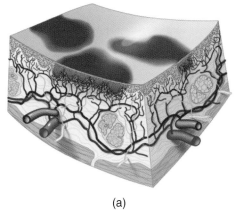

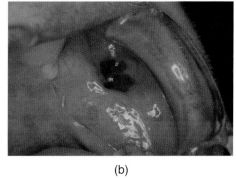

(a)   (b)

Figure 3.17 (a) and (b) Purpura.

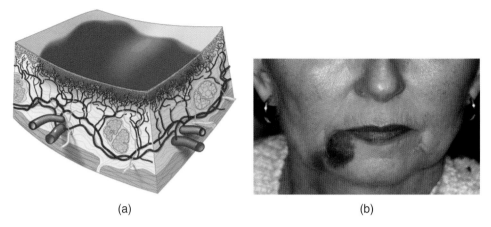

(a)   (b)

Figure 3.18 (a) and (b) Ecchymosis.

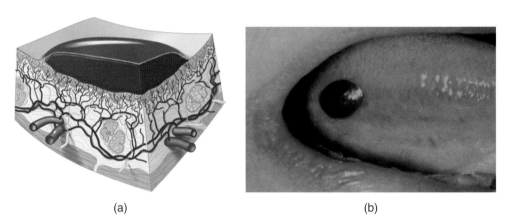

(a)   (b)

Figure 3.19 (a) and (b) Hematoma.

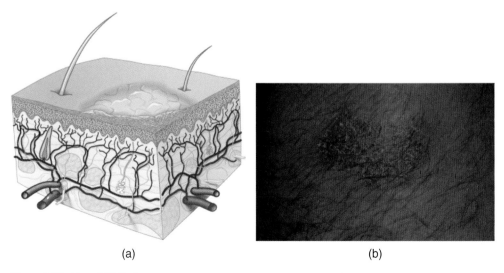

(a)   (b)

Figure 3.20 (a) and (b) Scale.

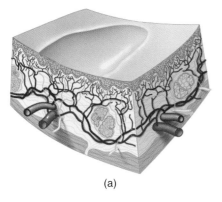

(a)

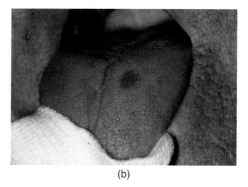

(b)

Figure 3.21 (a) and (b) Atrophy.

Atrophy

Atrophy (Figure 3.21a and b) is characterized by diminution in the size of cells, tissues, organs, or body parts. Figure 3.21b is an example of atrophy of the filiform papillae occurring on the dorsum of the tongue.

Erosion Erosion (Figure 3.22a and b), as it relates to skin and oral mucosa, is characterized by a breakdown (denudation) of the epithelium, which heals without scarring. Erosion, as it relates to oral hard tissues (enamel, dentin, cementum), is characterized by gradual loss of tooth substance by a chemical process that does not involve a known bacterial action. Figure 3.22b is an example of erosions affecting the marginal gingiva of the maxillary right premolar in a patient with erosive lichen planus.

Excoriation

Excoriation (Figure 3.23a and b) is a superficial, sometimes linear excavation of the epidermis usually associated with scratching. Figure 3.23b is an example of excoriation of the epidermis of the forearm.

Ulcer

An ulcer (Figure 3.24a and b) is an irregularly shaped excavation of the epithelium that extends below the basal cell layer and may heal with a scar. Figure 3.24b is an example of a recurrent aphthous ulceration occurring on the labial mucosa.

Fissure

A fissure (Figure 3.25a and b) is a linear crack or cleavage in epithelial tissue with sharply defined abrupt walls. Figure 3.25b is an example of a self-induced fissure occurring at the midline of the lower lip.

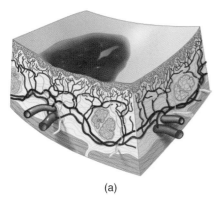

(a)

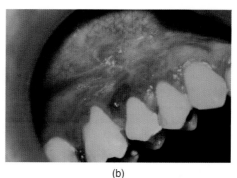

(b)

Figure 3.22 (a) and (b) Erosion.

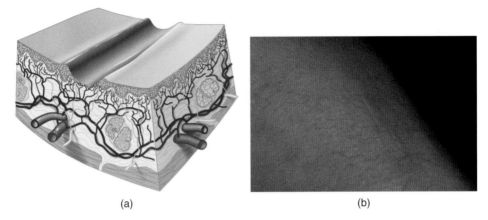

(a)   (b)

Figure 3.23 (a) and (b) Excoriation.

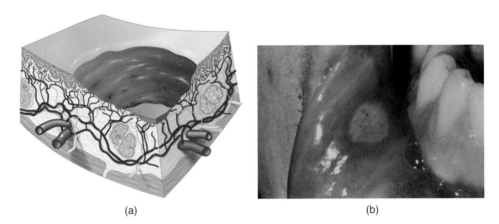

(a)   (b)

Figure 3.24 (a) and (b) Ulcer.

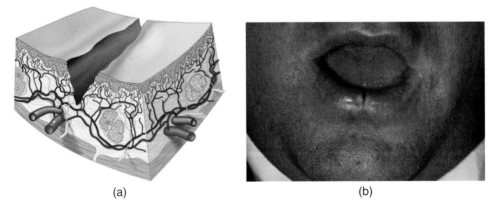

(a)   (b)

Figure 3.25 (a) and (b) Fissure.

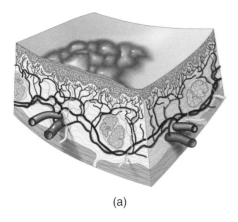

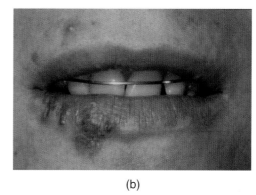

(a)

(b)

Figure 3.26 (a) and (b) Crust.

Crust

A crust (Figure 3.26a and b) is a hardened deposit of variable thickness consisting of dried blood, serum, or purulent exudate on skin and lip vermilion. Figure 3.26b is an example of crusting that has occurred after the rupturing of vesicles in a patient with recurrent herpes labialis.

Scar

A scar (Figure 3.27a and b) is a mark that remains after the healing of a wound, which may be atrophic or hypertrophic as a consequence of variable degrees of collagen proliferation. Figure 3.27b is an example of a scar affecting the middle of the lower lip after injury sustained from a fall.

Keloid

A keloid (Figure 3.28a and b) is a sharply elevated, irregularly shaped hypertrophic scar due to the formation of an excessive amount of collagen, which tends to extend and grow beyond the original site of injury during connective tissue repair. Figure 3.28b is an example of keloid occurring on the skin.

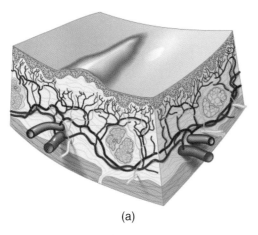

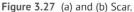

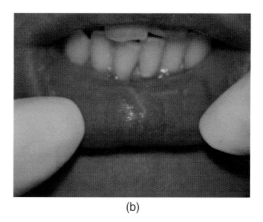

(a)

(b)

Figure 3.27 (a) and (b) Scar.

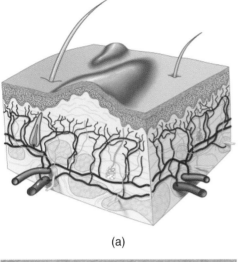

(a)

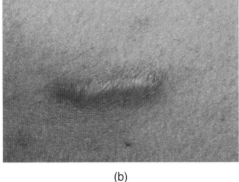

(b)

Figure 3.28 (a) and (b) Keloid.

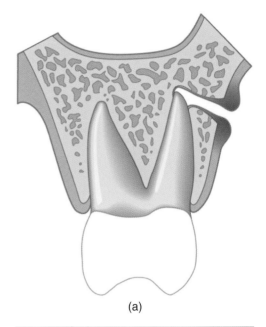

(a)

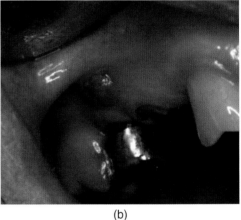

(b)

Figure 3.29 (a) and (b) Sinus tract.

Sinus

A sinus (Figure 3.29a and b) is an abnormal channel that leads from a pathological space to an anatomical space permitting the escape of pus. Figure 3.29b is an example of a sinus tract associated with an abscessed maxillary tooth.

Clubbing of the Nails and Fingers

Clubbing (Figure 3.30a and b) is characterized by curved overgrowth of the nail bed with bulbous enlarged fingertips. It is usually associated with congenital heart defects, congestive heart failure, chronic obstructive pulmonary disease, and carcinoma of the lung. Figure 3.30a and b represent clubbing of the fingernails in a patient who was diagnosed with cardiovascular disease.

Onycholysis

Onycholysis (Figure 3.31) is the result of keratin deposition beneath the nail bed, which produces opacification and irregular separation of the distal portion of the nail. Figure 3.31 is an example of onycholysis of the fingernails in a patient who had psoriasis.

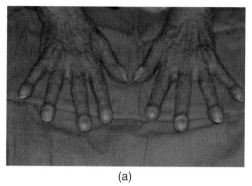 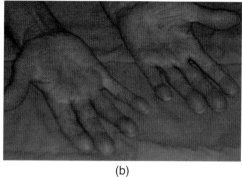

(a) (b)

Figure 3.30 (a) and (b) Digital clubbing.

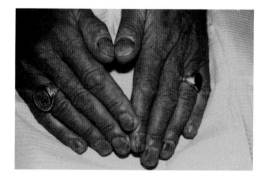

Figure 3.31 Onycholysis.

Table 3.1 Tissue characteristics noted upon palpation.

- Temperature – heat
- Tenderness or pain – superficial, deep, rebound, referred
- Muscle tones – increased resistance, spasm, rigidity
- Mass – nodule, tumor, and lymph node
  - Location – relation to other tissues
  - Architecture – size, shape, symmetry, discreteness
  - Consistency – soft, firm, hard (bony)
  - Mobility – attachment (bound or unbound)
  - Quality – pulsating or fluctuating

3.2 Palpation

Palpation is defined as the process of examination that relies on the sense of touch. The classic application of this technique is reflected in the process of assessing a patient's pulse pressure (reflecting the numerical difference between systolic and diastolic blood pressure [BP]), rate, and rhythm (see "Evaluation of Function").

In the head and neck area, palpation is invaluable in confirming and expanding upon the observations noted on inspection. It should be initiated as a light touch, followed by deep palpation. A light touch is useful to detect surface characteristics such as tissue texture and temperature, as well as qualities such as pulsation or fluctuation; deep palpation confirms the extent of nodules or tumors (Table 3.1).

Palpation of certain anatomical structures requires a bidigital or bimanual technique – for example, when palpating for cervical lymph nodes, the area being assessed is gently pinched between two fingers (bidigital palpation); when palpating the floor of the mouth, the structures being examined are trapped between the fingers of each hand (bimanual palpation). As palpation may cause the patient to experience tenderness or pain, judicious application of the technique is essential.

3.3 Percussion

Percussion is defined as the process of examination that relies on the technique of gently tapping an area of the body while noting the resonance or sound produced and the resistance encountered. It is the primary physical maneuver used in medicine to detect the presence or level of pleural effusion.

In the head and neck area, percussion is often used to provoke pain in an effort to identify teeth with periodontal or pulpal disease in patients who are unable to localize the discomfort or pain to a specific tooth. Similarly, percussion is useful to evaluate tenderness of the maxillary sinuses (maxillary sinusitis), which may be referred maxillary teeth.

3.4 Auscultation

Auscultation is defined as the process of examination that usually involves listening to the surface of the body with the aid of a stethoscope.

Auscultation is the time-tested technique used when determining BP (see Section 3.6) and breathing sounds such as inspiration, expiration, rales, rhonchi, stridor, and wheezing (see Section 3.6). When assessing sounds, such characteristics as intensity, pitch, duration, and quality should be also determined. In order to assess sounds adequately, these observations should be made in a quiet environment. Auscultation of the temporomandibular joint may reveal crepitus, the crackling or grating sound produced by bone rubbing on bone or roughened cartilage.

3.5 Olfaction

Olfaction is defined as the process of examination that relies on the sense of smell. It is useful to detect odors arising from the patient that may suggest the presence of local or systemic disease (Table 3.2).

3.6 Evaluation of Function

Pulse Rate and Rhythm

The pulse is a series of pressure waves within an artery caused by contractions of the left ventricle and corresponds to the heart rate.

Table 3.2 Common conditions associated with halitosis.

- Oral conditions
  - Oral sepsis associated with extensive caries, stomatitis, gingivitis, or periodontal disease
  - Fusospirochetal infections associated with ulcerative gingivitis, pharyngitis, or cancrum oris
- Systemic conditions
  - Upper respiratory tract infections
  - Lung abscess or bronchiectasis suggested by a fetid, foul putrefactive breath
  - Diet, gastrointestinal disturbances
  - Diabetic acidosis or hyperglycemic coma associated with a sweet, fruity acetone odor
  - Renal failure (uremia) associated with an odor of ammonia
  - Liver failure characterized by fetor hepaticus, a mousy, musty odor
  - Anxiety indicated by odor of alcohol resulting from self-medication on a sedative or compulsive basis

The pulse rate and rhythm vary with the demand for oxygen, age, and various disease states (Table 3.3). Consequently, it should be recorded for all new patients at the time of initial appointment, at all recall visits, and at all appointments for all patients with a history of cardiac arrhythmias, hypertension, cardiovascular diseases, diabetes mellitus, thyroid disorders, adrenal disease, renal dysfunction, and significant use of tobacco and coffee.

The normal pulse rate is 60–100 beats/minute for adults, 90–120 beats/minute for children, and 70–80 beats/minute in the aged.

Technique

To determine the pulse rate and rhythm, the patient's hand is grasped with the palm facing upward. The three middle fingers of the examiner are placed on the radial artery (located at the patient's wrist, lateral to the radius) with the index finger nearest to the heart (Figure 3.32). With the fingers in this position, gentle pressure is applied to feel the pulse rate and rhythm for a full minute.

Table 3.3 Alterations in pulse rate and rhythm and associated conditions.

Problem	Signs and symptoms	Causes

• Sinus bradycardia
  • Impulses originate from the SA node at a slow rate as a result of increased vagal tone.
    – HR is <60 beats/minute and the rhythm is regular
	• May be asymptomatic or cause light-headedness, fainting, chest discomfort, hypotension, and dyspnea	• Common in athletes and in patients with hypothyroidism and increased intracranial pressure; and during treatment with drugs with negative chronotropic action (e.g. β_1-adrenergic receptor antagonists, calcium channel blocking agents and digoxin).

• Atrial flutter
  • Impulses originate from a single abnormal focus in the atria resulting in the circular propagation of the impulses in the atria
    – Heart rate 250–350 beats/minute, and the rhythm is regular.
	• May be asymptomatic or cause palpitations, chest discomfort, dyspnea, weakness, and syncope.
	  • Because the AV node is unable to transmit all of the impulses only about half will get through resulting in a ventricular rate of 150 beats/minute.
		• Common causes include hypertension, cardiomyopathy, mitral or tricuspid valvular disorders, hyperthyroidism, and binge alcohol drinking.
		
		• Less common causes include pulmonary embolism, congenital heart defects, cardiopulmonary disease (COPD), myocarditis, and pericarditis

• Atrial fibrillation
  • Impulses originate from multiple atrial foci, which travel in a random manner in the atria
    – Heart rate 350–450 beats/minute, and the rhythm is irregular.
	• Symptoms include palpitations, vague chest discomfort, weakness, lightheadedness, dyspnea
	  • The ventricles respond to only about 120–180 of the impulses.
	• Stasis of blood in the fibrillating atrium can lead to blood clot formation and systemic embolism, which may present as stroke-like illness, i.e. sudden confusion; acute painful, pale, pulseless limbs; and an acute abdomen.	

• Atrioventricular (AV) blocks
  • Partial or complete interruption of impulse conduction from the atria to the ventricles
    – First degree – delay in impulse conduction
    – Second degree – intermittent failure in conduction
    – Third degree – permanent failure in conduction. Cardiac function is maintained by a ventricular pacemaker
	• First degree
	  • Asymptomatic
	• Second degree
	  • Asymptomatic or patient experiences lightheadedness and syncope,
	• Third degree
	  • Symptoms may include lightheadedness, fatigue, syncope, and heart failure
		• Common causes are idiopathic fibrosis and sclerosis of the conduction system (50 %) and ischemic heart disease (40 %).
		• Less commonly they are caused by drugs (e.g. β-blockers, digoxin), increased vagal tone, valvulopathy, and congenital heart disorders.

(Continued)

Table 3.3 (Continued)

Problem	Signs and symptoms	Causes

• Sinus tachycardia
  • Impulses originate from the SA node at a rapid rate under the influence of increased sympathetic tone or vagal blockade.
    – HR is 100–180 beats/minute and the rhythm is regular.
	• May be asymptomatic or cause palpitations (sensation of skipped beats or rapid forceful beats), symptoms of hemodynamic compromise (dyspnea, chest discomfort, syncope)	• Common in patients after exercise or smoking; in patients with hyperthyroidism, anxiety, toxic states, fever, anemia, severe hemorrhage, debilitation, and acute or chronic heart disease
		• May be precipitated by stimulants (e.g., tea, coffee), and medications with positive chronotropic effects.

• Premature ventricular contractions (PVCs)
  • Impulses originate from an ectopic ventricular focus.
    – Pronounced pause in an otherwise normal rhythm
	• May occur erratically or at predictable intervals,
	  • Every second beat (bigeminy)
	  • Every third beat (tigeminy).
		• PVCs may be an occasional finding in otherwise healthy adults and the incidence increases with age, fatigue, emotional stress, and the use of coffee and tobacco.
		• PVCs are significant in a patient with cardiovascular disease (coronary heart disease, valvular disease, and hypertension, congestive heart failure).

• Ventricular tachycardia (VT)
  • Usually evolves from an ectopic focus in the right or left ventricle
    – Rate 120–220 beats/minute
	• Sustained VT is almost always symptomatic causing palpitations, fatigue, lightheadedness, syncope, or sudden cardiac death	• It is a serious arrhythmia that occurs in patients with organic heart disease (prior MI and cardiomyopathy).
		• May be precipitated by drugs such as digoxin, serotonin reuptake inhibitors, and tricyclic antidepressants

• Ventricular fibrillation (VF)
  • The myocardium depolarizes in a chaotic manner and coordinated ventricular activity ceases
    – Heart rate 350–450 beats/minute and the rhythm is irregular
	• The heart ceases to pump, the blood pressure falls, and unconsciousness occurs.
	• VF is the presenting rhythm for about 70 % of patients in cardiac arrest
	• If left untreated, death will follow in about three to five minutes
		• Coronary artery disease is the most common cause of VF, followed by hypertrophic or dilated cardiomyopathy.

Blood Pressure

BP, defined as the lateral pressure exerted by the blood in a unit area of blood vessel wall, is a function of cardiac output and peripheral vascular resistance.

The BP is a reliable indicator of cardiovascular function and correlates well with a number of other systemic diseases and conditions (Table 3.4). Consequently, the BP should be recorded on all new patients at the time of initial appointment, at all recall appointments, and at all appointments for all patients with a history of hypertension, cardiovascular diseases, diabetes mellitus, thyroid disorders, adrenal disease, renal dysfunction,

Figure 3.32 Pulse pressure.

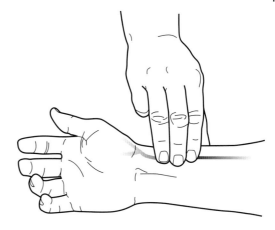

Table 3.4 Common conditions that affect BP.

Etiology of hypotension	Etiology of hypertension
• Anemia	• Physical or emotional stress
• Hypoaldosteronism	• Hyperaldosteronism
• Hypothyroidism	• Hyperthyroidism
• Syncope	• Dyslipidemia
• Shock	• Diabetes mellitus
• Heart failure	• Renal dysfunction
• Collagen vascular disorders	• Steroid therapy

and significant use of tobacco, coffee, and alcohol.

BP is classified as normal (<120/80 mm Hg), prehypertension (120 to 139/80 to 89 mm Hg), stage 1 hypertension (140–159 mm Hg systolic or 90–99 mm Hg diastolic), or stage 2 hypertension (≥160 mmHg systolic or ≥100 mmHg diastolic).

Technique

In the everyday practice of medicine (including medical dentistry), the BP is determined by sphygmomanometry, using a combination of the palpatory and auscultatory methods. A sphygmomanometer consists of a pressure manometer (mercury-gravity or aneroid type), a compressor cuff, and a pressure source. Automated readers that are available should be avoided, as they are often inaccurate.

The mercury-gravity manometer consists of a uniform diameter straight glass tube with a reservoir containing mercury. The pressure chamber of the reservoir communicates with the compression cuff through a rubber tube. When pressure is exerted on the mercury in the reservoir it falls, and the mercury in the glass tube rises. Since the weight of the mercury is dependent on gravity, which is constant, a given amount of pressure will always support a column of mercury of the same height. The mercury-gravity manometer is the most accurate, does not require recalibration, and is the standard for measuring BP.

The aneroid manometer consists of a metal bellows, which is connected to the compression cuff. Variations of pressure within the system cause the bellows to expand and collapse. The movement of the bellows rotates a gear that turns a needle, pivoted on bearings, across a calibrated dial. Since the BP recorded with the aneroid manometer depends upon the elasticity of the metal bellows, it is subject to errors inherent in the elastic properties of metals. For this reason, the aneroid manometer must be calibrated against a mercury manometer at regular intervals.

The compressor cuff consists of an inflatable rubber bladder enclosed in an inelastic covering and the pressure source consisting of a rubber hand bulb and pressure control valve. An appropriately sized cuff should cover two-thirds of the biceps; its bladder should be long enough to encircle more than 80 % of the arm and should have a width that equals at least 40 % of the arm's circumference. Thus, children require smaller cuffs and obese patients require larger cuffs (Table 3.5).

Ideally, the BP is measured after the patient has rested comfortably for at least five minutes in a sitting or recumbent position. The examiner's chair should be arranged so that the patient's right arm is always and inevitably presented for recording the BP. The arm should be abducted, slightly flexed, and supported by a smooth, firm surface. If the arm is unsupported, the BP may be elevated by 10–12 mm Hg due to added hydrostatic pressure induced by gravity. The brachial artery over which the BP is to be recorded should be at a level with the heart (Figure 3.33).

The deflated compression cuff is applied snugly around the right arm. The lower edge of the cuff should be 2–3 cm above the antecubital fossa. The radial pulse is palpated and the rate is noted. The compression cuff is then rapidly inflated to 70 mmHg and then steadily inflated in 10 mm increments (when the cuff is inflated it should not bulge nor become displaced) until the radial pulse disappears (an estimation of the systolic pressure). The cuff is then deflated.

The bell of the stethoscope is now applied lightly but snugly over the brachial artery to produce an airtight seal. The bell must not come in contact with the patient's clothing or with the compression cuff. The compression cuff is now inflated rapidly to about 20–30 mm Hg above the previously determined systolic estimated pressure. The cuff is then deflated at a rate of 2–3 mm Hg/heartbeat. While watching the meniscus of the mercury column of the mercury-gravity manometer or the needle of the aneroid manometer, the pressure at which

Table 3.5 Cuff selection.

Patient size	Arm circumference	Cuff bladder size
• Child or small adult	<23 cm	12 cm × 18 cm
• Standard adult	<33 cm	12 cm × 26 cm
• Large adult	<50 cm	12 cm × 40 cm

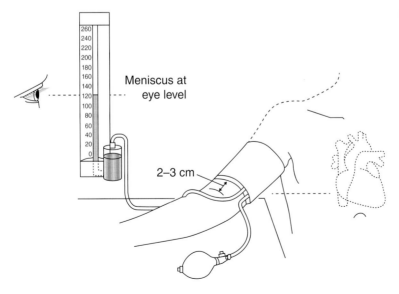

Figure 3.33 Blood pressure.

Meniscus at eye level

2–3 cm

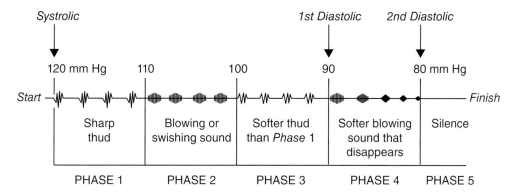

Figure 3.34 Korotkoff sounds.

characteristic changes in the Korotkoff sounds (Figure 3.34) occur is noted. From the changes in the quality of the sounds, the systolic and diastolic BP is determined.

The pressure within the compression cuff as indicated by the level of the mercury column (mercury-gravity manometer) or the position of the needle (aneroid manometer) at the moment the Korotkoff sounds are first heard represents the systolic BP. This is the start of Phase 1, which begins with faint, clear, and rhythmic tapping or thumping sounds that gradually increase in intensity.

The pressure within the compression cuff indicated by the level of the mercury column (mercury-gravity manometer) or the position of the needle (aneroid manometer) at the moment the Korotkoff sounds become muffled represents the first diastolic pressure (beginning of Phase 4). The second diastolic pressure is the pressure within the compression cuff at the moment the sounds finally disappear (beginning of Phase 5). Disappearance of the sound marks the diastolic BP.

The pulse pressure reflects the numerical difference between the systolic and the diastolic BP. The "hammering" or "pounding" effect of elevated pulse pressure (noted when palpating the radial artery) damages arterial walls, contributes to arteriosclerosis, and leads to target organ damage. The pulse pressure closely correlates with the systolic BP and is a reliable cofactor that will provide further evidence to either confirm or rule out significant cardiovascular disease.

Respiration

Respiration is the process of gaseous exchange between an organism and its environment wherein oxygen is taken up by the capillaries of the lungs and carbon dioxide is released from the blood.

The rate, rhythm, and depth of respiration are reliable indicators of respiratory function and correlate well with a number of other systemic diseases and conditions (Table 3.6). Consequently, the rate, rhythm, and depth of respiration should be recorded on all new patients at the time of initial appointment and at all subsequent appointments on all patients with a history of cardiovascular and respiratory abnormalities.

Respiration in men is primarily diaphragmatic and noticeable use of the chest muscles indicates air hunger (dyspnea, shortness of breath). Respiration in women is primarily costal and air hunger is indicated by pronounced use of the diaphragm. The use of the accessory muscles of respiration (neck, shoulders) indicates air hunger, as seen in cases of congestive heart failure, bronchial asthma, or advanced pulmonary emphysema.

Table 3.6 Abnormal rate and depth of respiration and associated conditions.

- Tachypnea
  - Increased rate and decreased depth of respiration
- Hyperpnea
  - Increased rate and depth of respiration typical of hyperventilation syndrome
- Kussmaul–Kien respiration
  - Hyperpnea, 30–40 breaths/minute, typical of profound diabetic acidosis and hyperglycemic coma
- Cheney–Stokes breathing
  - Hyperpnea alternating with periods of apnea typical of profound toxicity associated with heart disease, chronic nephritis, and advanced brain tumor
- Prolonged inspiration (sigh)
  - Typical of anxiety or a precursor to hyperventilation
- Prolonged expiration
  - Typical of moderate-to-advanced pulmonary emphysema

The normal respiration rate in adults is 16–20 breaths/minute and 24–28 breaths/minute in children. The rate typically increases by 4 breaths/minute for each Fahrenheit degree of body temperature elevation.

Technique

With the patient at rest, respiration is assessed by observing the rise and fall of the chest or upper abdomen over one minute. Patients may control respiration to some extent, so it is best determined without the patient's knowledge (awareness).

Temperature

Fever was a well-recognized sign of disease for centuries even before the introduction of the thermometer. Now it is also well-established that humans have a circadian temperature rhythm and this rhythm is difficult to disturb.

An awareness of this consistency assists clinicians with identifying disease or even factitious or self-induced illness (Table 3.7).

Table 3.7 Conditions affecting body temperature.

Hypothermia	Hyperthermia
<ul><li>Anemia</li><li>Alcoholism</li><li>Chronic debilitating disease</li><li>Hypothyroidism</li><li>Malignant hypothermia</li></ul>	<ul><li>Exercise</li><li>Infection</li><li>Ovulation</li><li>Hyperthyroidism</li><li>Factitious fever</li></ul>

Consequently, to establish a baseline value, the temperature of each patient should be recorded at the initial appointment and at all subsequent appointments when a patient presents with ominous signs of a serious odontogenic infection such as swelling (impending airway compromise, marked trismus), lymphadenopathy, chills, rapid respiration, hypotension, and tachycardia.

Factitious fever is an elevated temperature caused by some unnatural process (e.g. sipping a hot beverage right before having the temperature taken) that doesn't correlate with other presenting signs and symptoms. If a factitious fever is suspected, the patient should be closely observed while the temperature is retaken with a different thermometer. A factitious fever may be caused by a patient's desire to attract attention, gain sympathy, avoid work, or obtain a prescription for narcotics.

In health, the normal body temperature is about 37.0°C. The maximum circadian variation is about 0.6°C. Fever is defined as elevated body temperature of more than 38.2°C rectally or 37.8°C orally.

Technique

Prior to taking the temperature, the patient should be well rested and the medical history should have elicited information regarding the use of antipyretics that may have been taken within the past few hours.

Fever is most accurately diagnosed by rectal measurement; however, the technique is inappropriate in an oral healthcare setting.

Oral measurements, which are normally about 0.6°C lower than rectal measurements, are reproducible and convenient. Prior to determining the oral temperature, patients should not have smoked nor have had any hot or cold food or drink for at least 10 minutes. Other factors that may affect oral temperature include inadequate time of measurement (several minutes are required), mouth breathing, and hyperventilation. Measurement by tympanic membrane is the least accurate method of determining temperature.

3.7 Summary

Basic diagnostic procedures during initial and subsequent periodic limited physical examination of patients are of significant value in corroborating historical findings, formulating differential diagnoses, and determining the need for further diagnostic testing. Each procedure should be performed deliberately and systematically to permit the clinician maximum opportunity to detect and identify irregularities and abnormalities.

Suggested Reading

Beevers, G., Lip, G.Y., and O'Brien, E. (2001). ABC of hypertension. Blood pressure measurement. Part I – Sphygmomanometry: factors common to all techniques. *Br. Med. J.* 322 (7292): 981–985.

Dieterle, T. (2012). Blood pressure measurement – an overview. *Swiss Med. Wkly.* 142: w13517.

Goldsmith, L.A., Katz, S.I., Gilchrest, B. et al. (2012). The structure of skin lesions and fundamentals of diagnosis. In: *Fitzpatrick's Dermatology in General Medicine*, 8e (eds. L.A. Goldsmith et al.). McGraw-Hill.

Hodgkinson, J., Mant, J., Martin, U. et al. (2011). Relative effectiveness of clinic and home blood pressure monitoring compared with ambulatory blood pressure monitoring in diagnosis of hypertension: systematic review. *Br. Med. J.* 342: d3621.

Jarvis, C. (2012). General survey, measurement, vital signs. In: *Physical Examination and Health Assessment*, 6e, 127–158. Elsevier Saunders.

Little, J.W., Miller, C.S., and Rhodus, N.L. (2018). Cardiac arrhythmias. In: *Little and Falace's*

Dental Management of the Medically Compromised Patient, 9e (eds. J.A. Little et al.). Elsevier.

Medline Plus, U.S. National Library of Medicine and the National Institutes of Health. Measuring pulse. www.nlm.nih.gov/medlineplus/ency/article/003399.htm (accessed 16 December 2020).

Seidel, H.M., Ball, S.W., Dains, J.E. et al. (2011). Skin, hair, and nails. In: *Mosby's Guide to Physical Examination*, 7e, 150–212. Mosby Elsevier.

Whelton, P.K., Carey, R.M., Aronow, W.S. et al. (2018). 2017 ACC/AHA/AAPA/ABC/ACPM/AGS/APhA/ASH/ASPC/NMA/PCNA Guideline for the Prevention, Detection, Evaluation, and Management of High Blood Pressure in Adults: Executive Summary: A Report of the American College of Cardiology/American Heart Association Task Force on Clinical Practice Guidelines. *Hypertension.* 71 (6): 1269–1324.

4

Examination of the Head and Neck

A thorough examination of the head and neck is an essential component of the diagnostic process. Clinicians should be able to recognize normal variations and abnormalities. For maximum yield, the patient should be seated at eye level with the examiner. When an abnormality is noted, the following questions should be asked: (i) is the abnormality itself important, or is it an inconsequential finding; (ii) could the abnormality be related to a potential intraoral finding; and (iii) is the abnormality suggestive of an underlying systemic disorder?

4.1 Examine the Head and Face

Note Position and Observe Movement of the Head at Rest

Tilting of the head may indicate an attempt to compensate for defective vision or hearing or to minimize discomfort in the neck. An exaggerated forward thrust of the head may be associated with an abnormality of the cervical vertebrae. Sudden, unexpected movements of the head with facial grimaces may simply be

Physical Evaluation and Treatment Planning in Dental Practice, Second Edition.
Géza T. Terézhalmy, Michaell A. Huber, Lily T. García and Ronald L. Occhionero.
© 2021 John Wiley & Sons, Inc. Published 2021 by John Wiley & Sons, Inc.
Companion Website: www.wiley.com/go/terezhalmy/physical

a habitual spasm. A to-and-fro bobbing of the head may be secondary to aortic insufficiency. A subtle but steady rhythmic tremor of the head may suggest Parkinson's disease (PD). Constant licking of the corners of the mouth or smacking of the tongue is suggestive of tardive dyskinesia (TD), a condition often associated with neuroleptic drug therapy.

Parkinson's Disease

PD is a degenerative central nervous system (CNS) disorder, which may be either primary or secondary. Primary PD is characterized by degeneration of dopaminergic neurons of the substantia nigra and other brainstem dopaminergic cell groups. The loss of substantia nigra neurons results in depletion of the neurotransmitter dopamine. Secondary PD is associated with loss of, or interference with, the action of dopamine in the basal ganglia due to other degenerative CNS diseases, exogenous toxins, or drugs.

Clinical Features Regardless of its etiology, striatal dopamine deficiency leads to an impaired ability to control the smooth movement of skeletal muscle. The term TRAP has been used to refer to the characteristic findings of tremor at rest, rigidity, akinesia, and postural instability. The most common initial symptom is a resting tremor of the hands, often observed as the classic "pill-rolling" motion of the fingers. Tremor is often unilateral, usually decreases with voluntary movement, is absent during sleep, and may be exacerbated during emotional stress and fatigue. The hands, arms, and legs are affected in decreasing order of frequency.

As PD progresses, the face becomes mask-like, the mouth remains open, and blinking is diminished. The patient may experience difficulty swallowing and tends to drool. Speech becomes slurred, monotonous, stuttering, and soft (hypophonia). Cognitive and emotional symptoms of PD include depression, memory impairment, and an inability to make executive decisions. Approximately 25% of patients with PD meet the criteria for dementia.

Diagnosis The diagnosis of PD is suggested by unilateral hand tremor, infrequent blinking, lack of facial expression, decreased movement, impaired postural reflexes, and a characteristic gait. The strongest support for the diagnosis of PD is provided by a positive clinical response to carbidopa and levodopa.

Treatment Treatment protocols focus on increasing dopamine availability in the CNS and/or inhibiting the effects of acetylcholine. Levodopa, combined with carbidopa, remains the most effective symptomatic treatment for PD. Dental management of the patient with PD requires an awareness and accommodation of its progressive nature, which leads to physical, cognitive, and behavioral changes.

Tardive Dyskinesia

TD is a potentially irreversible, involuntary hyperkinetic disorder affecting the orofacial, limb, trunk, and respiratory musculature. The etiology of TD is not completely understood. One hypothesis suggests the possibility of dopamine receptor supersensitivity, while another contends that it is due to gamma-aminobutyric acid insufficiency. Advancing age is the most consistently established risk factor for TD, and there appears to be a linear correlation between age and both the prevalence and the severity of TD. Some ethnic differences, with higher rates in African Americans and lower rates in Chinese and other Asian populations, have been reported. Patients with diabetes mellitus are at a greater risk for developing TD, as are alcohol or drug abusers.

Numerous drugs have been implicated in TD. Prolonged treatment with neuroleptics such as risperidone, olanzapine, and haloperidol increase dopamine metabolism, which in turn results in increased free radical production. It is postulated that free radicals and other toxic agents damage the basal ganglia. A type of delayed-onset TD has also been reported in patients taking dopamine antagonists (e.g. metoclopramide, prochlorperazine), L-dopa, and amphetamines. Other drugs reported to be associated with acute TD include anticonvulsants (phenytoin, carbamazepine), oral contraceptives, chloroquine-based antimalarials, lithium, and tricyclic antidepressants. In patients taking these latter drugs, the symptoms of TD are reversible upon dose reduction or discontinuation of the offending drug.

Clinical Features TD is characterized by rapid, jerky, writhing (twisting and turning), and involuntary movements that most often affect the orofacial region along with distorted tonicity of arm, leg, and trunk muscles. Involvement of the arm, leg, and trunk muscles occurs chiefly during walking. The movements are highly complex and appear to be well coordinated, but are senseless. Dyskinetic blinking is an early sign.

Puckering or pouting, lip smacking, chewing, jaw clenching or mouth opening, facial grimacing, and blowing are common features. As the condition progresses, writhing of the tongue is characterized by thrusting of the tongue out of the mouth as if "fly catching." Repeated licking of the lips or pressing the tongue against the cheeks may produce an obvious bulge of the cheek.

Diagnosis The characteristic dyskinetic movements and their occurrence following exposure to neuroleptic drugs should suggest the presumptive diagnosis and mandate a medical consultation. The diagnosis is established following a complete neuropsychiatric evaluation.

Treatment The best chance to induce remission, or at the least to minimize the progression of TD, is to discontinue the offending neuroleptic drug. In moderate-to-severe TD, drug therapy to treat involuntary movements may be necessary.

Note the Color of the Face

Pallor may be seen in patients with anemia or edema, and as a transient phenomenon in association with vasopressor syncope. Cyanosis may be evident in patients who have a congenital heart defect, heart failure, or chronic obstructive pulmonary disease. Increased concentration of bilirubin in the blood leads to jaundice of the skin, sclera of the eyes, and mucous membranes. It may be indicative of excessive red blood cell destruction, hepatitis, cirrhosis, hepatocellular carcinoma, cholelithiasis, or pancreatic cancer. Port-wine nevi, or capillary or cavernous malformations affecting the cutaneous/mucosal distribution of the trigeminal nerve, may represent a manifestation of Sturge–Weber angiomatosis or Klippel–Trenaunay syndrome. Deep bronzing of the face may be associated with Addison's disease (AD).

Pallor

Pallor refers to the abnormally pale appearance of the skin and/or mucous membranes and is a principal sign of anemia. Anemia reflects a reduction of oxygen in blood due to an abnormality in the quantity or quality of red blood cells and is characterized by a reduction in hemoglobin concentration and the volume of erythrocytes in a unit volume of whole blood (hematocrit). Anemia may be due to (i) defective proliferation of red blood cells; (ii) defective maturation of red blood cells; (iii) increased destruction of red blood cells; or (iv) acute or chronic blood loss.

Edema of the skin may also produce pallor. The structural elements of the integument are rendered more distant from each other as they are separated by fluid. Light penetrating the skin meets a diminished quantity of pigment, more rays are reflected, and the skin appears paler than normal.

A common cause of transient pallor is vasodepressor syncope due to the dilatation of resistance vessels. This form of fainting is likely to occur in the oral healthcare setting in response to sudden emotional stress

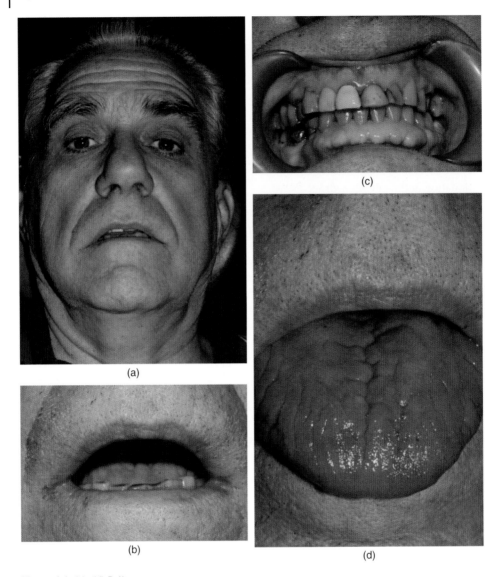

Figure 4.1 (a)–(d) Pallor.

brought on by pain, surgical manipulation, sight of blood, or heat. Cerebral blood flow becomes significantly reduced, precipitated by a generalized, progressive, autonomic (adrenergic followed by compensatory cholinergic) discharge.

Clinical Features Pallor is a physical sign. While there is a wide variability in skin color among individuals due to the size of capillaries and their depth below the skin surface, the clinical appearance of the conjunctivae, lips,

and oral mucosae, which demonstrate less of a variation in color, provide a more reliable indication of pallor (Figure 4.1a–d). Similarly, the color of the nail bed and a well-delineated lunula are also good indicators of pallor.

Diagnosis The diagnosis of pallor is based on a careful inspection of the skin, conjunctivae, lips, oral mucosa, and nail beds. Establishing the etiology of persistent pallor is the responsibility of the patient's physician.

Treatment An appreciation for the extent and duration of pallor, along with any associated symptoms, may lead to the establishment of a specific etiology followed by appropriate treatment that will correct both the clinical signs and the underlying cause.

Cyanosis

Cyanosis is a physical finding characterized by a bluish discoloration due to an excess amount of reduced hemoglobin in the sub-papillary venous plexus. It may be peripheral or central. Peripheral cyanosis may be seen following exposure to low ambient temperatures, anxiety-induced vasoconstriction, Raynaud's disease-associated vasospasm, other obstructive peripheral vascular abnormalities, and low cardiac output. Central cyanosis results from arterial hypoxemia and may result from serious cardiac and/or pulmonary abnormalities.

Clinical Features Peripheral cyanosis tends to affect the upper and/or lower extremities, particularly the palms of the hands, the soles of the feet, and the nail beds. When cyanosis is caused by heart or lung disease, in addition to the extremities, it affects the "central" parts of the body, that is, the torso, face, lips, and oral mucosae (Figure 4.2a and b).

Diagnosis Cyanosis is best recognized under natural, bright daylight in regions where the skin is thick, unpigmented, and flushed, such as the ear lobes, cutaneous surfaces of the lips, and the nail beds. Cyanosis is less apparent in the oral mucosae of patients with light complexion when compared to patients with dark skin. Overall, the visual perception of "blueness" varies greatly among clinicians and it is believed that most clinicians do not perceive cyanosis until the oxygen saturation has fallen to less than 80%.

Treatment A careful history and physical examination by a physician are warranted to determine the specific etiology and, consequently, the most appropriate treatment.

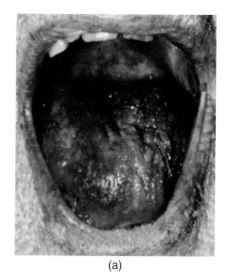

(a)

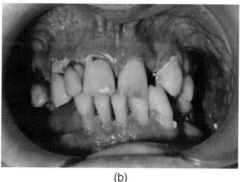

(b)

Figure 4.2 (a) and (b) Cyanosis.

Jaundice

Jaundice is the result of increased concentrations of bilirubin in blood. Red blood cells, when destroyed, release hemoglobin, and bilirubin is a by-product of subsequent hemoglobin catabolism. The bilirubin molecule is attached to albumin and is conjugated with glucuronic acid in the liver, rendering it water-soluble. Conjugated bilirubin becomes a constituent of the bile and is transported to the duodenum where it gives the fecal matter its characteristic color. The predominance of conjugated or unconjugated bilirubin can pinpoint the metabolic problem as prehepatic (destruction of red blood cells), hepatic (acute viral, drug-induced, or alcoholic

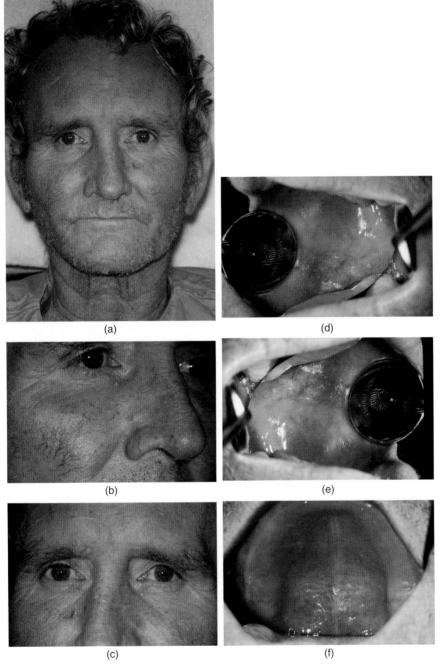

Figure 4.3
(a)–(f)
Jaundice.

(a)

(b)

(c)

(d)

(e)

(f)

hepatitis; subacute or chronic hepatitis; cirrhosis; hepatocellular carcinoma), or posthepatic (biliary tract obstruction by duct stones, duct stricture, or pancreatic cancer).

Clinical Features Jaundice is a sign that typically affects the skin, oral mucosa, and sclera of the eyes (Figure 4.3a–f). When associated with spider angiomas of the face, it may suggest acute or chronic hepatitis. Vascular spiders seldom occur in patients with jaundice resulting from obstruction secondary to bile duct stones or neoplasia.

Diagnosis The diagnosis is based on visual inspection. While the skin is easily observed, the peripheral portion of the conjunctivae and the oral mucosae represent highly sensitive areas that may manifest jaundice before the skin. Medical consultation for further evaluation is warranted.

Treatment The treatment of jaundice falls under the purview of the physician and is targeted at removing or controlling the underlying cause.

Port-Wine Nevi

A port-wine nevus is a characteristic form of a capillary hemangioma affecting the head and neck. While it often occurs as an isolated entity, its presence may be indicative of a more serious condition such as Sturge–Weber syndrome (encephalotrigeminal angiomatosis) or Klippel–Trenaunay syndrome.

Clinical Features Port-wine nevi are purplish, diffuse macules with irregular borders that are sharply demarcated from the adjacent normal skin. They occur unilaterally on the face and follow the first, second, third, or all three divisions of the trigeminal nerve (Figure 4.4a–e).

Diagnosis Port-wine nevi are easily diagnosed based on their characteristic appearance and history. A differential diagnosis should include Sturge–Weber syndrome and Klippel–Trenaunay syndrome (Table 4.1).

Treatment Isolated port-wine nevi rarely require treatment and often involute during puberty. No consistently effective treatment is available to remove a port-wine nevus. Laser therapy may improve the cosmetic appearance of some lesions, but the improvement may only be temporary.

Table 4.1 Syndromes associated with port-wine nevi.

Sturge–Weber syndrome	Klippel–Ternaunay syndrome
Port-wine nevus	Port-wine nevus
Seizures	Venous malformation (varicosities)
Mental impairment	Bony and soft tissue hypertrophy
"Tramline" calcifications of the cerebral cortex	

Hyperpigmentation

Hyperpigmentation results from excess melanin deposition, most typically as a response to excess sunlight exposure. Other potential causes include inflammation or exposure to medications (e.g. hydroxychloroquine, amiodarone, oral contraceptives). Diseases associated with excess adrenocorticotropic hormone (ACTH) and/or melanocyte-stimulating hormone (MSH) production such as Cushing's syndrome and AD may also produce hyperpigmentation, which is classically referred to as bronzing.

AD is a potentially life-threatening endocrine disorder characterized by chronic adrenocortical hypofunction. The resultant lack of cortisol impairs the patient's ability to respond to physiologic stress. The cause of AD may be primary, secondary, or tertiary. Most cases of primary AD are caused by a gradual autoimmune destruction of the adrenal cortex. Less frequent causes of primary AD include glandular destruction by tuberculosis and human immunodeficiency virus (HIV) infection, histoplasmosis, primary or metastatic malignancies, amyloidosis, sarcoidosis, and drugs.

The incidence of primary AD in the general population is about 1/100 000. Secondary AD results from deficient ACTH secretion, usually due to the presence or treatment of a pituitary or hypothalamic

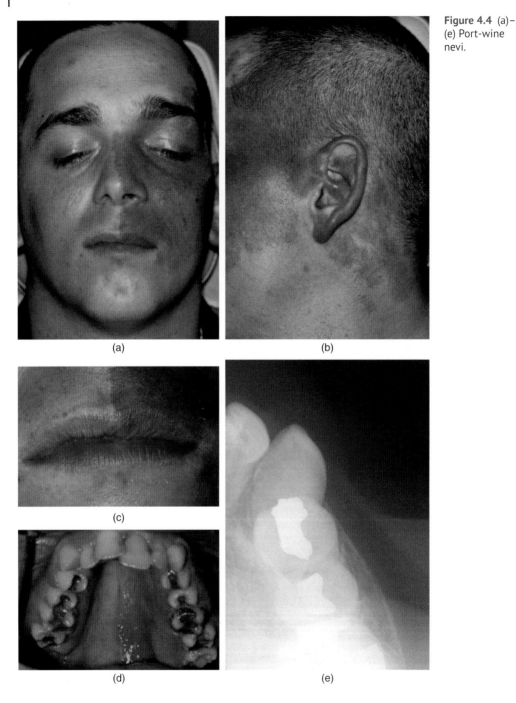

Figure 4.4 (a)–(e) Port-wine nevi.

(a)

(b)

(c)

(d)

(e)

tumor. Tertiary AD is the most frequently observed type and develops as a consequence of long-term high-dose therapeutic corticosteroid administration, which leads to suppression of the hypothalamic–pituitary–adrenal axis.

Clinical Features The clinical manifestations of AD include fatigue, weakness, listlessness, orthostatic hypotension, weight loss, and anorexia. Patients may also report a craving for salt and experience periods of hypoglycemia.

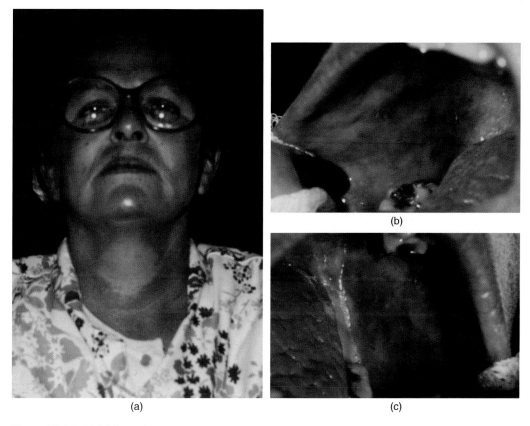

(a) (b) (c)

Figure 4.5 (a)–(c) Addison disease.

The distinguishing sign of primary AD is hyperpigmentation, or bronzing, most evident on sun-exposed areas of the skin, and patchy brown pigmentation of the buccal mucosae, tongue, and less frequently the lips and gingivae (Figure 4.5a–c). The cause of these pigmentations is thought to be an increased compensatory pituitary synthesis of ACTH and MSH.

Diagnosis The suspicion of AD is based on the presenting clinical signs and symptoms. Medical referral for further evaluation is warranted. Both passive (e.g. serum cortisol and ACTH levels) and provocative (e.g. insulin tolerance test) laboratory testing, combined with appropriate imaging tests, are required to establish the specific diagnosis.

Treatment Both primary and secondary adrenocortical hypofunction require life-long glucocorticoid, and if necessary, mineralocorticoid replacement therapy. Therapy is empirically individualized to maintain normal weight and sense of well-being. Commonly prescribed glucocorticoid agents include hydrocortisone, prednisone, or dexamethasone. The chosen agent is often administered in the morning and evening to mimic the normal diurnal release of these hormones.

The impaired innate ability to respond to excess physiologic stress places a patient with AD at risk for developing an Addisonian crisis. During an Addisonian crisis, the patient becomes dangerously hypotensive and experiences hypoglycemia. Precipitating factors may include stress, infection, trauma, surgery, and the use of general anesthesia. Treatment of an Addisonian crisis is a medical emergency and includes prompt intravenous administration of saline and glucocorticoid.

Observe Facial Characteristics

A massive face, craggy eyebrows, prominent nose, enlarged mandible, and macroglossia are characteristic of acromegaly. A puffy edematous face; dry, coarse, and scaly skin; and slowed speech and mentation are characteristic signs of hypothyroidism. A moon facies (fat deposition in the face), hirsutism, and acne may represent Cushing's syndrome associated with excess corticosteroids either from an endogenous or an exogenous source. Bell's palsy (BP), characterized by unilateral paralysis of the facial muscles, may reflect transient or permanent seventh nerve damage.

Acromegaly

Acromegaly results from an overproduction of growth hormone (GH) after closure of the epiphyseal plates, and is usually due to an adenoma of the anterior lobe of the pituitary gland (Figure 4.6a). It is a rare condition with a prevalence of approximately 50–70 cases per million and an incidence of three cases per million per year. Acromegaly progresses slowly and insidiously and is most often diagnosed during the fourth decade of life, typically 10 years after initial onset. Untreated acromegaly is associated with a 30% reduction in life-span, usually as a consequence of cardiovascular, cerebrovascular, and pulmonary dysfunction.

Clinical Features Clinical signs and symptoms include hyperhidrosis, muscle weakness, paresthesia, sleep apnea, hypertension, and heart disease. Skeletal growth can lead to prognathism, frontal bossing, nasal bone hypertrophy, and large hands and feet; coarsening of facial features, prominent lips, and macroglossia are common (Figure 4.6b–g). An anterior open bite reflects supereruption of posterior and flaring of anterior teeth.

Diagnosis The characteristic clinical presentation of acromegaly should alert the clinician and prompt a medical referral. Reviewing previous photographs of a patient may help to confirm the clinical impression. Laboratory testing to establish the presence of elevated levels of GH insulin-like growth factor 1 (IGF-1) confirms the diagnosis. Radiographic imaging often reveals ballooning of the sella turcica, an indicator of pituitary enlargement. Other potential head and neck radiographic findings include enlargement of the paranasal sinuses, thickening of the outer table of the skull, increased condylar growth, and hypercementosis.

Treatment Measures to abolish or obtund excess GH production include microsurgery, radiation therapy, and medical therapy combined with routine follow-up examinations. The skeletal and to some degree soft-tissue changes are permanent.

Hypothyroidism

Hypothyroidism is the most common form of thyroid dysfunction encountered in medical practice. If the condition occurs in infants and young children, it leads to cretinism. In adults it causes myxedema. Approximately 95% of cases occur as a consequence of primary thyroid disease or it management. The three most common causes of primary hypothyroidism are autoimmune thyroiditis (Hashimoto thyroiditis), thyroidectomy for Graves' disease or nodular goiter, and radioactive iodine therapy for Graves' disease. Secondary hypothyroidism is due to inadequate production of thyroid-stimulating hormone (TSH) by the pituitary gland. Other infrequent causes of hypothyroidism include radiation to the neck, postpartum thyroiditis, and exposure to drugs such as iodine, lithium, and amiodarone.

Clinical Features The thyroid gland may be normal, nonpalpable, or diffusely enlarged. The classic features of hypothyroidism include

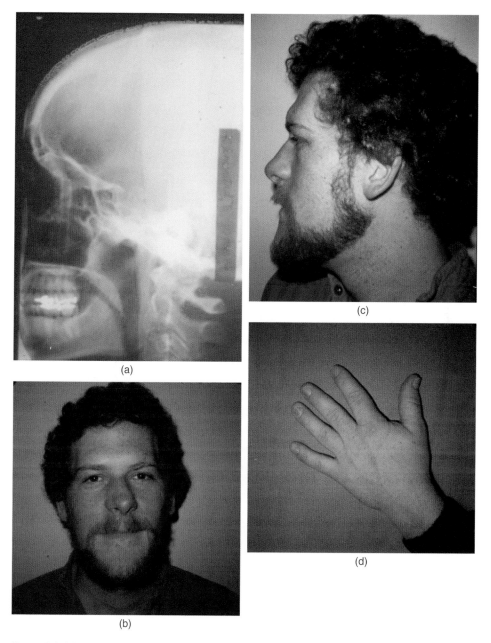

(a)

(b)

(c)

(d)

Figure 4.6 (a)–(g) Acromegaly.

sinus bradycardia, hoarseness, nonpitting edema (myxedema) of the skin, periorbital edema, dryness of the skin, brittleness of the scalp hair, and an enlarged tongue and mouth breathing (Figure 4.7). Other signs and symptoms such as lethargy, depression, memory loss, cognitive impairment, modest weight gain, intolerance to cold, constipation, and neuromuscular dysfunction (vague aches and pains) are common.

Diagnosis The diagnostic workup for a patient suspected of having hypothyroidism should include a thorough historical, clinical, and

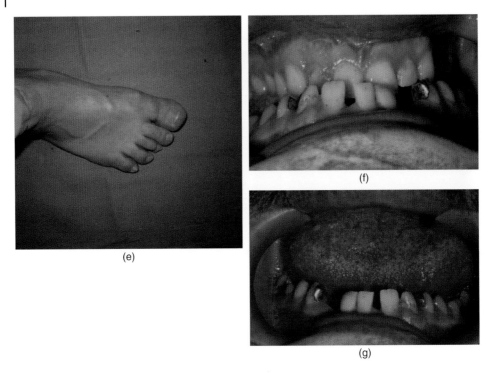

(e)

(f)

(g)

Figure 4.6 (*Continued*)

laboratory assessment. The laboratory hallmark of primary hypothyroidism is an increased compensatory serum TSH concentration with low free-thyroxine (FT4).

Treatment The treatment of hypothyroidism involves lifelong thyroid hormone replacement, most commonly with levothyroxine. Once a euthyroid state is attained, follow-up at regular intervals is recommended to avoid over-treatment (iatrogenic hyperthyroidism). Mild to moderate hypothyroidism is not a contraindication to dental care, but patients with severe hypothyroidism have an impaired ability to respond to physiologic stress and are at risk for myxedema coma. Patients with hypothyroidism, to a variable degree, are hypersensitive to CNS depressants.

Cushing's Syndrome
Corticotropin-releasing hormone (CRH) synthesized in the hypothalamus stimulates pituitary ACTH secretion. ACTH stimulates

the adrenal cortex to release cortisol. Cortisol, the body's main glucocorticoid, exerts a negative feedback to help modulate further CRH and ACTH secretion. Chronic glucocorticoid excess, regardless the cause, leads to the development of Cushing's syndrome. The annual incidence is estimated at about 2.3 per million and most cases are iatrogenic, occurring as a consequence of medically prescribed glucocorticoid therapy. The pathogenic mechanisms of endogenous Cushing's syndrome can be divided into those that are ACTH-dependent and those that are ACTH-independent. A pituitary adenoma represents the most common type of ACTH-dependent Cushing's syndrome and accounts for 60–80% of all cases. The most common form of ACTH- independent Cushing's syndrome is due to adrenal hyperplasia.

Clinical Features The clinical signs and symptoms of Cushing's syndrome include truncal obesity, glucose intolerance, muscle weakness,

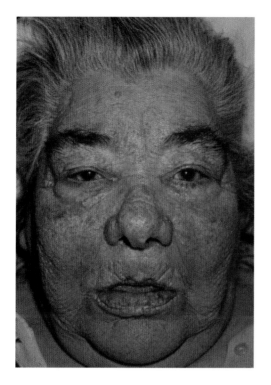

Figure 4.7 Hypothyroidism.

hypertension, osteoporosis, easy bruising, and edema (Figure 4.8a). Head and neck and oral manifestations of Cushing's syndrome include red cheeks, moon face, hirsutism, acne, and retarded dental age (Figure 4.8b and c). It should be noted that ACTH-dependent cases may be associated with hyperpigmentation.

Diagnosis Patients presenting with signs and symptoms suggestive of Cushing's syndrome should be referred for medical evaluation. The most common tests used for screening for Cushing's syndrome are 24-hour urinary free cortisol (UFC), 1-mg overnight dexamethasone suppression test (DST), and the late night salivary cortisol assay. More specific laboratory tests are often necessary to determine the specific cause of the Cushing syndrome and imaging techniques (computerized tomography [CT]; magnetic resonance imaging [MRI]) are useful to localize pituitary or ectopic ACTH-producing tumors and adrenal masses.

Treatment Surgical treatment, depending on the etiology, may include trans-sphenoidal selective pituitary adenomectomy or bilateral adrenalectomy. Pituitary irradiation may be used in adult patients in whom a surgical approach is contraindicated. Depending on the extent of the therapeutic intervention, some patients will require lifelong hormonal replacement therapy. During periods of extreme stress (e.g. infection, surgery, and trauma), patients on replacement glucocorticoid therapy may require supplemental glucocorticoid administration to prevent adrenal insufficiency. Because of an increased susceptibility to infection and possible delayed wound healing, the postoperative status of surgical patients should be monitored closely.

Bell's Palsy

BP is a common, acute, neurological disorder characterized by the sudden onset of facial nerve (C.N. VII) paresis or paralysis. The average annual incidence of BP is estimated at 20 cases per 100 000. It is more common in those aged 15–40 years. The right and left sides are affected equally, and there is no gender predominance. Bilateral facial palsy is rare, with a frequency of less than 1%.

The cause of BP remain an enigma. Proposed etiologies include infectious, neoplastic, traumatic, and idiopathic causes. Edema and subsequent nerve entrapment of the facial nerve secondary to infection remains one of the most plausible causes. Reactivated herpes viruses (e.g. herpes simplex and herpes zoster) in the geniculate ganglion of c.n. VII are often implicated in BP, but, no specific virus has been consistently demonstrated.

Clinical Features The onset of BP is usually acute and peaks after a few days. The affected side of the face lacks expression during normal conversation. The inability to close the eyes places the patient at risk for corneal/conjunctival dryness and ulceration. The eyeball may be turned upward in an attempt to block entering light; other common

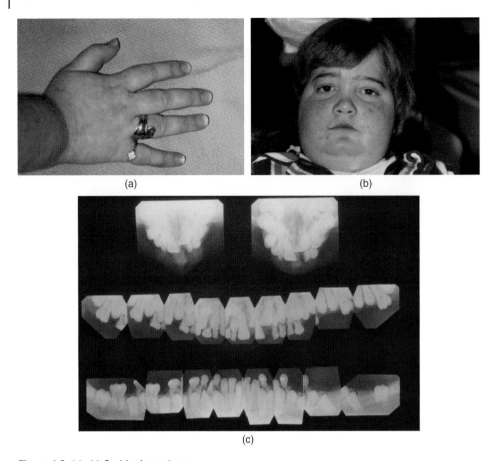

(a)

(b)

(c)

Figure 4.8 (a)–(c) Cushing's syndrome.

findings include an inability to whistle, smile, or grimace (Figure 4.9a–c). Hypersensitivity to sound (hyperacusis), loss of taste (ageusia), and pain near the mastoid area may also be present.

Diagnosis The diagnosis of BP is relatively straightforward. However, a careful clinical history must be obtained to rule out other forms of facial nerve dysfunction such as trauma, otologic disease, and intracranial mass. A thorough examination of the head and cervical spine, including cranial nerve testing (i.e. eye closure, elevation of the eyebrows, smiling, frowning, and pursing of the lips) should be performed. Evidence of involvement of other cranial nerves should alert the clinician to consider other causes.

Treatment The management of BP often requires a multidisciplinary approach. Overall, about 70% of BP patients fully recover within 30 days and 30% experience delayed or incomplete recovery. The risk of incomplete recovery is increased by a multitude of factors including initial disease severity, older age (>60 years), delayed onset of recovery (>3 weeks), pregnancy, and the presence of other comorbidities such as diabetes mellitus and herpes zoster infection.

Supportive treatment includes a temporary patch to protect the exposed eye, ocular antibiotics and artificial tears to prevent corneal ulceration, and physical therapy to prevent contracture of the paralyzed muscles. The use corticosteroid and antivirals in managing BP remains controversial. However, recent

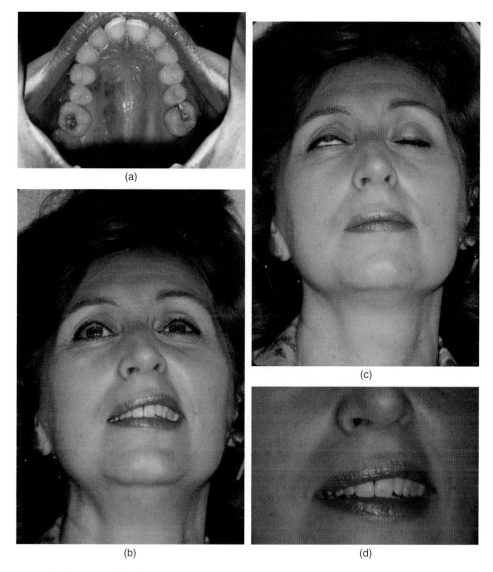

Figure 4.9 (a)–(d) Bell's palsy.

studies have shown corticosteroid therapy, with or without concurrent antiviral therapy, initiated within 72 hours of onset appears to be beneficial.

Note Facial Architecture

Facial asymmetry may be caused by a neurofibroma, an intramuscular hemangioma (IMH), a lymphangioma, fibrous dysplasia, progressive hemifacial atrophy, osteosarcoma, chondrosarcoma, or by rare genetic disorders such as focal dermal hypoplasia. Subcutaneous emphysema may present as an acute, spontaneous form of facial asymmetry. A pronounced enlargement of the cranial vault is characteristic of Paget's disease. Multiple sebaceous or dermoid cysts and osteomas involving the skull may indicate Gardner's syndrome.

Neurofibroma

A neurofibroma is a benign tumor derived from the nerve sheath and is composed of

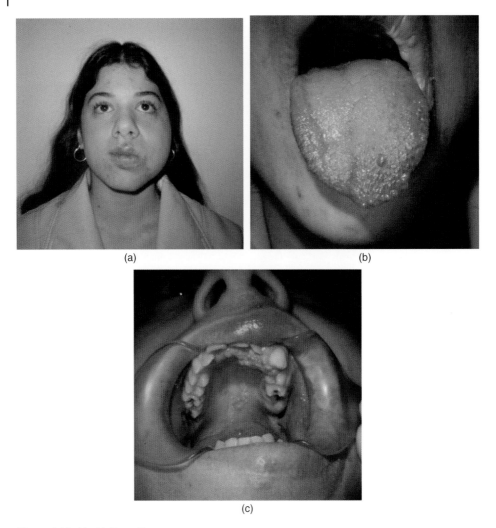

(a) (b)

(c)

Figure 4.10 (a)–(c) Neurofibroma.

a proliferation of Schwann cells, perineural fibroblasts, and axons intermixed with mast cells. Most are discovered in adulthood and there is no gender predilection.

Clinical Features Some neurofibromas are discrete and well circumscribed, whereas others are diffuse and infiltrating. Neurofibromas are commonly found on the skin. Intraorally, neurofibromas are most commonly found in the tongue, buccal mucosa, and lips; less commonly they may affect the alveolar bone (Figure 4.10a–c). Neurofibromas arising in the tongue tend to be diffuse, while those arising

in other locations tend to present as relatively well-demarcated, freely moveable, submucosal nodules. Depending on the degree of collagenization, neurofibromas may be soft or firm on palpation. Intraosseous neurofibromas typically present as a swelling without pain or parasthesia. Radiographically, the intraosseous neurofibroma is relatively well demarcated, radiolucent, and may be either unilocular or multilocular. Root divergence may be evident.

Diagnosis A definitive diagnosis of a neurofibroma is established by biopsy. The presence of more than two neurofibromas and six or more café-au-lait macules each greater than 15 mm in diameter should prompt the practitioner to consider the possibility of neurofibromatosis type 1 (von Recklinghausen's disease of the skin). It is a hereditary neurological disorder with an incidence of about 1 per 3500. No racial or sex predilection is noted. Patients with neurofibromatosis type 1 are at an increased risk for developing cognitive deficits, epilepsy, and malignant nerve sheath tumors.

Treatment There is no cure for neurofibromatosis. Treatment consists of routine monitoring and surgery when required to remove painful or disfiguring tumors. While the overall prognosis is good, malignant transformation of tumors occurs in 3–5% of the cases.

Intramuscular Hemangioma

IMHs are benign congenital neoplasms believed to evolve from an abnormally differentiated endothelial primordial network. This network is characterized by endothelial hyperplasia and malformations that enlarge by rapid cellular proliferation during the neonatal period, followed by a slow involution phase. IMH account for less than 1% of all hemangiomas, of which approximately 14% occur in the head and neck area.

Clinical Features In the head and neck area, the masseter muscle represents the most common site (36%) for an IMH, followed by the trapezius, sternocleidomastoid, periorbital, and temporalis muscles. IMH are usually asymptomatic until a growth spurt begins in the second or third decades of life, at which time pain occurs in about 50% of the cases. A palpable, fluctuant or firm mass is present in up to 98% of the cases (Figure 4.11a). The size of an intramasseter hemangioma may increase with sustained masticatory pressure (clinching of teeth) and decrease subsequent to relaxation of the masticatory muscles. Radiographically, the presence of soft-tissue calcifications or phleboliths (spherical lamellar structures with irregular radiopaque and radiolucent areas) is seen in more than 15% of cases (Figure 4.11b–d). Phleboliths are "stones" that appear to form within benign vascular lesions (hemangiomas, vascular malformations) secondary to a thrombotic episode.

Diagnosis Sonography is the first-line imaging procedure for patients with soft-tissue swellings. Magnetic resonance imaging may be more reliable in detecting and delineating deeply situated and large IMHs. Angiography is diagnostic in most cases. The finding of a phlebolith is pathognomonic for a benign hemangioma. In many cases, a biopsy is required to confirm the diagnosis.

Treatment Management of IMHs should be individualized according to the size and anatomic accessibility of the tumor, rate of growth, age of the patient, and cosmetic and functional considerations. If indicated, complete surgical excision is the treatment of choice. Local recurrence has been reported in about 18% of the cases.

Lymphangioma

Lymphangiomas are benign nonencapsulated tumors of lymphatic vessels. The majority of lymphatic malformations are present at birth and 80% become clinically evident before two years of age. However, lymphangiomas have been known to suddenly manifest in older children, adolescents, and adults. There is no gender predilection.

Clinical Features Facial lymphangiomas are the most common cause for enlarged lips (macrocheilia), enlarged ears (macrotia), and enlarged cheeks (macromala); cervicofacial lymphangiomas are associated with overgrowth of the mandibular body, which may lead to malocclusion (Figure 4.12a–c).

Intraoral lymphangiomas most commonly occur on the tongue but are also seen on the palate, buccal mucosa, gingiva, and lips. Superficial microcystic lesions are manifested

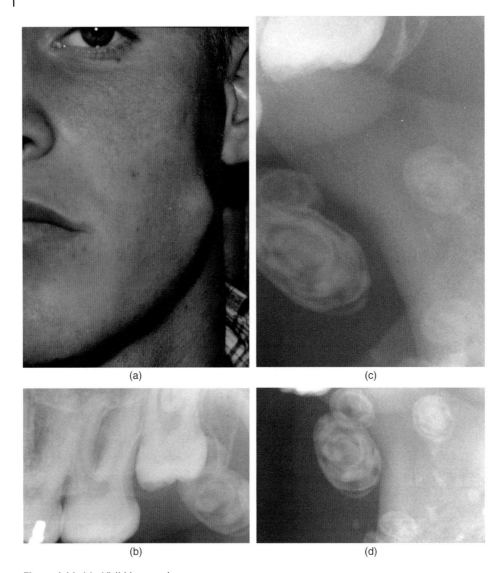

(a)

(b)

(c)

(d)

Figure 4.11 (a)–(d) IM hemangioma.

as papillary lesions, which may be the same color as the surrounding mucosa, or may be slightly erythematous. Deeper macrocystic lesions appear as diffuse nodules or masses without any significant change in surface texture or color. If the tongue is affected, considerable enlargement may occur.

Diagnosis A lymphangioma should be considered in the differential diagnosis of all head and neck masses or swellings. Magnetic resonance

imaging and a biopsy are often utilized to help confirm the diagnosis.

Treatment Surgical excision is the treatment of choice since a lymphangioma is radioresistant and insensitive to sclerosing agents. Spontaneous regression is rare and lesions tend to recur after removal.

Fibrous Dysplasia

Fibrous dysplasia is a developmental abnormality of bone characterized by replacement

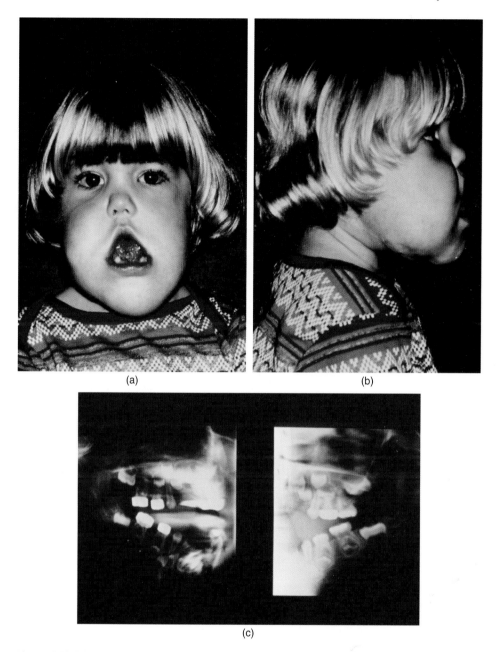

Figure 4.12 (a)–(c) Lymphangioma.

of normal bone with benign fibro-osseous tissue. Fibrous dysplasia represents 2% of all bone abnormalities, and there are two recognized variants: monostotic (single bone) and polyostotic (multiple bones).

The monostotic form is more common and accounts for approximately 80% of cases. It occurs primarily during the second decade of life with 75% of patients younger than 30 years of age at the time of diagnosis and the most

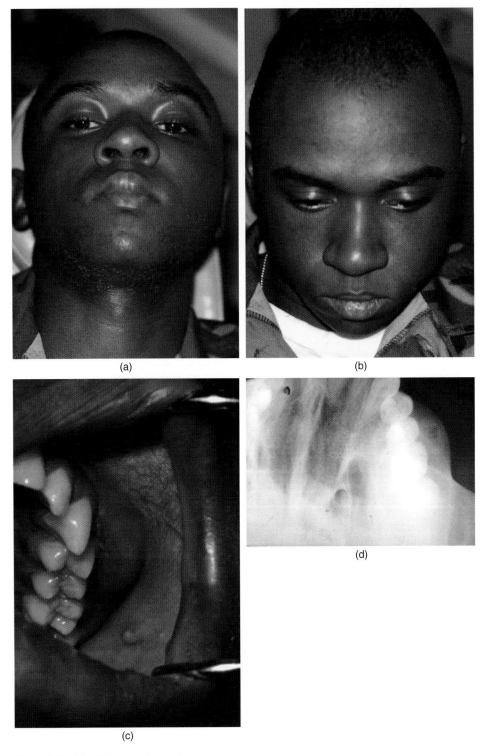

Figure 4.13 (a)–(d) Fibrous dysplasia.

Table 4.2 Differential diagnosis of fibrous dysplasia and central cemento-ossifying fibroma.

Fibrous dysplasia	Central cemento-ossifying fibroma
<40 years of age	Third and fourth decade
Maxilla or multiple bones	Body of mandible
Poorly defined, diffuse margins	Well-demarcated
Ground-glass appearance	Nodular opacities

commonly affect bones are the thigh bone, shinbone, ribs, and skull. The male–female ratio is approximately equal, and the maxilla is more commonly involved than the mandible.

Polyostotic fibrous dysplasia often presents as a more serious form called McCune–Albright syndrome, which is characterized by polyostotic fibrous dysplasia, café-au-lait dermal macules, and precocious puberty or other endocrine disturbances.

Clinical Features Fibrous dysplasia involving the bones of the craniofacial complex usually presents as a slowly progressive unilateral facial swelling (Figure 4.13a and b). Displacement of teeth may be present, along with abnormal occlusion due to jaw enlargement. Bone expansion typically causes buccal swelling as opposed to lingual swelling (Figure 4.13c). Maxillary lesions may extend into the sinuses, zygoma, sphenoid bone, and floor of the orbit.

Radiographically, the lesions appear radiolucent to radiopaque; the classic description is that of a smooth "ground-glass" appearance (Figure 4.13d). The lamina dura is often absent along with narrowing of the periodontal ligament space. Superior displacement of the mandibular canal strongly suggests fibrous dysplasia. Lesions may be unilocular or multilocular but generally are characterized by margins that blend into the surrounding normal bone.

Diagnosis The diagnosis of fibrous dysplasia is based on correlating the characteristic histological findings with the clinical presentation and medical history. Histologically, fibrous connective tissue proliferation interspersed with trabecular woven bone has been described as resembling "Chinese characters." A primary consideration in the differential diagnosis is a central cemento-ossifying fibroma (Table 4.2).

Treatment The treatment of fibrous dysplasia consists of conservative surgical resection since the condition tends to be self-limiting. Recontouring procedures generally are delayed until after puberty, when the lesions tend to become static. Radiation treatment is ineffective and may promote malignant transformation. The polyostotic form may undergo spontaneous malignant transformation.

Progressive Hemifacial Atrophy

Progressive hemifacial atrophy (Parry–Romberg syndrome) is a rare pathologic process characterized by slowly progressive but self-limited unilateral atrophy of the face. It is thought to represent a focal or localized form of scleroderma. The etiology is unknown. Symptoms usually begin in the first or second decade of life, but onset has also occurred in patients older than 60 years. Progression of the disease tends to persist for 2–20 years, followed by a period of burn-out or stability.

Clinical Features Hemifacial atrophy variably involves skin, subcutaneous tissues, fat, muscles, and less commonly the underlying osseous tissues along one or more of the trigeminal dermatomes. Many patients demonstrate normal neurological function,

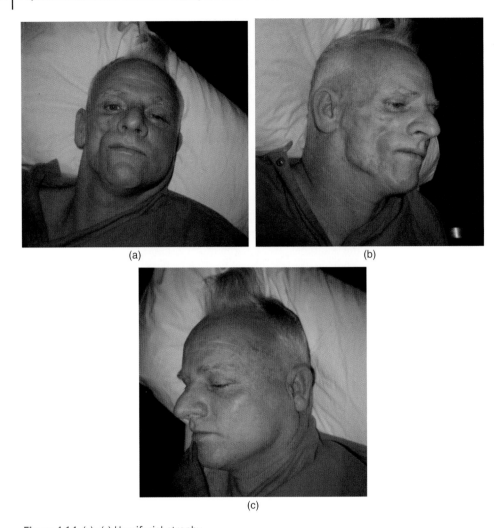

Figure 4.14 (a)–(c) Hemifacial atrophy.

although symptoms attributable to ipsilateral cerebral hemispheric dysfunction are not uncommon. Neurological involvement may result in seizures, migraine headaches, cranial nerve deficits, masticatory spasms, cognitive abnormalities, and fixed focal deficits.

Affected areas may demonstrate pigment changes, alopecia, and a change from normal hair color to white (Figure 4.14a–c). Ophthalmic defects such as ipsilateral Horner syndrome, blepharophimosis, chronic cyclitis, iritis, cataract, and secondary glaucoma may occur. Oral manifestations may include hemiatrophy of the lips, tongue, jaws, and buccal fat pad. Corresponding radiographic changes may include hemispheric calcifications, leptomeningeal enhancement, loss of cortical gyration, increased density of deep white and gray matter structures, and atrophy.

Diagnosis The diagnosis of progressive hemifacial atrophy is based on clinical presentation, neurological findings, and computed tomography and magnetic resonance imaging.

Treatment There is no cure for this disease. Treatment is limited to surgical reconstruction of the affected areas.

Osteosarcoma

Osteosarcoma is a rare bone tumor with an annual incidence of about two to three per million and the knee region is the most frequently affected site. It is a true malignant neoplasm of bone, which may occur as a central, juxtacortical, or peripheral lesion. Primary osteosarcoma of the jaws is uncommon, accounting for about 10% of all osteosarcomas reported. It is less aggressive and less likely to metastasize than osteosarcoma arising in long bones. Predisposing etiologic factors include a history of fibrous dysplasia, Paget's disease, radiation therapy, or trauma to the bone. The mean age at presentation in the maxilla/mandible is 30–34 years, which is 10 years younger than the age of presentation for long bone osteosarcoma. Men and

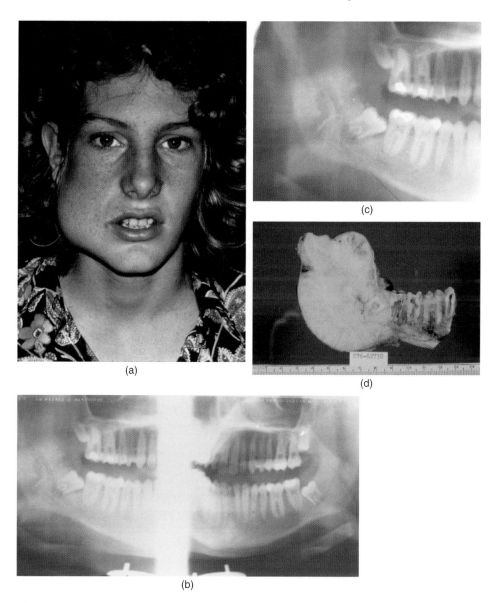

(a)

(c)

(d)

(b)

Figure 4.15 (a)–(d) Osteosarcoma.

women appear equally affected and the maxilla and mandible are affected about equally.

Clinical Features A patient typically presents with loose teeth in the area of the tumor, localized swelling, and, at times, significant facial asymmetry (Figure 4.15a). The overlying mucosa is usually normal in appearance, but may be red with small telangiectatic surface vessels. Paresthesia and/or pain are late features of the disease, as are nasal obstruction, blurred vision, and headache.

Radiographically, the lesions may appear radiolucent, radiopaque, or mixed. Mixed lesions exhibit the characteristic lamellar pattern of ossification, classically described as a "sunburst" or a "sunray" (Figure 4.15b–d). Other characteristic radiographic signs include a uniform widening of the periodontal ligament space and an increase in height of the alveolar process when compared to unaffected areas. Periosteal reactions may include the deposition of irregular new bone or lamellar new bone (onion skin).

Diagnosis The diagnosis of osteosarcoma is established by a biopsy.

Treatment Most cases of osteosarcoma are treated with chemotherapy (neoadjuvant) before radical surgical resection, at times followed by adjuvant chemotherapy. With early detection and treatment, longtime survival rates can be as high as 60%.

Chondrosarcoma

Chondrosarcoma accounts for about 15% of all skeletal malignancies and most typically affects the long bones, pelvis, and ribs. Only about 1–4% of cases occur in the head and neck area and most cases occur between the fourth and sixth decade of life. It has been postulated that chondrosarcoma is more likely to develop in individuals who have a specific pre-existing genetic condition, such as Ollier's disease, Maffucci syndrome, and multiple hereditary exostoses or osteochondromatoses. Individuals affected by these conditions manifest pre-existing benign bone tumors that are postulated to undergo malignant degeneration. Adults with Paget's disease may be at increased risk for osteosarcoma or chondrosarcoma.

Clinical Features Chondrosarcomas are more common in the maxilla than in the mandible. Although some tumors may follow an aggressive clinical course, chondrosarcoma is usually slow-growing and may lead to subtle facial asymmetry (Figure 4.16a). Symptoms vary depending on the location and size of the tumor. A chondrosarcoma most commonly presents as a painless swelling or mass and expansion into oral cavity may lead to tooth separation and mobility (Figure 4.16b–d). Radiographically, lesions in the jaws may vary from radiolucent to radiolucent/radiopaque, while a tumor that invades the sinuses usually appears radiopaque (Figure 4.16e–g).

Diagnosis The diagnosis of chondrosarcoma is established by a biopsy.

Treatment The most common therapeutic approach is surgical excision. The overall five-year survival rate for chondrosarcoma affecting the head and neck region is about 81%.

Subcutaneous Emphysema

Subcutaneous emphysema of the head and neck region and thorax is caused by the introduction of air into fascial planes. Because of the relative looseness of mucosal connective tissue, air can accumulate in these areas as a result of increased intraoral pressure associated with coughing, sneezing, blowing the nose, rinsing the mouth, playing a musical instrument, air-generating dental instruments (dental handpiece or an air–water syringe), and the release of oxygen from hydrogen peroxide. This can create spaces of considerable size. Along with air, the introduction of bacteria

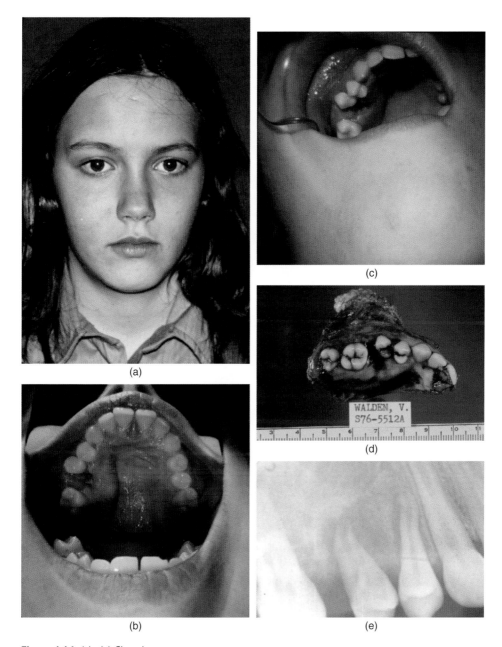

Figure 4.16 (a)–(g) Chondrosarcoma.

and foreign bodies into the fascial planes can lead to infection.

Clinical Features A sudden onset of facial swelling with a sensation of fullness of the face may be the first clinical sign of subcutaneous emphysema (Figures 4.17a–c, 4.18a and b). The patient may also complain of intraoperative tingling in the periorbital area, which may lead to closure of the eyelids on the affected side. Crepitation, pain, and tenderness may be noted when palpating the swelling.

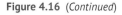

Figure 4.16 *(Continued)*

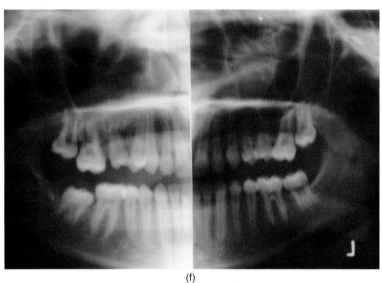

(f)

(g)

Radiographically, subcutaneous emphysema may appear as a large multilocular soft-tissue radiolucency displacing the posterior pharyngeal wall forward. Chest X-rays and soft-tissue films of the neck may display interstitial air emphysema of the retropharynx on the involved side of the face and neck.

Diagnosis Early recognition is the most important aspect in the diagnosis of subcutaneous emphysema. Crepitation upon auscultation with a stethoscope is almost pathognomonic for subcutaneous emphysema. A sudden swelling of the neck, difficulty breathing, a brassy quality to the voice, and crackling when the swollen region is palpated are characteristic features of mediastinal emphysema. A crunching noise may be heard on auscultation, and air spaces may be noted in anteroposterior and lateral chest radiographs. An allergic reaction, a hematoma, angioedema, and an esophageal rupture should be considered in the differential diagnosis.

Treatment The treatment of subcutaneous emphysema is mainly supportive. Broad-spectrum antibiotics should be prescribed for 10 days as a precaution to prevent secondary

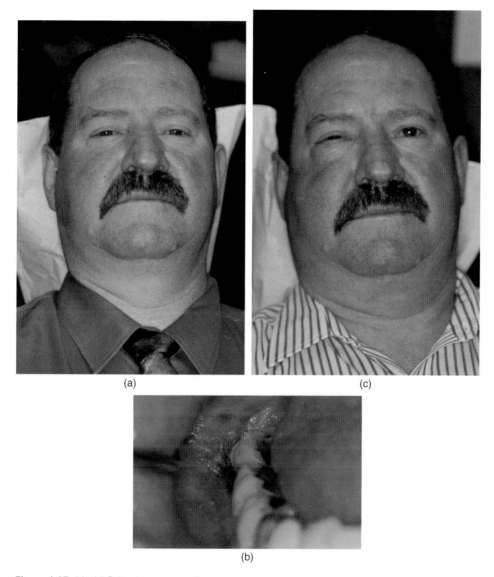

(a)

(c)

(b)

Figure 4.17 (a)–(c) Subcutaneous emphysema.

infection. Cough suppressants may be prescribed to prevent further entry of air into the fascial planes. A follow-up appointment within 48 hours is imperative to monitor for resolution and signs of infection. Severe cases mandate medical referral. Serious complications include meningitis when the maxilla is involved and mediastinitis when the mandible is affected. In severe cases, a pneumothorax or air embolism may occur.

Paget's Disease

Paget's disease (osteitis deformans) is a heterogenous, progressive bone disease characterized by brisk haphazard bone remodeling. It is the second most common metabolic bone disorder after osteoporosis and affects an estimated 1% of patients over the age of 55 years. Men are at slightly greater risk than women. The etiology is unknown, but autoimmunity and a variety of environmental factors

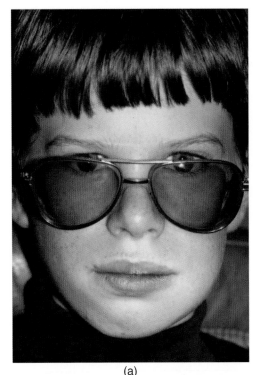

(a)

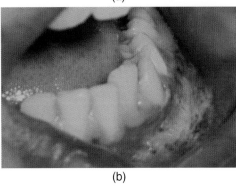

(b)

Figure 4.18 (a) and (b) Subcutaneous emphysema.

have been postulated as contributing to the disease.

Clinical Features Paget's disease may affect one (monostotic) or several (polyostotic) bones, and most cases are asymptomatic and discovered incidentally. The most commonly affected sites include the pelvis, skull, vertebra, femur, and tibia. Common clinical signs and symptoms include osseous distortion or expansion and mild-to-moderate bone pain.

Skull involvement is estimated to occur in about 27% of cases and may result in hearing loss and vestibular problems in up to 89% of those affected. While osteosarcoma is a rare complication, most cases of adult osteosarcoma occur in patients with Paget's disease.

The characteristic radiographic findings of Paget's disease include lytic changes, characterized by osteoporosis; and sclerotic changes, characterized by a cotton-wool appearance. An overall mosaic of lytic and sclerotic findings is frequently noted. Numerous dental abnormalities, such as malocclusion, hypercementosis, tooth mobility, root resorption, pulp calcification, osteomyelitis, poor fitting prostheses, and excessive postsurgical bleeding have been associated with Paget's disease.

Diagnosis The diagnosis of Paget's disease is confirmed by correlating the presenting signs and symptoms with appropriate laboratory tests. The characteristic laboratory finding is an elevated serum alkaline phosphatase. A bone scan is useful to determine the extent of bone involvement.

Treatment Therapy is dictated by the extent of the disease and associated symptoms. Bisphosphonates are powerful inhibitors of bone resorption and have been shown to be highly effective in stabilizing bone turnover and reducing disease-related symptoms. However, these drugs are not curative.

Gardner's Syndrome

Gardner's syndrome is a variant of familial adenomatous polyposis (FAP). FAP is a hereditary autosomal dominant disorder characterized by development of tens to thousands of adenomatous polyps in the rectum and colon by the second decade of life. These polyps exhibit a 100% risk of malignant transformation, typically between the ages of 40–50 years. Potentially malignant polyps may also develop in the stomach, duodenum, and small bowel.

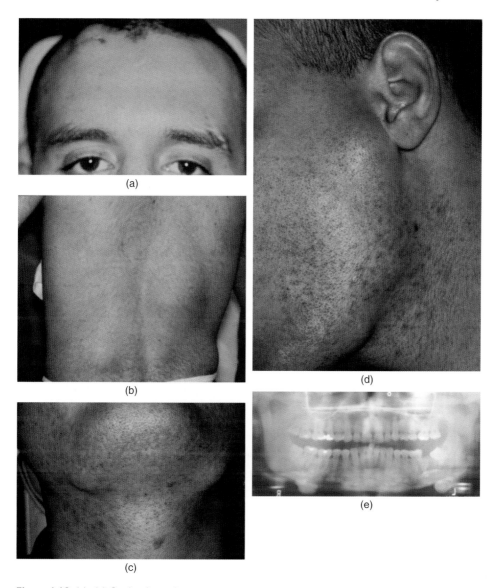

Figure 4.19 (a)–(g) Gardner's syndrome.

Gardner's syndrome is characterized by the presence of FAP plus a variety of bone, cutaneous, and soft-tissue tumors. Although the reported incidence of FAP is 1 in 13 000, Gardner's syndrome is much less common, affecting about one individual per million in the general population.

Clinical Features Epidermoid cysts, which develop before puberty, are present in approximately 50–65% of patients (Figure 4.19a and b). Other commonly observed cutaneous neoplasms include fibromas, lipomas, leiomyomas, neurofibromas, and pigmented skin lesions. Desmoid tumors and multifocal, pigmented lesions of the ocular fundus have been described. Osteomas are an essential component of Gardner's syndrome, and the mandible is the most common location (Figure 4.19c–g). Other oral findings may include congenitally

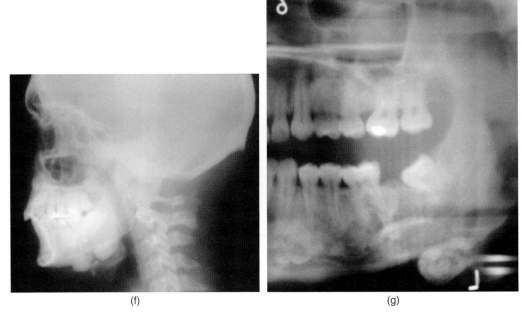

(f)   (g)

Figure 4.19 (*Continued*)

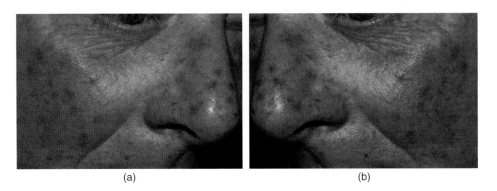

(a)   (b)

Figure 4.20 (a) and (b) Rosacea.

absent teeth, hypercementosis, dentigerous cysts, impacted teeth, supernumerary teeth, and fused or unusually long roots. Long bones may demonstrate cortical hyperostosis or the formation of osteomas. Osteomas generally precede the clinical and radiographic evidence of colonic polyps.

Diagnosis The presence of the characteristic stigmata of Gardner's syndrome should prompt referral for a thorough medical evaluation. Panoramic radiographs are particularly useful to screen for Gardner's syndrome.

Treatment Medical management of FAP is usually accomplished with prophylactic cancer preventive colorectal surgery followed by life-long close surveillance. Since siblings and children of patients with Gardner's syndrome have a 50% chance of being affected, all first-degree relatives must be screened for the disorder.

Assess the Character and Integrity of the Skin

A variety of skin lesions may be noted on the face. Acne is a common finding in teenagers, and is characterized by multiple pustules and comedons. Rosacea is an acne-like condition that typically affects older individuals. Psoriasis is a common skin disorder that often affects the eyebrows and anterior scalp and presents as scaly plaques. Seborrheic keratoses are discrete, rough-surfaced, and brown to black papules that typically occur in patients over 40 years of age. Important malignancies that commonly affect the face are basal cell carcinoma (BCC), squamous cell carcinoma (SCC), and melanoma. BCC initially presents as a persistent papule with surface telangiectatic blood vessels and evolves into an umbilicated ulcer. SCC typically appears as a persistent, rapidly growing ulcer with raised borders. A melanoma may arise de novo or from a pre-existing nevus. Any nevus that demonstrates bleeding, growth, a change in color, or the development of satellite lesions should be biopsied in order to rule out potential malignant transformation to melanoma.

Rosacea

Rosacea is a chronic and progressive cutaneous vascular disorder affecting the nasal and malar areas of the face. It appears to be inflammatory in nature, but the specific etiology is unknown. There is a slight female predilection, and patients with fair complexion who flush or blush easily or have a family history of rosacea are most susceptible. Specific triggers such as sunlight or cosmetics may contribute to the disease process. Most patients are diagnosed between the ages of 30 and 50.

Clinical Features Classic signs of rosacea include flushing, persistent erythema, papules, pustules, and telangiectasia (Figure 4.20a and b). Four subtypes of rosacea are recognized: erythematotelangiectatic, papulopustular, phymatous, and ocular. The phymatous subtype has a predilection for men and is characterized

by rhinophyma, large lobulated masses affecting the tip and wings of the nose. The ocular subtype affects over 50% of rosacea patients. Typical ocular signs and symptoms include blepharitis, dry eyes, burning, soreness, and grittiness. In severe cases, corneal involvement may lead to blindness.

Diagnosis When rosacea is suspected, the patient should be referred to a dermatologist for definitive diagnosis and subsequent management. Other conditions to consider in the differential include acne vulgaris, seborrheic dermatitis, chronic contact dermatitis, and lupus erythematosus.

Treatment Therapeutic options for rosacea include topical and oral agents, laser and light treatments, and surgical interventions. Patients with rosacea should avoid known triggers such as sun exposure and any offending cosmetic products. The most commonly prescribed topical agents are metronidazole, azelaic acid, and sodium sulfacetamide⁻ sulfur. The most commonly prescribed oral agent is low-dose doxycycline monohydrate. Surgical or laser therapy may be necessary to ablate cosmetically unacceptable rhinophyma.

Psoriasis

Psoriasis is a common chronic, recurrent, inflammatory skin disorder. It is characterized by hyperproliferation of the epidermis and inflammation secondary to a T-cell (CD4)-mediated autoimmune process. The pool of proliferating keratinocytes is expanded, their migration from the basal cell layer to the surface is more rapid, and the cell cycle is shortened. Prevalence rates range from 2 to 4.7% and a bimodal age grouping has been noted, specifically 20–30 years and 50–60 years.

Clinical Features The most commonly observed form of psoriasis is the plaque form, which presents as circumscribed, thickened, silvery,

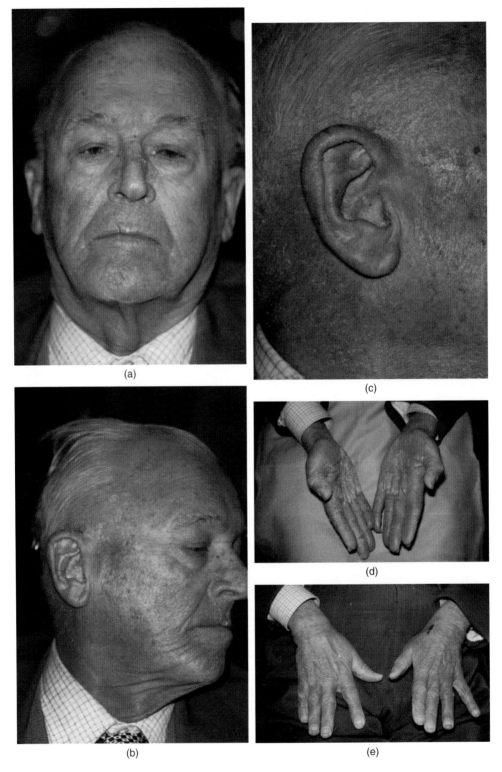

Figure 4.21 (a)–(j) Psoriasis.

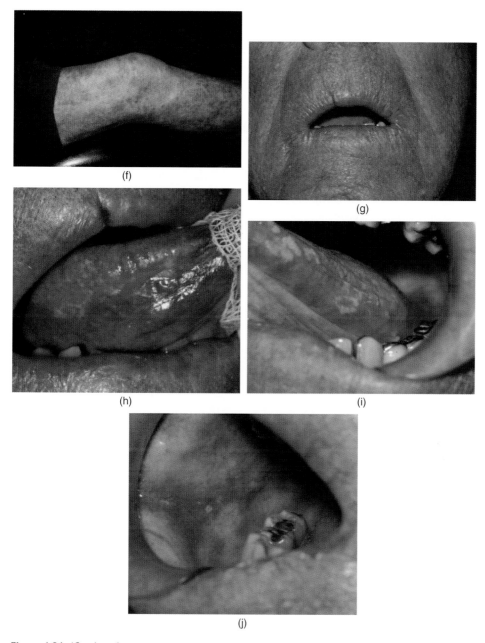

(f)

(g)

(h)

(i)

(j)

Figure 4.21 (*Continued*)

scaly papules and plaques that may be pruritic. They occur most often on the scalp, face, nails, eyebrows, elbows, knees, buttocks, and sites of local trauma (Koebner phenomenon) (Figure 4.21a–j). Psoriatic arthritis is a related condition in which the joint tissues are targeted by the autoimmune process underlying psoriasis. Psoriasis is a dynamic disease that often appears to wax and wane over time. Numerous factors such as infection, stress, climate changes, and certain medications may contribute to disease flares.

Diagnosis The diagnosis of psoriasis is based on clinical findings, which may be supplemented by a skin biopsy.

Treatment At present, there is no cure for psoriasis. The extent of care is determined on a case-by-case basis with the target of decreasing disease severity and improving the patient's quality of life. The number of therapeutic agents available to manage psoriasis is vast and can generally be divided into three groups: (i) topical agents; (ii) light therapies; and (iii) systemic agents. Newly developed biologic therapies that target specific cytokine networks in the disease process may prove useful.

Seborrheic Keratosis

Seborrheic keratosis is a benign skin growth surfaced by loose adherent scales. The etiology of seborrheic keratosis is unknown but has been suggested to include genetic predisposition, exposure to sunlight, human papillomavirus, and hyperplasia of melanocytes. Men and women are equally affected and the incidence increases with age. Seborrheic keratosis is not contagious.

Clinical Features Seborrheic keratosis is commonly seen in Caucasians and rarely identified in African Americans and Native Americans. The lesions initially present as flat, well-demarcated tan to brown to black macules that gradually become greasy papules or plaques with a verruca-like surface, which appears to be stuck to the skin. The look is often compared to brown candle wax that was dropped onto the skin. They are usually located on the face, trunk and limbs.

Diagnosis The diagnosis of seborrheic keratosis is primarily clinical. In some cases, differentiating between pigmented seborrheic keratosis, malignant melanoma, and other cutaneous lesions might be difficult. Such equivocal cases warrant referral to a dermatologist for further evaluation. Any seborrheic keratosis that presents with an atypical appearance or undergoes dramatic change should be biopsied.

Treatment The management of seborrheic keratosis is usually considered to be cosmetic. When necessary, most seborrheic keratoses are treated by one of three methods: (i) liquid nitrogen cryotherapy; (ii) curettage or excision; and (iii) electrosurgery.

Basal Cell Carcinoma

BCC is the most common skin cancer and up to 90% of lesions present in the head and neck. Although metastasis rarely occurs, it is locally invasive. BCC accounts for 75–80% of all skin cancers in whites and more than 2.2 million new cases occur each year in the United States. Despite its prevalence in adults, it is extremely rare in children. The primary established risk factor for BCC is ultraviolet radiation and fair-complexioned individuals are at highest risk for developing this neoplasm.

Clinical Features BCC is fairly typical in appearance and can usually be diagnosed by an experienced observer on clinical grounds alone. The classic form presents as an indurated nodule with a rolled edge, often associated with surface telangiectasias or a pearly appearance (Figures 4.22a, b, 4.23, and 4.24). Some tumors may ulcerate (Figures 4.25 and 4.26). BCC in children has been associated with familial syndromes such as nevoid BCC syndrome (Gorlin's syndrome) and xeroderma pigmentosum. It has also been reported in children previously treated with ionizing radiation therapy.

Diagnosis Although BCC can usually be diagnosed by an experienced observer on clinical grounds alone, verification by excisional biopsy is necessary.

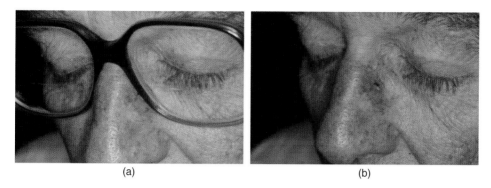

(a)

(b)

Figure 4.22 (a) and (b) BCC.

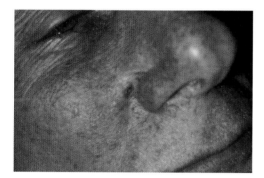

Figure 4.23 BCC.

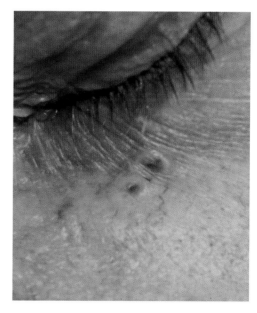

Figure 4.24 BCC.

Prevention Patients must be educated about the importance of reducing unprotected exposure to ultraviolet radiation. Sensible measures include sun avoidance, wearing tightly woven clothing, and the use of sunscreens. Patients should be further educated about the early signs and symptoms of cutaneous malignancies and the importance of skin self-examination, with assistance if necessary from hand mirrors or family members in viewing inaccessible areas. Patients with one BCC of the skin are at increased risk of developing new tumors and also are at increased risk for various noncutaneous types of cancer.

Treatment Surgical excision is the treatment of choice for most primary BCCs. Micrographic surgery is recommended for larger BCCs of the face and those with more aggressive growth patterns.

Assess Trigeminal Nerve Function

The trigeminal nerve is the sensory nerve of the face, teeth, and mucous membranes. It also provides motor function to the mylohyoid, anterior belly of the digastric, tensor veli palatini, tensor tympani, and muscles of mastication. Branches of the trigeminal nerve convey pain associated with diseases of the teeth and oral soft tissues, eyes, and paranasal sinuses.

Facial and oral trauma may result in paresthesia, an abnormal sensation variably

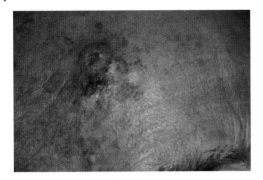

Figure 4.25 BCC.

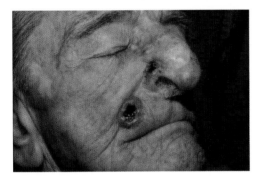

Figure 4.26 BCC.

described as tingling, pins and needles, burning, coldness, or a sense of water running over the skin. In addition, the trigeminal nerve may be affected by a disorder known as paroxysmal trigeminal neuralgia.

Sensory Evaluation

With the patient's eyes closed, test for touch (cotton wisp or applicator stick), temperature (warm and cold objects), and pain (pointed object) over the distribution of the ophthalmic, maxillary, and mandibular divisions of the trigeminal nerve. A lack of response (anesthesia), altered response (paresthesia), or increased response (hyperesthesia) may be noted.

Motor Evaluation

Have the patient clench his or her teeth while biting on a tongue blade. The examiner should not be able to pull the tongue blade from the mouth. The left and right sides should be tested separately.

Assess Facial Nerve Function

The facial nerve (VII) is the motor nerve of the face (muscles of facial expression), the posterior belly of the digastric, stylohyoid, and stapedius muscles. It also provides secretory motor function to the parotid, submandibular, sublingual, and lacrimal glands. In addition, the facial nerve provides the sense of taste on the anterior two-thirds of the tongue.

Facial trauma and neoplasms in the parotid glands may damage branches of the facial nerve and result in paralysis of the muscles supplied by the affected branches. In addition, transient or permanent seventh nerve damage may result in BP characterized by unilateral paralysis of the facial muscles.

Motor Evaluation

Have the patient implement movements of the muscles of facial expression, including smiling, frowning, raising the eyebrows, and closing the eyelids. While the eyes are closed, apply upward pressure to raise the eyebrows. The attempt should be unsuccessful.

Secretory Motor Evaluation

The secretory motor function of the facial nerve is difficult to evaluate, but signs and symptoms of xerostomia, in the absence of other etiologies, warrant consideration.

Evaluate Taste

Have the patient protrude his/her tongue and apply sugar or salt to one side of the anterior two-thirds of the tongue. The patient should experience the taste before retruding the tongue. After a rinse with water, the other side should be tested in a similar fashion.

4.2 Examine the Ears and Temporomandibular Joints

Hard nodules on the helix may represent sodium biurate deposits suggestive of gout.

Eroded areas on the ears may be associated with BCC or SCC, both of which may cause distortion or destruction of the auricle. Developmental deformities are rare, but when encountered, they may be associated with malformations of the genitourinary tract with head and neck/facial manifestations (e.g. Treacher–Collins syndrome).

A hematoma along the mastoid process is indicative of a temporal bone fracture. A bloody but watery discharge from the ears and nose is likely to represent cerebrospinal fluid that has escaped through a meningeal tear caused by a skull fracture. Palpation of the temporomandibular joint as the patient attempts to move the mandible may reveal a dislocation. Limitation of movement may indicate other pathological conditions.

Assess Acoustic Nerve Function

The acoustic nerve (VIII) provides the special sense of hearing (auditory) and the special sense of balance (vestibular). Vestibular lesions cause vertigo (dizziness) and unbalance. Deafness may either be due to faulty conduction or nerve damage. Conduction deafness is usually a sequela of to inflammatory middle ear disease. It may also be secondary to obstruction of the Eustachian tube, otosclerosis, or Paget's disease. Nerve deafness may be congenital, drug-induced, or caused by fractures of the temporal bone. Ménière's disease, a gross distention of the labyrinth by fluid, is characterized by deafness, tinnitus (ringing in the ears), and vertigo. It occurs most often in middle-aged women.

Evaluate Air Conduction

A simple yet effective way to quickly assess air conduction is to hold a ticking watch about 8 in. from the patient's ear (in a quiet room). Repeat on the opposite side. The perception should be the same in each ear.

Evaluate Bone Conduction

Hold a ringing tuning fork against the top of the patient's head. It should be heard equally in both ears. Alternatively, the struck tuning fork should be held against the mastoid process until the patient can no longer hear it. It should then be held next to the ear and the patient should hear it again (air conduction is about three times more efficient than bone conduction). Repeat on the opposite side.

4.3   Examine the Nose

Respiratory abnormalities may be associated with dilation of the nostrils upon inspiration and contraction of the nostrils upon expiration. A deviated septum, allergies, or nasal polyps may cause chronic nasal obstruction. BCC is the most common malignancy affecting the skin of the nose. A "butterfly" lesion on the skin of the nose extending out over the cheeks is characteristic of lupus erythematosus.

Note a deviated or depressed nasal bone or cartilage, which along with extraocular movements may indicate a fractured or displaced facial bone. A bloody but watery discharge from the nose and ears is likely to reflect cerebrospinal fluid that has escaped through a meningeal tear caused by a skull fracture.

Lupus Erythematosus

Systemic lupus erythematosus (SLE) is a B-cell mediated autoimmune disease. It is characterized by the presence of circulating immune complexes and activation of the complement system, which can affect the joints, skin, lungs, heart, and kidneys. In North America and northern Europe, SLE occurs in about 40 persons per 100 000. Women are nine times more likely to be affected by SLE than men, and blacks are more commonly affected than Caucasians. The etiology of SLE remains unclear, although a genetic predisposition is likely. Other etiologic risk factors include environmental exposures (e.g. infectious, dietary, or toxic), ultraviolet light, and exposure to certain drugs (e.g. procainamide).

The autoantibodies in SLE are predominantly of the immunoglobulin G (IgG) type.

These autoantibodies can react with a variety of cellular and extracellular constituents, including DNA and other nucleic acids, nucleoproteins, cytoplasm components, cell surface antigens, and matrix components, and initiate an inflammatory response that often leads to cell death and failure of affected organs.

Clinical Features SLE can strike suddenly and severely but is more likely to cause mild, chronic illness for a long period of time before being diagnosed. Skin rashes in lupus come in all shapes and sizes and can be divided into three categories. Acute cutaneous LE is characterized by the classic photosensitive "butterfly" rash of SLE (Figure 4.27). Subacute cutaneous LE (SCLE) is characterized by non-scarring, photosensitive annular (red rings) or papulosquamous (red scaly) lesions. About 10% of these cases progress to full-blown SLE. The most common form, chronic cutaneous LE, also termed discoid LE (DLE), is characterized by scarring usually localized to the scalp, face, and ears (Figure 4.28a–c).

Other manifestations include flu-like symptoms with fever, tiredness, headaches, muscle and joint pain, transient hair loss, arthritis, vasculitis, cardiac and renal involvement, blood disorders (anemia, leukopenia, and thrombocytopenia), and emotional disturbances.

Oral lesions specific to LE represent the mucosal equivalent of their cutaneous counterparts. However, the moist environment of the oral cavity mucosa alters the clinical appearance of these lesions (e.g. no scales, no follicular plugging, and less scarring). Typical sites of occurrence are the palate and buccal mucosa. Lesions are generally described as annular leukoplakic areas or erythematous erosions.

Diagnosis Due to its widely variable presentation, the diagnosis of SLE may be difficult. It should be suspected in any patient who has features affecting two or more organ systems. The diagnosis of SLE is based on correlating the presenting signs and symptoms with

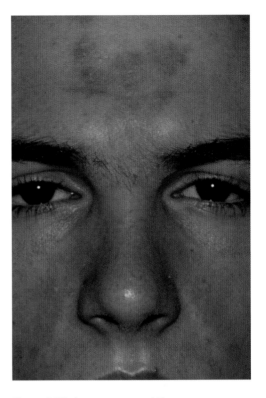

Figure 4.27 Acute cutaneous LE.

appropriate laboratory testing. The presence of anti-double-stranded DNA antibodies is a specific diagnostic test, and is also used to monitor lupus activity.

Treatment There is currently no cure for SLE. Therapy is aimed at relieving symptoms with the hope of controlling the disease so that patients can lead a normal life. Patients should avoid sunlight and wear a broad-spectrum sunscreen, when necessary. Medications prescribed to manage patients with SLE may include NSAIDs, antimalarials (hydroxychloroquine), anticoagulants, corticosteroids, immunosuppressants (azathioprine, cyclophosphamide), and biologics.

Assess Olfactory Nerve Function

The olfactory nerve (I) provides the special sense of smell. The sense of smell may be impaired with age, upper respiratory tract

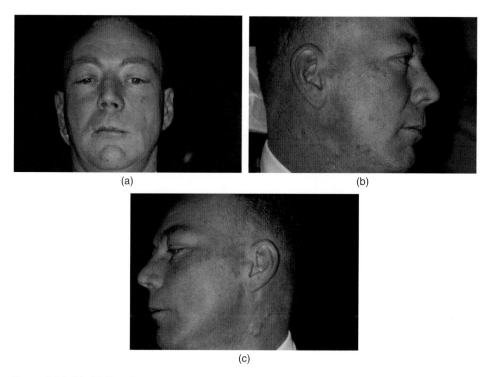

Figure 4.28 (a)–(c) Chronic cutaneous LE.

infections, allergies, smoking, and medications. Loss of the sense of smell (anosmia) may also occur as a result of a fracture of the base of the skull or pressure on the olfactory nerve by a tumor.

Evaluate Smell

Occlude one nostril and with the patient's eyes closed ask him or her to identify familiar substances (coffee, tobacco) by smell. Repeat on the opposite side.

4.4 Examine the Eyes

Increased monocular blinking often follows physical irritation of the eye, while bilateral blinking is often associated with the wearing of contact lenses. Decreased monocular blinking is seen in patients with BP or a facial nerve deficit. Conjunctivitis occurs in response to physical irritants, specific allergens, or infections. Focal lid edema is often due to contact allergy. Xanthelasmic plaques, most frequently seen on the lower lids, suggest dyslipidemia. Ptosis, unilateral or bilateral drooping of the eyelids, may be an early manifestation of myasthenia gravis (MG). Blue sclera may be associated with osteogenesis imperfecta. A yellow sclera suggests icterus. Exophthalmia is an abnormal protrusion of the eyes. When only one eye is affected, the likely cause is a tumor. When both eyes are affected, the most likely cause is Graves' disease. Compare the orbital rims and zygomatic arches for symmetry and note extraocular movements. Abnormalities may indicate a fractured or displaced facial bone.

Myasthenia Gravis

MG is a rare but potentially debilitating autoimmune disease of the neuromuscular junction characterized by an impaired transmission of the neuron-to-muscle impulse.

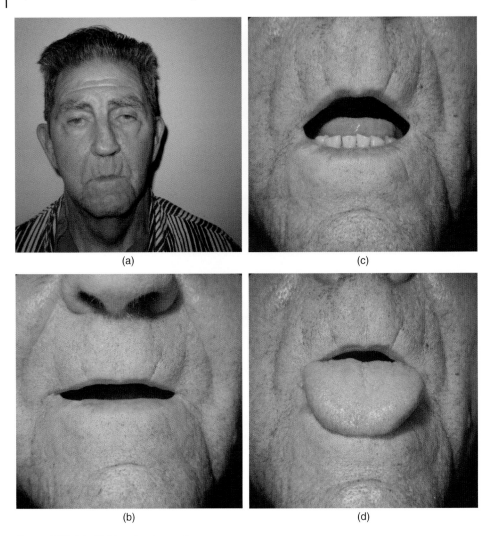

(a)

(c)

(b)

(d)

Figure 4.29 (a)–(d) Myasthenia gravis.

In MG, the acetylcholine receptors at the postsynaptic nerve membrane are blocked by acetylcholine receptor antibodies. The estimated prevalence of MG varies from 50 to 150 cases per million. Approximately 80% of patients with MG have hyperplasia of the thymus and 10% have thymomas. MG may also be associated with other disorders such as rheumatoid arthritis, pernicious anemia, or SLE. Certain medications, including aminoglycosides, ciprofloxacin, lithium, phenytoin, procainamide, quinidine sulfate, and beta-adrenergic receptor-blocking drugs (including eye drops) may exacerbate MG.

Clinical Features MG is characterized by progressive fatigue with exercise. The signs and symptoms may range from isolated ptosis (Figure 4.29a), diplopia, or mild proximal muscle weakness to severe generalized weakness. More generalized disease usually affects muscles that control neck movement, facial movement, mastication, and the tongue (Figure 4.29b–d). A smile resembles a snarl, chewing is impaired, and swallowing or speaking becomes difficult. Involvement of the vocal cords gives speech a nasal quality. Disease involving the muscles in the limbs, neck, shoulders, hands, diaphragm, and abdomen may lead to difficulty walking, sitting up, and breathing.

Diagnosis The diagnosis of MG should be considered in all patients with ptosis or ocular motor weakness without pupillary involvement or in older patients presenting with any bulbar or skeletal muscle weakness and a history of recurrent falls. Testing for acetylcholine-receptor antibodies is specific and detectable in 80–95% of patients with generalized MG and in 34–56% of patients with isolated ocular involvement. MG should be differentiated from a stroke and other motor neuron diseases.

Treatment Therapy for MG is directed at reducing the degradation of acetylcholine with cholinesterase inhibitors, thereby increasing its duration of activity in the neuromuscular junction. Drugs implicated in possibly exacerbating MG should be avoided. Therapeutic interventions include acetylcholinesterase inhibitors, thymectomy, and immunosuppression (corticosteroids, azathioprine, methotrexate, tacrolimus, mycophenolate mofetil, and cyclosporine).

About 20% of MG patients experience a myasthenia crisis, a medical emergency requiring ventilator support. Such patients may also require short-term immunotherapy, including plasma exchange and intravenous immune globulin to establish disease control. Signs and symptoms of pending myasthenia crisis include rapid worsening of MG symptoms, rapid progression of bulbar weakness, tachypnea, tachycardia, reduced forced vital capacity, and respiratory infection.

Dentinogenesis Imperfecta

DI is a genetic disorder of tooth development and affects an estimated 1 in 6000–8000 individuals. Three forms of DI are recognized. DI Type I occurs in association with osteogenesis imperfecta, a disease caused by a type 1 collagen defect. DI Types II and III exist as isolated dentition-related diseases attributed to mutations affecting the dentin sialophosphoprotein (DSPP) gene. DSPP encodes two tooth matrix proteins (dentin sialoprotein [DSP] and dentin phosphoprotein [DPP]) that are associated with tooth mineralization. Recent studies have shown that DI Types II and III are associated with DSPP mutations affecting DSP and DPP production, respectively.

Clinical Features All three forms of DI manifest an amber-brown to blue-gray hue to the teeth with an opalescent sheen, cracking/loss of enamel, and attrition (Figure 4.30a–c). Radiographically, the teeth in DI Type I exhibit bulbous crowns, cervical constrictions, short roots, obliteration of pulp chambers, and periradicular radiolucencies (Figure 4.30d and e). In Type III DI the pulp is normal or nonmineralized (shell-teeth).

Diagnosis The dentist will often be the first to recognize the characteristic clinical presentation of DI. The presence of blue sclera and/or a history of increased bone fragility, in association with DI, should raise the suspicion of osteogenesis imperfecta, and an appropriate medical referral should be initiated to rule it out.

Treatment DI Types II and III pose no threat to longevity but may present significant challenges in terms of restoring esthetics and function.

Hyperthyroidism

Hyperthyroidism is a condition caused by overactivity of the thyroid gland. In contrast, thyrotoxicosis refers to any state of thyroid hormone excess, including ingestion of exogenous thyroid hormone and thyroiditis (inflammatory changes within the thyroid gland). Hyperthyroidism is common, affecting approximately 4.5 million Americans, and there is

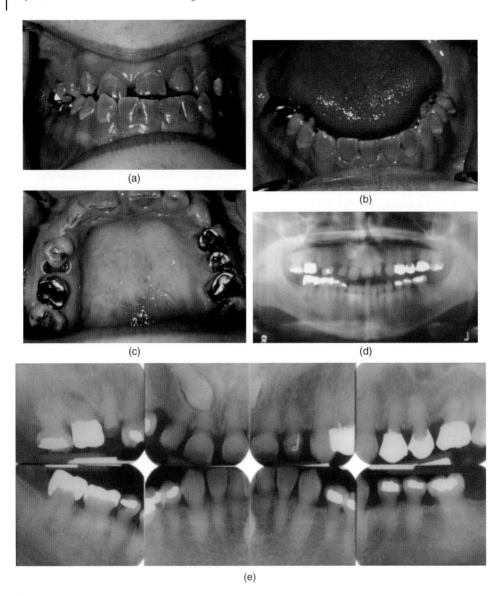

Figure 4.30 (a)–(e) Dentinogenesis imperfecta.

a clear predilection for women (5–10 : 1). The most frequent cause of hyperthyroidism is Graves' disease, an autoimmune disease caused by the production of autoantibodies that target the TSH receptor. Other causes of hyperthyroidism include toxic nodular goiter and thyroiditis.

Clinical Features Common signs and symptoms of hyperthyroidism include nervousness,

increased sweating, heat intolerance, palpitations, dyspnea, fatigue, weight loss, exophthalmos, and unilateral or bilateral enlargement of the thyroid gland (Figure 4.31a–c). Unfortunately, hyperthyroidism may develop insidiously over time, and the classic signs and symptoms may be easily overlooked.

Diagnosis A diagnosis of hyperthyroidism is suggested by the presence of the classic

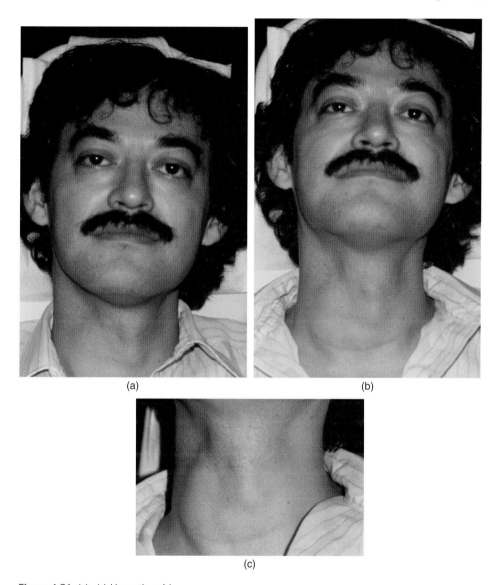

(a)

(b)

(c)

Figure 4.31 (a)–(c) Hyperthyroid.

signs and symptoms, which occur in 50% of patients. Appropriate laboratory testing is essential and is characterized by low levels of TSH and high levels of free thyroxin (T_4).

Treatment Treatment of hyperthyroidism is aimed at attaining a state of euthyroidism by decreasing circulating thyroid hormone levels. Current options include antithyroid medications, radioactive iodine (^{131}I), or subtotal thyroidectomy. The type of treatment rendered is determined by the underlying cause, the age of the patient, the size of the goiter, and the presence of coexisting morbidities. A potential side effect of any therapy, but especially ^{131}I, is hypothyroidism. Hypothyroid patients will require supplemental thyroid hormone replacement therapy to obtain a euthyroid state.

Assess Optic Nerve Function

The optic nerve provides the special sense of vision. Changes in visual acuity may be associated with diseases such as hypertension, renal disease, blood dyscrasias, glaucoma, and diabetes mellitus. Visual field impairment may be caused by optic nerve impingement associated with a pituitary tumor or Paget's disease. Acute oculomotor palsy and/or visual disturbances may develop as a complication of the injection of local anesthesia into the infraorbital region. Oculomotor palsy manifests as diplopia, strabismus, eye deviation, impaired ocular movement, and ptosis. Visual disturbances include blurred vision, central vision loss, and altered color vision.

If an ocular complication develops secondary to infraorbital injection, the patient should be reassured that this complication is usually transient, and the affected eye should be covered with a gauze dressing to protect it until the anesthesia wears off. Because monocular vision limits distance perception, an adult should escort the patient home. If the complication lasts for more than six hours, a referral to an ophthalmologist is mandatory.

Evaluate Visual Acuity

Test visual acuity by asking the patient to read a passage from a newspaper. This test is performed with both eyes uncovered and then with each eye covered in turn.

Evaluate Visual Field

The patient is instructed to stare at the examiner's nose. The examiner moves his or her index finger into the patient's visual field from the extreme periphery to the center starting at each quadrant around the circle. The patient is instructed to indicate initial sighting of the finger as well as any loss of visual continuity. Normal visual fields are 60° to the medial (nasal) side, 100° to the lateral (temporal) side, and 130° vertically.

Assess Oculomotor, Trochlear, and Abducens Nerve Function

The oculomotor nerve (III) controls the papillary sphincters and ciliary muscle and provides motor function to the superior, inferior and medial rectus, inferior oblique, and levator palpebrae muscles. The trochlear nerve (IV) provides motor function to the superior oblique muscle. The abducens nerve (VI) provides motor function to the lateral rectus muscle.

Evaluate the Pupils

Using a point source light in a somewhat darkened room, test each eye to ensure that the pupils are equal, round, reactive to light, and accommodation (PERRLA). The pupils may be constricted, as in a drug overdose; unequal, as in a stroke; or dilated, as in shock and unconsciousness. Coloboma is a congenital ocular malformation presenting as an out-of-round pupil. Less commonly, it may result from injury or surgery to the eye.

Evaluate Ocular Movement

The patient should be instructed to follow the examiner's index finger vertically, horizontally, and diagonally. If the oculomotor nerve is damaged, the patient will exhibit ptosis, pupillary dilation, and an inability to move the eye up, down, and medially. If the trochlear nerve is damaged, the patient will be unable to rotate the eye diagonally, downward, and laterally. If the abducens nerve is damaged, the eye will not abduct. A neurological deficit in any of these nerves will manifest as diplopia. Strabismus, or deviation of the eyes in relation to one another, may be indicative of muscle paresis. Ptosis may be an early sign of MG. Nystagmus, or oscillation of the eyes, is a pathologic sign of a neurological disorder. Any of these findings warrant referral to an ophthalmologist.

4.5 Examine the Hair

Male-pattern baldness is inevitable in the presence of a genetic predisposition. Distinct patches of baldness may result from chemical or radiation burns and are common in ringworm infestations of the scalp. Sudden, patchy, idiopathic loss of hair (alopecia areata [AA]), may be related to stress. Sparse hair may be noted in patients with pituitary insufficiency and ectodermal dysplasia (ED). Scant, coarse, dry, and lusterless hair should suggest hypothyroidism.

Alopecia Areata

AA is a remitting, recurring loss of hair with an unpredictable prognosis. There is growing evidence to suggest that AA is a tissue-restricted autoimmune disease, mediated by a T-lymphocyte response to a follicular autoantigen. A family history of AA occurs in 10–42% of cases and in identical twins, the concordance rate of AA is as high as 55%. Other conditions associated with AA are allergic diseases (atopy, asthma, and eczema). Overall, an estimated 1.7% of the population has AA, there is no sex predilection, and it is most common in children and young adults.

Clinical Features AA usually presents as small, round patches of hair loss on the scalp (Figure 4.32a–c). In about one-fifth of patients with AA, the condition evolves into complete scalp hair loss (alopecia totalis), and in some cases the loss of all body hair may occur (alopecia universalis). Other associated clinical changes may include nail dystrophy, which usually presents as fine pitting or ridges on the surface of the nail. The course of AA is unpredictable, with periods of remission and exacerbation. The rate and pattern of hair loss is variable. New hair growth may show loss of pigment.

Diagnosis The diagnosis of AA is usually made on the basis of clinical history and physical examination. A biopsy may be helpful

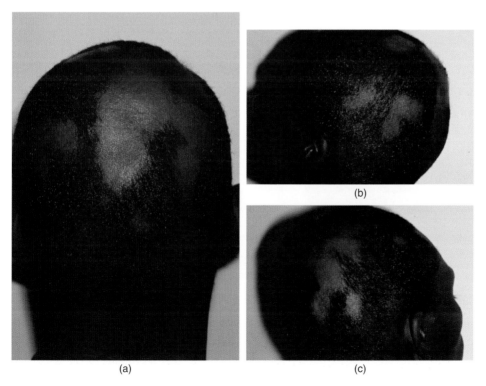

(a)

(b)

(c)

Figure 4.32 (a)–(c) Alopecia areata.

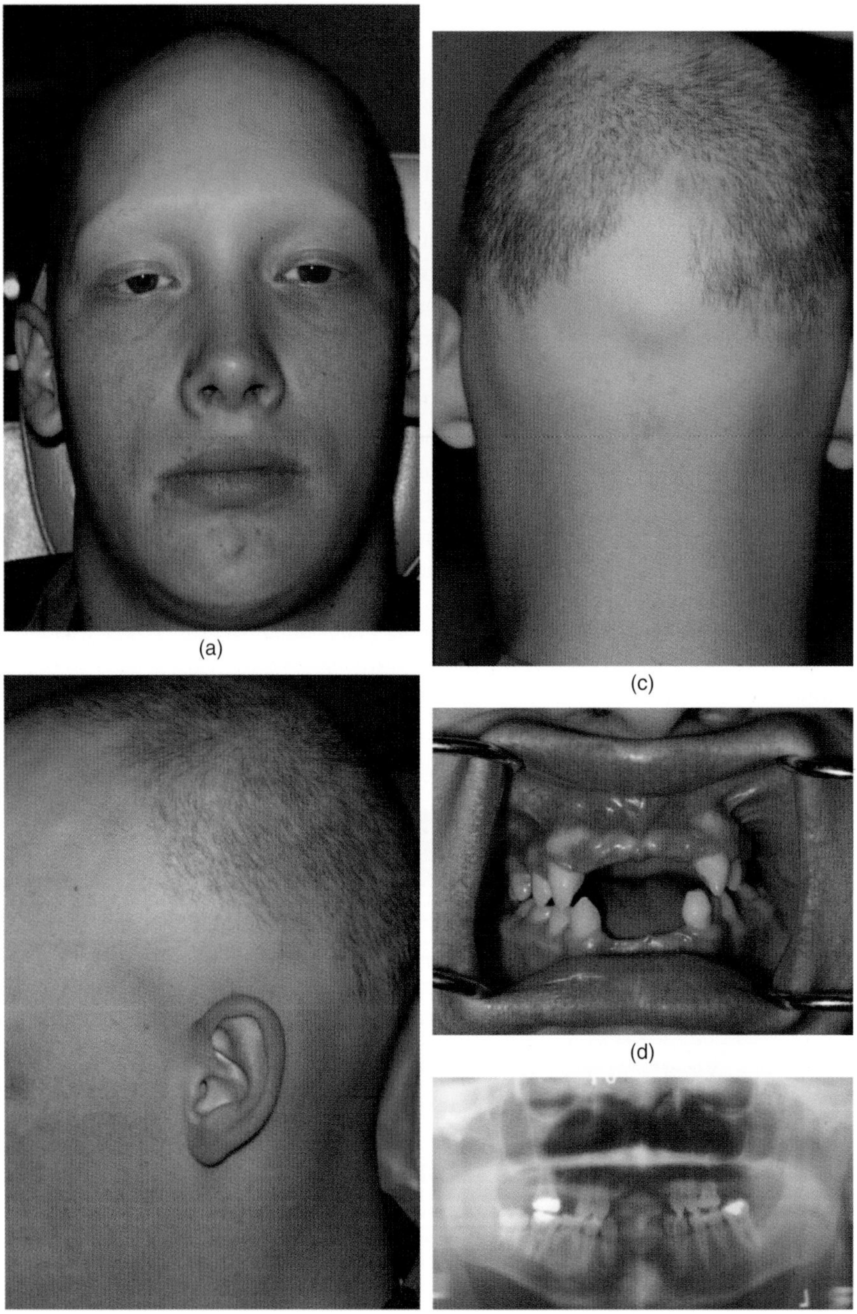

Figure 4.33 (a)–(e) Ectodermal dysplasia.

(a)

(b)

(c)

(d)

(e)

to rule out other conditions. A differential diagnosis should include infection, traction (e.g. tight braids, pony tails), stress, hormonal disturbances, and psychiatric illness (trichotillomania).

Treatment About half of AA patients experience spontaneous return of hair growth without therapy. Treatment for AA includes steroids (topical, intralesional, and systemic), minoxidil, anthralin, and immunotherapy.

However, in some cases, AA progressively worsens in spite of therapy.

Ectodermal Dysplasia

ED represents a rare group of inherited disorders characterized by aplasia or dysplasia of ectodermally derived tissues. Hair, nails, teeth, and skin are often affected. The mode of inheritance varies among the different types of ED. ED may be inherited as an X-linked recessive trait (hypohidrotic ED), in which case the gene is carried by the female and manifested in the male. However, there are reports of multiple siblings being affected and of females suffering from this condition. It is likely that most of these cases are examples of the autosomal-recessive form (hidrotic ED) of the disease. The prevalence in the general population has been assessed as between 1 in 10 000 and 1 in 100 000 live male births.

Clinical Features The X-linked hypohidrotic form (Christ–Siemens–Touraine syndrome) of ED is the most common and is characterized by the classic triad of hypohidrosis (abnormal or missing sweat glands), hypotrichosis (abnormal hair), and hypodontia. The facial manifestations of ED include a prominent forehead, sparse and fine blonde hair, depressed nasal bridge, high/broad cheekbones, pointed chin, and protuberant lips (Figure 4.33a–c). The less common hidrotic form (Clouston syndrome) does not typically involve sweat glands but does affect teeth, hair, and nails.

Other signs and symptoms may include rhinitis, pharyngitis, asthma, epistaxis, and hearing loss (resulting from an accumulation of wax in the auditory canal). Xerostomia is an uncommon complaint because complete absence of the salivary glands is rare. Dental findings in ED may range from anodontia, to, more commonly, hypodontia of the primary or permanent teeth (Figure 4.33d and e). Teeth that are present often have conical crowns. Other defects include high palatal arch or even a cleft palate, reduced vertical dimension because of the absence of teeth, and enamel hypoplasia.

Diagnosis The diagnosis of ED is typically straightforward and established in early childhood. At least two clinical features of the components (hypodontia, hypotrichosis, and hypohidrosis) must be present in order to establish the diagnosis of ED. Conditions to consider in the differential include sporadic oligodontia, exposure to head and neck irradiation during childhood, chondroectodermal dysplasia, and cleidocranial dysplasia.

Treatment The dental management of ED is both complex and challenging. The major goal is to provide the patient with optimal esthetics and function to foster normal physical and emotional growth. Implant-supported prostheses may offer the best opportunity for successful rehabilitation. The major advantage of implant-supported prostheses is increased retention and stability of the prostheses, leading to improvement in function and esthetics. It has been suggested that dental and skeletal maturity, not chronological age, should be the determining factor if implants are to be considered. When feasible, fixed restorations allow ED patients to avoid social problems that are associated with partial or full dentures, particularly in younger patients.

4.6   Examine the Neck

Inspect the neck for asymmetry, unusual pulsations, or limitations of motion. By simply extending and turning the neck, tension of the sternocleidomastoid muscle brings into view the boundaries of the anterior and posterior triangles. The carotid arteries often visibly pulsate if there is aortic insufficiency, or they may throb in patients who have severe anemia, atherosclerosis, arteriosclerosis, or hyperthyroidism.

Upon palpation, enlargement of the thyroid gland or abnormalities of the vascular structures may become apparent. Normally, the thyroid gland is a firm, smooth, midline mass that moves upward with swallowing. A thyroglossal duct cyst (TDC) typically presents as a fluctuant midline swelling and represents residua of the thyroglossal tract following descent of the thyroid gland from the base of the tongue. A branchial cleft cyst appears in the upper lateral neck just anterior to the sternocleidomastoid muscle. Anatomically, the inferior lobe of the submandibular gland lies inferior to the posterior attachment of the mylohyoid muscle. Inflammation or a sialolith associated with the inferior lobe of the sub-mandibular gland may become apparent in the neck.

Thyroglossal Duct Cyst

The TDC is the most common developmental nonodontogenic cyst to occur in the neck. It accounts for approximately 40% of cervical malformations in children and has a peak incidence during the first three decades of life. Men and women are equally affected. It usually presents as an asymptomatic midline mass in the anterior neck at the level of the thyroid gland. However, it may arise anywhere along the thyroglossal tract, from the base of the tongue (lingual thyroid) to the anterior neck.

Clinical Features The TDC usually presents as a painless, well-defined, smooth, asymptomatic midline swelling in the neck (Figure 4.34). About 25% of cases are present at birth and another 30% are diagnosed by the age of 10 years. They may be found anywhere in the midline from the submental region to the suprasternal notch, but most are found near the hyoid bone. Only 1% of TDCs are lateral to the midline. With swallowing or protrusion of the tongue, a TDC classically rises in the neck as a result of the cyst being anchored to the hyoid bone and the muscles of the tongue. If a TDC is secondarily infected, drainage to the overlying skin through a sinus tract may occur. Approximately 1% of TDCs undergo neoplastic change, usually to form a papillary adenocarcinoma.

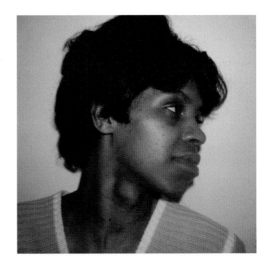

Figure 4.34 Thyroglossal duct cyst.

Diagnosis The presence of a midline mass that undergoes upward movement upon swallowing is highly suggestive of a TDC. The diagnosis is usually confirmed with a fine needle aspiration biopsy. Radiographic studies are useful to delineate extent of the lesion and the presence of ectopic functioning thyroid tissue. Other lesions to consider in a differential diagnosis include a dermoid cyst, ectopic thyroid tissue, lipoma, sebaceous cyst, lymph node, branchial cleft cyst, and autoimmune thyroiditis.

Treatment Treatment of a TDC is complete surgical excision. It is often recommended that the central portion of the hyoid bone be removed in an effort to eliminate any residual thyroglossal tract epithelium and avoid recurrence. Indications for excision may include cosmetic appearance, recurrent infections, sinus tract formation, and the risk of malignant transformation. Routine follow-up care is recommended to monitor for recurrence.

Branchial Cleft Cyst

Branchial cleft cyst is a congenital developmental defect that arises from the primitive branchial apparatus (usually the second branchial arch). It is believed to reflect incomplete closure of clefts and pouches or a failure

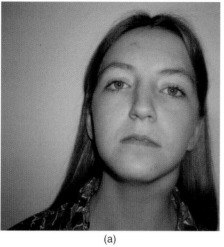
(a)

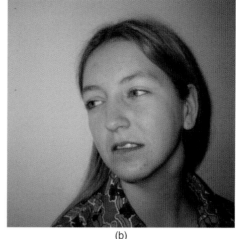
(b)

Figure 4.35 (a) and (b) Branchial cleft cyst.

of obliteration of the cervical sinus. It is an epithelial lined cavity, which may be associated with a draining sinus tract.

Clinical Features The branchial cleft cyst typically presents as a soft, round mass located along the anterior border of the sternocleidomastoid muscle (Figure 4.35a and b). It can increase in size during an upper respiratory tract infection. It may also appear in the submandibular area, adjacent to the parotid gland, or around the sternocleidomastoid muscle. A branchial cleft cyst usually becomes clinically apparent in late childhood or early adulthood. Computed tomography is useful to delineate the extent of the lesion.

Diagnosis The typical lateral presentation of a branchial cleft cyst is highly suggestive of the correct diagnosis. However, a definitive diagnosis is usually obtained after histological examination of the excised tissue. Differential diagnosis should include cervical lymphadenitis, dermoid cyst, retropharyngeal abscess, skin inclusion cyst, lymphangioma, and primary or metastatic parotid tumor.

Treatment Complete excision is the treatment of choice. The overall recurrence rate is about

3–5%, with a slightly increased risk of recurrence when a sinus tract is present.

Sialolith

Sialoliths are a major cause of salivary gland dysfunction. They are spherical, calcareous deposits within the ductal system or parenchyma of major or minor salivary glands. It is believed that they are derived from intracellular microcalculi that when excreted into the ductal system provide a platform for further calcification. Other theories suggest that "mucous plugs" within the ductal system or bacteria from the oral cavity that migrated into the ductal system become the nidus for further calcification. Multiple sialoliths occur in approximately 25% of patients.

Clinical Features The most characteristic complaint is a painful swelling within the affected gland just before, during, and immediately after meals (Figure 4.36a and b). The submandibular gland is most frequently affected (92%), followed by parotid gland (6%), and sublingual gland (2%). In a minority of cases, symptoms are absent. Some sialoliths may be detected by bidigital palpation of Wharton's or Stensen's ducts, while others may be revealed by radiographic or ultrasonic examination

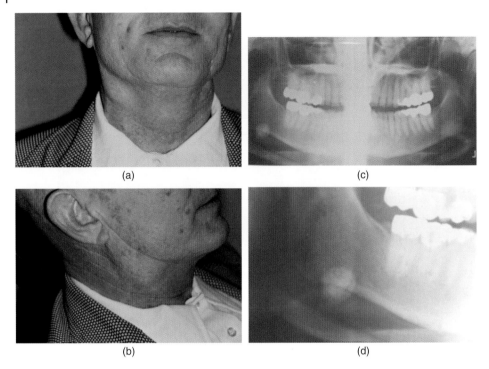

(a)

(b)

(c)

(d)

Figure 4.36 (a)–(d) Sialolith.

(Figure 4.36c and d). If the duct (usually Wharton's duct) becomes completely occluded, retrograde movement of oral bacteria in the duct may result in acute sialadenitis. Untreated sialadenitis may lead to fibrosis and atrophy of the affected gland.

Diagnosis The most important considerations in the diagnosis of obstructive salivary gland disease are patient history and clinical examination. Palpation of the affected gland may reveal reduced flow from the affected duct. The presence of cloudy or purulent flow usually indicates the presence of secondary infection. Radiographs and ultrasonography may be useful to demonstrate a sialolith. However, while submandibular sialoliths are usually radiopaque, parotid blockages are usually caused by mucous plugs and often not visible on radiographs.

Treatment Management of a sialolith within the submandibular gland depends on the duration of the symptoms, the size of the stone, and the location of the stone. Small sialoliths may be successfully excreted or removed while preserving the gland and associated duct. Larger sialoliths necessitate surgical removal of the affected gland. Newer, less invasive techniques include interventional sialendoscopy and ultrasound-guided piezoelectric extracorporeal lithotripsy.

Assess Spinal Accessory Nerve Function

The spinal accessory nerve (XI) provides motor function to the sternocleidomastoid and trapezius muscles. Injury to the nerve may manifest as paralysis of these muscles.

Evaluate Motor Function
Ask the patient to rotate the head to one side and palpate the sternocleidomastoid muscle while applying counter-rotational pressure to the head. Repeat on the opposite side. In a similar manner, the size and strength of

the trapezius muscles may be palpated as the patient shrugs the shoulders against resistance provided by the examiner. The muscles should not yield to the examiner's downward pressure.

4.7 Examine the Lymph Nodes

After a general evaluation of the head and neck has been completed, but before the oral cavity is examined, the various lymph nodes in the head and neck region should be palpated (Figure 4.37) Lymphadenopathy associated with intraoral pathoses primarily involves the submandibular, submental, and anterior cervical nodes.

Lymphadenopathy is an indication of an abnormality that must be identified (Table 4.3). Pathological changes in cervical lymph nodes may represent an inflammatory, degenerative, or neoplastic process. Neoplastic involvement of cervical nodes may occur as a primary process of lymphoma. Secondary involvement of lymph nodes in the neck may be seen in association with intraoral SCC.

Table 4.3 General conditions suggested by palpable nodes.

Condition	Nodal characteristics
Acute inflammatory disease	Smooth, firm, movable, and tender node
Past or present chronic disease with fibrosis	Discrete, firm, movable, and nontender node
Neoplasm	Matted, nontender, usually firm and fixed node
Systemic disease	Variably palpable, usually nontender node

Lymphoma

Lymphoma is a neoplasm of lymphoid cells found in the lymph nodes, spleen, liver, and bone marrow. It is defined by uncontrolled growth of a specific lymphocyte lineage. While there are several specific types of lymphoma, all are classified as either being a Hodgkin's or a non-Hodgkin's lymphoma. Over 79 000 cases of lymphoma are diagnosed in the United

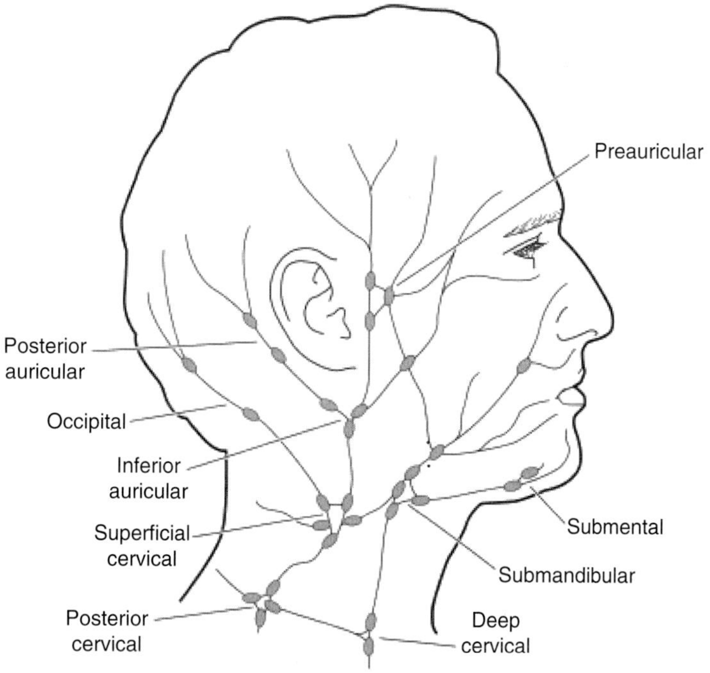

Figure 4.37 Lymph nodes.

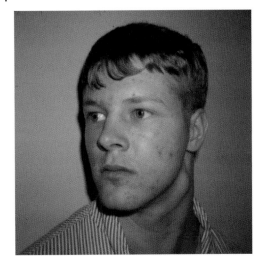

Figure 4.38 Hodgkin's lymphoma.

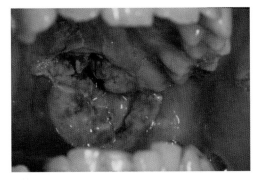

Figure 4.39 Hodgkin's lymphoma.

States each year, and over 88% of these cases are of the non-Hodgkin's type. Both types of lymphoma demonstrate a slight male predilection. Like most other malignancies, the etiology of lymphoma is only partially understood, and numerous genetic and environmental factors likely contribute to the disease. As many cases of lymphoma initially present in the head and neck, the dental practitioner is often in a unique position to be the first to suspect its presence and initiate a medical referral.

Clinical Features The signs and symptoms of lymphoma are often indolent and include swollen, painless lymph nodes in the neck (Figure 4.38), armpits, or groin; unexplained weight loss; fever; soaking night sweats; chronic cough and breathing difficulties; persistent fatigue; pruritis; and fullness or pain in the abdomen. Oral involvement is rare, but if present, typically manifests as a progressive swelling or mass that may undergo ulceration (Figure 4.39).

Diagnosis Lymphoma should be considered in any patient with the signs and symptoms listed above. A biopsy of a suspicious lymph node is required to establish a definitive diagnosis.

This may be accomplished by performing either a simple excisional biopsy or a fine needle aspiration. Once the diagnosis is obtained, an extensive medical workup is undertaken to determine the stage (spread) of the lymphoma.

Treatment The treatment and prognosis of a patient with lymphoma is dependent on both the type and the stage of the disease. Potential therapeutic measures include surgery, chemotherapy, radiation therapy, immunotherapy, and bone marrow or stem cell transplantation. Overall, the survival rate of lymphoma has gradually improved over the past few decades and now exceeds 65%.

Squamous Cell Carcinoma

SCC is an invasive tumor with metastatic potential. It is derived from the thin, flat squamous cells that are found on the skin surface; and the mucosal lining of hollow organs such as the respiratory and digestive tracts, including the oral cavity.

In the United States, the number of new cancer cases for 2020 reached 1,806,590. Oral cancer consistently ranks as one of the top 10 cancers worldwide, with broad differences in geographic distribution. In 2020, there were approximately 53,260 malignancies of the oral cavity and pharynx. While this represents less than 3% of all malignant neoplasms diagnosed annually in the United States, in developing countries the incidence is much higher. Oral cancer remains predominantly a disease of males; but the male to female ratio has steadily shifted from about 6 : 1 in 1950 to about 2.5 : 1 in 2020. The changing ratio is likely the result of the increase in smoking among women in the past three decades. Most cases of oral cancer in the United States are diagnosed in the sixth and seventh decades of life, with the highest prevalence noted in patients over 65 years of age. A recent study in the United States reported an alarming increase in the incidence of oral cancer, particularly tongue cancer, in young white males under the age of 40 years.

Over 90% of oral and pharyngeal cancers are SCCs. There are three major risk factors that contribute to the development of oral and pharyngeal cancer: tobacco, alcohol, and oncongenic human papilloma viruses. Tobacco, particularly cigarette smoking, remains the major risk factor associated with the development of oral SCC. However over the past few decades the burden of tobacco associated oral and pharyngeal SCC has been declining, while the burden of oncogenic HPV associated oral pharyngeal SCC has been steadily increasing. The most frequently implicated HPV strains are 16 and 18. Alcohol is an independent risk factor for oral and pharyngeal SCC and a synergistic relationship between tobacco and alcohol use and the development of oral and pharyngeal SCC has been noted. Additional risk factors such as living in rural areas, socioeconomic status, age, gender, and humoral and cellular immune mechanisms may play less well understood roles. Chronic periodontal disease, poor oral hygiene, ill-fitting dentures, sharp teeth, electrogalvanism, and edentulism have been suggested as cofactors.

Clinical Features SCC may appear as a flat leukoplakia, erythroplakia, or speckled leukoplakia, which may evolve into a persistent nodule, tumor, or indurated ulcer (Figure 4.40a and b). Symptoms are uncommon in earlier stages of the disease but become more frequent with local invasion. In particular, paresthesia and anesthesia in the absence of a history of trauma are highly suggestive of invasive SCC. Metastatic dissemination occurs through the submandibular, cervical (Figure 4.40c), and jugular lymphatic pathways, and distant metastases most commonly spread to the lungs. The majority of oral SCCs originate from nonkeratinized mucosa. The three most common sites of involvement are the tongue (30%), lip (17%), and floor of the mouth (14%). Recently, a trend toward an increased number of lesions arising on both the dentate and edentulous gingiva has been reported. While tobacco associated oral and pharyngeal SCC predominantly occurs in easily visualized oral cavity structures (e.g. lateral tongue, floor of mouth), HPV-associated oral and pharyngeal SCC predominately affects the oropharynx which includes the palatine and lingual tonsils, the posterior one-third (base) of the tongue, the soft palate and the posterior pharyngeal wall. These lesions may be more difficult to visually detect and symptoms often mimic pharyngitis or tonsillitis.

Diagnosis The responsibility to identify any suspicious oral and pharyngeal lesion clearly falls under the purview of a dental professional. A biopsy remains the gold standard by which oral cancer is diagnosed and any unusual or suspicious lesion lasting more than two weeks must be regarded with suspicion, and a biopsy should be considered to rule out malignancy. To safeguard and advance the welfare of the patient, a clinician who is uncomfortable performing a biopsy has the obligation to refer the patient to a respected peer or specialist with the skills, knowledge, and experience in managing oral cancer (e.g. head and neck surgeon, oral and maxillofacial surgeon).

Treatment Once the diagnosis of SCC has been established, the patient will need to undergo a thorough medical evaluation to stage the

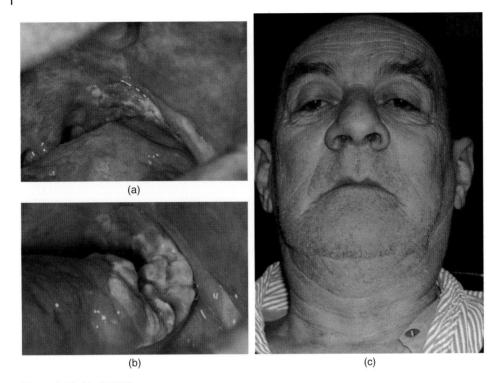

Figure 4.40 (a)–(c) SCC.

neoplasm. Staging is an essential component in the management scheme and helps to determine prognosis and guide therapy. Typically, head and neck cancer is treated by one or more of a combination of the three principal therapeutic modalities: surgery, radiotherapy, and chemotherapy. The use of one treatment over another depends on the size, location, and stage of the primary tumor; the patient's ability to tolerate treatment; and the patient's desires.

Surgical excision is the preferred modality for most well-defined and accessible solid tumors. However, it has its limitations for inaccessible or more advanced tumors demonstrating lymph node involvement and/or metastasis. For such cases, radiotherapy may be either an effective alternative to surgery or a valuable adjunct to surgery and/or chemotherapy in the loco-regional control of SCC. While the benefit of neoadjuvant (induction) chemotherapy has been recently scrutinized, several studies have shown that concomitant chemo-radiotherapy improves both loco-regional control and survival.

4.8 Conclusion

Physical signs are produced by physical causes. Since physical problems are the determinants of physical signs, these signs and symptoms must be recognized before the physical problems can be diagnosed and treated.

Suggested Reading

Ali, S. and Sarwari, A.R. (2007). A patient with a painless neck swelling. *Clin. Infect. Dis.* 45 (1): 87, 131–132.

Alvares, L.C., Capelozza, A.L., Cardoso, C.L. et al. (2009). Monostotic fibrous dysplasia: a 23-year follow-up of a patient with spontaneous bone remodeling. *Oral Surg. Oral Med. Oral Pathol. Oral Radiol. Endod.* 107 (2): 229–234.

Aly, H. (2004). Respiratory disorders in the newborn: identification and diagnosis. *Pediatr. Rev.* 25: 201–208.

Andretta, M., Tregnaghi, A., Prosenikliev, V., and Staffieri, A. (2005). Current opinions in sialolithiasis diagnosis and treatment. *Acta Otorhinolaryngol. Ital.* 25 (3): 145–149.

Baykul, T., Heybeli, N., Oyar, O., and Dogru, H. (2003). Multiple huge osteomas of the mandible causing disfigurement related with Gardner's syndrome: case report. *Auris Nasus Larynx* 30: 447–451.

Bensenor, I.M., Olmos, R.D., and Lotufo, P.A. (2012). Hypothyroidism in the elderly: diagnosis and management. *Clin. Interv. Aging* 7: 97–111.

Bezerra Júnior, G.L., Silva, L.F., Pimentel, G.G. et al. (2017). Treatment of large thyroglossal duct cyst. *J Craniofac Surg.* 28 (8): e794–e795.

Bianchi, S.D. and Boccardi, A. (1999). Radiological aspects of osesarcome of the jaws. *Dentomaxillofac. Radiol.* 28: 42–47.

Bishop, K. and Wragg, P. (1997). Ectodermal dysplasia in adulthood: the restorative difficulties and management. *Dent. Update* 24: 235–240.

Boland, D.F. and Stacy, M. (2012). The economic and quality of life burden associated with Parkinson's disease: a focus on symptoms. *Am. J. Manag. Care* 18 (7 Suppl): S168–S175.

Boscaro, M. and Arnaldi, G. (2009). Approach to the patient with possible Cushing's syndrome. *J. Clin. Endocrinol. Metab.* 94 (9): 3121–3131.

Boyd, K.P., Korf, B.R., and Theos, A. (2009). Neurofibromatosis type 1. *J. Am. Acad. Dermatol.* 61 (1): 1–14. quiz 15–16.

Braun, R.P., Rabinovitz, H.S., Oliviero, M. et al. (2005). Dermoscopy of pigmented skin lesions. *J. Am. Acad. Dermatol.* 52: 109–121.

Bull, P.D. (2001). Salivary gland stones: diagnosis and treatment. *Hosp. Med.* 62 (7): 396–399.

Clayton, P.T. (2003). Diagnosis of inherited disorders of liver metabolism. *J. Inherit. Metab. Dis.* 26: 135–146.

Cleveland, J.L., Junger, M.L., Saraiya, M. et al. (2011). The connection between human papillomavirus and oropharyngeal squamous cell carcinomas in the United States: implications for dentistry. *J. Am. Dent. Assoc.* 142 (8): 915–924.

Colao, A., Grasso, L.F.S, Giustina, A. et al. (2019). Acromegaly. *Nat. Rev. Dis. Primers.* 5 (1): 20. https://doi:10.1038/s41572-019-0071-6.

Comi, A.M. (2007). Update on Sturge-weber syndrome: diagnosis, treatment, quantitative measures, and controversies. *Lymphat. Res. Biol.* 5: 257–264.

Cornblath, W.T. (2018). Treatment of ocular myasthenia gravis. *Asia Pac. J. Ophthalmol (Phila).* 7 (4): 257–259.

Crowson, A.N. (2006). Basal cell carcinoma: biology, morphology and clinical implications. *Mod. Pathol.* 19 (Suppl 2): S127–S147.

Dhanrajani, P.J. and Jiffry, A.O. (1998). Management of ectodermal dysplasia: a literature review. *Dent. Update* 25: 73–75.

Dirks, S.J., Paunovich, E.D., Terézhalmy, G.T., and Chiodo, L.K. (2003). The patient with Parkinson's disease. *Quintessence Int.* 34: 379–393.

El-Kehdy, J., Abbas, O., and Rubeiz, N. (2012). A review of Parry-Romberg syndrome. *J. Am. Acad. Dermatol.* 67 (4): 769–784.

Eversole, R., Su, L., and El Mofty, S. (2008). Benign fibro-osseous lesions of the craniofacial complex. A review. *Head Neck Pathol.* 2 (3): 177–202.

Fargo, M.V., Grogan, S.P., and Saguil, A. (2017). Evaluation of jaundice in adults. *Am Fam Physician.* 95 (3): 164–168.

Farmakidis, C., Pasnoor, M., Dimachkie, M.M. et al. (2018). Treatment of myasthenia gravis. *Neurol. Clin.* 36 (2): 311–337.

Fonseca, L.C., Kodama, N.K., Nunes, F.C. et al. (2007). Radiographic assessment of Gardner's syndrome. *Dentomaxillofac. Radiol.* 36: 121–124.

Frei, F. (2018). Tardive dyskinesia: Who gets it and why. *Parkinsonism Relat Disord.* 59: 151–154.

Guaraldi, F. and Salvatori, R. (2012). Cushing syndrome: maybe not so uncommon of an endocrine disease. *J. Am. Board Fam. Med.* 25 (2): 199–208.

Gupta, M., Kaste, S.C., and Hopkins, K.P. (2002). Radiologic appearance of primary jaw lesions in children. *Pediatr. Radiol.* 32 (3): 153–168.

Gupta, M., Singh, S., and Gupta, M. (2011). Lingual thyroglossal duct cyst treated by intraoral marsupialisation. *BMJ Case Rep.* 8: 2011.

Gupta, P., Bhalla, A.S., Karthikeyan, V., and Bhutia, O. (2012). Two rare cases of craniofacial chondrosarcoma. *World J. Radiol.* 4 (6): 283–285.

Ha, P.K., Eisele, D.W., Frassica, F.J. et al. (1999). Osteosarcoma of the head and neck: a review of the Johns Hopkins experience. *Laryngoscope* 109: 964–969.

Half, E., Bercovich, D., and Rozen, P. (2009). Familial adenomatous polyposis. *Orphanet J. Rare Dis.* 4: 22. https://doi.org/10.1186/1750-1172-4-22.

Helfrich, M.H. (2003). Osteoclast diseases. *Microsc. Res. Tech.* 61: 514–532.

Hessel, A.C., Vora, N., Koutakis, S.E., and Chang, C.Y.J. (1999). Vascular lesion of the masseter presenting with phlebolith. *Otolaryngol. Head Neck Surg.* 120: 545–548.

Himes, C.P., Ganesh, R., Wight, E.C. et al. (2020). Perioperative evaluation and management of endocrine disorders. *Mayo Clin. Proc.* 95 (12): 2760–2774.

Holland, J. and Bernstein, J. (2014). Bell's palsy. *BMJ Clin Evid* 7: 1204.

Huber, M.A. and Tantiwongkosi, B. (2014). Oral and oropharyngeal cancer. *Med. Clin. N Am.* 98: 1299–1321.

Huber, M.A. and Terézhalmy, G.T. (2007). Risk stratification and dental management of patients with adrenal dysfunction. *Quintessence Int.* 38 (4): 325–338.

Huber, M.A. and Terézhalmy, G.T. (2008). Risk stratification and dental management of the patient with thyroid dysfunction. *Quintessence Int.* 39 (2): 139–150.

Imhof, H., Czerny, C., Hörmann, M., and Krestan, C. (2004). Tumors and tumor-like lesions of the neck: from childhood to adult. *Eur. Radiol.* 14: 155–165.

Inoue, Y., Nemoto, Y., Tashiro, T. et al. (1997). Neurofibromatosis Type 1 and Type 2. Review of the central nervous system and related structures. *Brain Dev.* 19: 1–12.

Inwards, C.Y. (2007). Update on cartilage forming tumors of the head and neck. *Head Neck Pathol.* 1 (1): 67–74.

Johnson-Huang, L.M., Lowes, M.A., and Krueger, J.G. (2012). Putting together the psoriasis puzzle: an update on developing targeted therapies. *Dis. Model. Mech.* 5 (4): 423–433.

Jouhilahti, E.M., Peltonen, S., Heape, A.M., and Peltonen, J. (2011). The pathoetiology of neurofibromatosis 1. *Am. J. Pathol.* 178 (5): 1932–1939.

Kalantri, A., Karambelkar, M., Joshi, R. et al. (2010). Accuracy and reliability of pallor for detecting anaemia: a hospital-based diagnostic accuracy study. *PLoS One* 5 (1): e8545.

Kemp, S., Gallagher, G., Kabani, S. et al. (2008). Oral non-Hodgkin's lymphoma: review of the literature and World Health Organization classification with reference to 40 cases. *Oral*

Surg. Oral Med. Oral Pathol. Oral Radiol. Endod. 105: 194–201.

Khanna, G., Smith, R.J.H., and Bauman, N.M. (2006). Causes of facial swelling in pediatric patients: correlations of clinical and radiologic findings. *Radiographics* 26: 155–171.

Koch, B.B., Karnell, L.H., Hoffman, H.T. et al. (2000). National cancer database report on chondrosarcoma of the head and neck. *Head Neck* 22: 408–425.

Lee, L., Yan, Y.H., and Pharoah, M.J. (1996). Radiographic features of the mandible in neurofibromatosis: a report of 10 cases and review of the literature. *Oral Surg. Oral Med. Oral Pathol. Oral Radiol. Endod.* 81: 361–367.

Leet, A.I., Chebli, C., Kushner, H. et al. (2004). Fracture incidence in polyostotic fibrous dysplasia and the McCune-Albright syndrome. *J. Bone Miner. Res.* 19 (4): 571–577.

Longo, D., Fauci, A., Kasper, D. et al. (2013). Cyanosis. In: *Harrison's Manual of Medicine*, 18e, 229–230. McGraw Hill.

Lowes, M.A., Bowcock, A.M., and Krueger, J.G. (2007). Pathogenesis and therapy of psoriasis. *Nature* 445: 866–873.

Luba, M.C., Bangs, S.A., Mohler, A.M., and Stulberg, D.L. (2003). Common benign skin tumors. *Am. Fam. Physician* 67 (4): 729–738.

Lustman, J., Regev, E., and Melamed, Y. (1990). Sialolithiasis. A survey on 245 patients and a review of the literature. *Int. J. Oral Maxillofac. Surg.* 19 (3): 135–138.

MacDonald-Jankowski, D. (1999). Fibrous dysplasia in the jaws of a Hong-Kong population: radiographic presentation and systematic review. *Dentomaxillofac. Radiol.* 28: 195–202.

Madani, S. and Shapiro, J. (2000). Alopecia areata update. *J. Am. Acad. Dermatol.* 42 (4): 549–565.

Malmgren, B. and Lindskog, S. (2003). Assessment of dysplastic dentin in osteogenesis imperfecta and dentinogenesis imperfecta. *Acta Odontol. Scand.* 61: 72–80.

Malmgren, B., Lindskog, S., Elgadi, A. et al. (2004). Clinical, histopathologic, and genetic investigation in two large families with dentinogenesis imperfecta type II. *Hum. Genet.* 114: 491–498.

Mather, A.J., Stoykewych, A.A., and Curran, J.B. (2006). Cervicofacial and mediastinal emphysema complicating a dental procedure. *J. Can. Dent. Assoc.* 72: 565–568.

Mattioni, J., Azari, S., Hoover, T. et al. (2019). A cross-sectional evaluation of outcomes of pediatric branchial cleft cyst excision. *Int. J. Pediatr. Otorhinolaryngol.* 119: 171–176.

McGuire, J.F., Ge, N.N., and Dyson, S. (2009). Nonmelanoma skin cancer of the head and neck I: histopathology and clinical behavior. *Am. J. Otolaryngol.* 30 (2): 121–133.

Melmed, S. (2009). Acromegaly pathogenesis and treatment. *J. Clin. Invest.* 119 (11): 3189–3202.

Mendenhall, W.M., Fernandes, R., Werning, J.W. et al. (2011). Head and neck osteosarcoma. *Am. J. Otolaryngol.* 32 (6): 597–600.

Michou, L. and Brown, J.P. (2011). Emerging strategies and therapies for treatment of Paget's disease of bone. *Drug Des. Devel. Ther.* 5: 225–239.

Miller, C.S., Little, J.W., and Falace, D.A. (2001). Supplemental corticosteroids for dental patients with adrenal insufficiency. *JADA* 132: 1570–1575.

Miteva, L.G., Dourmishev, A.I., Schwartz, R.A., and Mitev, V.I. (1998). Oral vascular manifestations of Klippel-Trenaunay syndrome. *Cutis* 62: 171–174.

Muthalagu, R., Bai, V.T., Gracias, D. et al. (2018). Developmental screening tool: accuracy and feasibility of non-invasive anaemia estimation. *Technol. Health Care.* 26 (4): 723–727.

Narayanan, C.D., Prakash, P., and Dhanasekaran, C.K. (2009). Intramuscular hemangioma of the masseter muscle: a case report. *Cases J.* 18 (2): 7459.

Neuhaus, I.M., LeBoit, P.E., and McCalmont, T.M. (2006). Seborrheic keratosis with basal clear cells: a distinctive microscopic mimic of melanoma in situ. *J. Am. Acad. Dermatol.* 54: 132–135.

Nico, M.M., Vilela, M.A., Rivitti, E.A., and Lourenço, S.V. (2008). Oral lesions in lupus erythematosus: correlation with cutaneous lesions. *Eur. J. Dermatol.* 18 (4): 376–381.

Nicollas, R., Guelfucci, B., Roman, S., and Triglia, J.M. (2000). Congenital cysts and fistulas of the neck. *Int. J. Pediatr. Otorhinolaryngol.* 55 (2): 117–124.

Paczona, R., Jori, J., and Czigner, J. (1998). Pharyngeal localization of branchial cysts. *Eur. Arch. Otorhinolaryngol.* 255 (7): 379–381.

Papaleontiou, M. and Haymart, M.R. (2012). Approach to and treatment of thyroid disorders in the elderly. *Med. Clin. North Am.* 96 (2): 297–310.

Parkar, A., Medhurst, C., Irbash, M., and Philpott, C. (2009). Periorbital oedema and surgical emphysema, an unusual complication of a dental procedure: a case report. *Cases J.* 2: 8108.

Patel, H., Thakkar, C., and Patel, K. (2010). Parry-romberg syndrome: a rare entity. *J. Maxillofac. Oral Surg.* 9 (3): 247–250.

Pigno, M.A., Blackman, R.B., Cronin, R.J. Jr., and Cavazos, E. (1996). Prosthodontic management of ectodermal dysplasia: a review of the literature. *Prosthe.t Dent.* 76: 541–545.

Pinsolle, V., Rivel, J., Michelet, V. et al. (1998). Treatment of fibrous dysplasia of the cranio-facial bones. Report of 25 cases. *Ann. Chie Plast. Esthet.* 43: 234–239.

Pratt, C.H., King, L.E. Jr, Messenger, A.G. et al. (2017). Alopecia areata. *Nat. Rev. Dis. Primers.* 3: 17011. https://doi:10.1038/nrdp.2017.11.

Rahman, A. and Isenberg, D.A. (2008). Systemic lupus erythematosus. *N. Engl. J. Med.* 358 (9): 929–939.

Rahman, I. and Sadiq, S.A. (2007). Ophthalmic management of facial nerve palsy: a review. *Surv. Ophthalmol.* 52: 121–144.

Ralston, S.H. (2013). Clinical practice. Paget's disease of bone. *N Engl J Med.* 368 (7): 644–650.

Ricciardi, L., Pringsheim, T., Barnes, T.R.E. et al. (2019). Treatment recommendations for tardive dyskinesia. *Can J Psychiatry.* 64 (6): 388–399.

Rivero, A.L. and Whitfeld, M. (2018). An update on the treatment of rosacea. *Aust Prescr.* 41 (1): 20–24.

Romeo, U., Galanakis, A., Lerario, F. et al. (2011). Subcutaneous emphysema during third molar surgery: a case report. *Braz. Dent. J.* 22 (1): 83–86.

Rubin, A.I., Chen, E.H., and Ratner, D. (2005). Basal cell carcinoma. *N. Engl. J. Med.* 353 (21): 2262–2269.

Sarment, D.P. and Weisgold, A.S. (1998). The importance of dentistry in the differential diagnosis of a medical disorder. *Compend. Contin. Educ. Dent.* 19: 124–126, 128–129.

Sclar, A.G., Kannikal, J., Ferreira, C.F. et al. (2009). Treatment planning and surgical considerations in implant therapy for patients with agenesis, oligodontia, and ectodermal dysplasia: review and case presentation. *J. Oral Maxillofac. Surg.* 67 (11 Suppl): 2–12.

Shapiro, J. and Price, V.H. (1998). Hair regrowth: therapeutic agents. *Dermatol. Clin.* 16: 341–356.

Siegel, R., Miller, K.D., and Jemal, A. (2020). Cancer statistics. *CA Cancer J. Clin.* 70 (1): 7–30.

Silberbach, M. and Hannon, D. (2007). Presentation of congenital heart disease in the neonate and young infant. *Pediatr. Rev.* 28: 123–131.

Spillane, J., Higham, E., and Kullmann, D.M. (2012). Myasthenia gravis. *Br. Med. J.* 21;345: e8497. https://doi.org/10.1136/bmj.e8497.

Steelman, R.J. and Johannes, P.W. (2007). Subcutaneous emphysema during restorative dentistry. *Int. J. Paediatr. Dent.* 17: 228–229. Paget's Disease.

Stoltzfus, R.J., Edward-Raj, A., Dreyfuss, M.L. et al. (1999). Clinical pallor is useful to detect severe anemia in populations where anemia is prevalent and severe. *J. Nutr.* 129 (9): 1675–1681.

Sullivan, F.M., Swan, I.G.C., Donnan, P.T. et al. (2007). Early treatment with prednisolone or acyclovir in Bell's palsy. *N. Engl. J. Med.* 357 (16): 1598–1607.

Suskauer, S.J., Trovato, M.K., Zabel, T.A., and Comi, A.M. (2010). Physiatric findings in individuals with Sturge-Weber syndrome. *Am. J. Phys. Med. Rehabil.* 89 (4): 323–330.

Tarakad, A. and Jankovic, J. (2017). Diagnosis and management of Parkinson's disease. *Semin Neurol.* 37 (2): 118–126.

Thiele, O.C., Freier, K., Bacon, C. et al. (2008). Interdisciplinary combined treatment of craniofacial osteosarcoma with neoadjuvant and adjuvant chemotherapy and excision of the tumour: a retrospective study. *Br. J. Oral Maxillofac. Surg.* 46 (7): 533–536.

Vaienti, L., Soresina, M., and Menozzi, A. (2005). Parascapular free flap and fat grafts: combined surgical methods in morphological restoration of hemifacial progressive atrophy. *Plast. Reconstr. Surg.* 116: 699–711.

Van Sickels, J.E., Raybould, T.P., and Hicks, E.P. (2010). Interdisciplinary management of patients with ectodermal dysplasia. *J. Oral Implantol.* 36 (3): 239–245.

Villaseñor-Park, J., Wheeler, D., and Grandinetti, L. (2012). Psoriasis: evolving treatment for a complex disease. *Cleve. Clin. J. Med.* 79 (6): 413–423.

Walther, S. and Strik, W. (2012). Motor symptoms and schizophrenia. *Neuropsychobiology* 66 (2): 77–92.

Wehner, M.R., Shive, M.L., Chren, M.M. et al. (2012). Indoor tanning and non-melanoma skin cancer: systematic review and meta-analysis. *Br. Med. J.* 345: e5909. https://doi.org/10.1136/bmj.e5909.

Wenzel, J. (2019). Cutaneous lupus erythematosus: new insights into pathogenesis and therapeutic strategies. *Nat. Rev. Rheumatol.* 15 (9): 519–532.

Whitt, J.C., Dunlap, C.L., and Martin, K.F. (2007). Oral Hodgkin lymphoma: a wolf in wolf's clothing. *Oral Surg. Oral Med. Oral Pathol. Oral Radiol. Endod.* 104: e45–e51.

Woolfeden, A.R., Tong, D.C., Norbash, A.M., and Albers, G.W. (1998). Progressive facial hemiatrophy: abnormality of intracranial vasculature. *Neurology* 50: 1915–1917.

Yang, W.T., Ahuja, A., and Metreweli, C. (1997). Sonographic features of head and neck hemangiomas and vascular malformations. *J. Ultrasound Med.* 16: 39–44.

Yavuz, I., Baskan, Z., Ulku, R. et al. (2006). Ectodermal dysplasia: retrospective study of fifteen cases. *Arch. Med. Res.* 37: 403–409.

Young, M.S. (2006). The morbidity of psoriatic disease. *Dermatol. Nurs.*: 4–6.

5

Examination of the Oral Cavity

Dentists should have a special interest in the physical examination of the oral cavity since the mouth is the anatomical area of the body for which they are the ultimate authority. Therefore, the organization of this section is more detailed and provides greater emphasis on possible findings and interpretation of data. Basic instrumentation for the oral examination includes a good light source, a mouth mirror, an explorer, a periodontal probe, dry gauze sponges, and an air syringe. The need for specialized instrumentation and additional diagnostic procedures will vary with the findings and differential diagnoses developed.

5.1 Examine the Vermilion of the Lips

The mouth begins at the mucocutaneous junction of the vermilion border of the lips. The vermilion border, a zone of specialized non-mucus-producing tissue, is bounded by the facial skin and the moist labial mucosa of the mouth. With age and exposure to the elements, the color of the vermilion border may change from a pink or red (vermilion) to a bluish hue. This region is a common site for physiological pigmentation, ephelides, or freckles, and rarely, pigmentation suggestive

Physical Evaluation and Treatment Planning in Dental Practice, Second Edition.
Géza T. Terézhalmy, Michaell A. Huber, Lily T. García and Ronald L. Occhionero.
© 2021 John Wiley & Sons, Inc. Published 2021 by John Wiley & Sons, Inc.
Companion Website: www.wiley.com/go/terezhalmy/physical

of Peutz–Jeghers syndrome (PJS). Varices, hemangiomas, and rarely, telangiectasias (hereditary hemorrhagic telangiectasia [HHT] and CREST syndrome) may be noted.

Swelling of the lip may indicate cellulitis of dental origin or angioedema (AE). Vesicular lesions of the lip may represent the initial phase of recurrent herpes labialis (RHL) (see "Herpetic Infections"). Serohemorrhagic crusting of the lips is highly suggestive of erythema multiforme (EM), an acute vesiculoulcerative disorder. Thickening of the vermilion border with the development of vertical fissures and/or the loss of distinction of the mucocutaneous junction may be indicative of actinic cheilosis. The upper and lower lips join at the commissures. Crusting or weeping erosion in this area is characteristic of angular cheilitis.

Peutz–Jeghers Syndrome

PJS is a rare autosomal dominant disorder characterized by mucocutaneous melanin pigmentation and unique hamartomatous polyps (Peutz–Jeghers polyps) affecting the gastrointestinal tract. These polyps have a predilection for the small intestine. Mutations of the *LKB1* tumor suppressor gene have been demonstrated in up to 80 % of cases. PJS patients are at an increased risk of cancer, especially cancer of the colon, stomach, small intestine, pancreas, breast, and ovary. The incidence of PJS is estimated to be less than 1 per 100 000.

Clinical Features The characteristic mucocutaneous pigmentation presents as 1–5 mm dark brown or blue macule affecting the lip vermilion (Figure 5.1a), buccal mucosa, hands (Figure 5.1b), and feet. These macules typically develop in infancy, but may fade with age. Since these areas of pigmentation are asymptomatic, their presence is often underappreciated. Underlying gastrointestinal symptoms, such as intestinal obstruction, abdominal pain, and bloody stools, often prompt the patient to seek medical attention.

Diagnosis The diagnosis of PJS is straightforward and established by the presence of either two or more Peutz–Jeghers polyps, one Peutz–Jeghers polyp and mucocutaneous pigmentations, or one Peutz-Jeghers polyp and a positive family history for PJS.

Treatment There is no cure for PJS. The increased cancer risk associated with PJS mandates earlier and more frequent screening for malignant disease. The mucocutaneous pigmentation requires no treatment.

Hereditary Hemorrhagic Telangiectasia

HHT is an uncommon autosomal dominant fibrovascular disorder. Also known as Rendu–Osler–Weber disease, HHT is characterized by the triad of mucocutaneous telangiectasias, arteriovenous malformations (AVMs), and recurrent hemorrhagic episodes. The morbidity and mortality of HHT is mainly

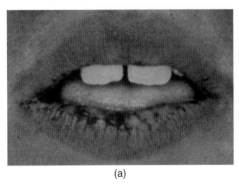
(a)

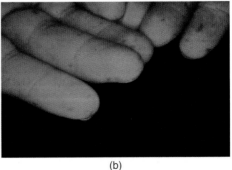
(b)

Figure 5.1 (a) and (b) Peutz-Jeghers syndrome.

attributable to the AVMs, which may occur in the lungs, skin, brain, liver, and gastrointestinal tract. Mutations underlying HHT have been identified in two different genes: edoglin (ENG) and activin-receptor-like-kinase (ALK1). For either case, homozygous forms of HHT are considered lethal. The incidence of HHT is estimated to be 1 in 5000 to 1 in 8000.

Clinical Features The most common presenting feature of HHT is recurrent epistaxis, which usually occurs between the ages of 10 and 20 years and may progress in frequency and severity with age. The telangiectasias become apparent in the third to fourth decade of life and usually progress both in size and number with age. They present as small flat or slightly raised bright red-purple lesions. These lesions blanch upon pressure and may be found on the face (Figure 5.2a), conjunctivae, lips (Figure 5.2b), tongue, palate, gingivae (Figure 5.2c and d), fingers (Figure 5.2e), arms, and trunk. Gastrointestinal involvement may result in severe blood loss leading to severe anemia with pallor (Figure 5.2f). AVMs are associated with pulmonary shunting, transient ischemic attacks, brain abscess, and hepatic shunting.

Diagnosis The diagnosis is based on the presence of three of the following four findings: spontaneous recurrent epistaxis, mucocutaneous telangiectasia, visceral involvement, and an affected first-degree relative.

Treatment There is no cure for HHT, and current treatment strategies entail close monitoring to identify and treat a potentially lethal AVM. Symptomatic treatment of epistaxis is often required, as is iron supplementation to manage anemia.

Angioedema

AE is a reversible localized swelling of the deep subcutaneous or submucosal tissues secondary to increased vascular permeability caused by

Table 5.1 Causes of angioedema.

Mechanism of disease	Precipitating factors
IgE mediated allergic response	Insect venom, shellfish, peanuts, antibiotics, NSAIDs
Pseuodoallergic response	Opioids, polymyxin, ACE inhibitors
Autoimmune disease	Hashimoto thyroiditis
C1 esterase inhibitor (C1-INH) deficiency	Hereditary, acquired, idiopathic
Trauma	Mechanical, chemical, thermal

locally produced vasoactive substances such as histamine, tryptase, prostaglandin $F_{2\alpha}$, and bradykinin. While there are many established causes for AE (Table 5.1), the cause in most cases remains unknown. The true incidence of AE is unknown, but it is postulated that up to 25 % of the population will experience at least one episode of AE in a lifetime.

Clinical Features While any part of the body may be affected, most cases are characterized by edema of the face and/or pharyngeal tissues (Figure 5.3a and b). The affected skin or mucosa may be tender and warm and the patient may complain of a burning sensation. Severe AE affecting the head and neck may spread to the larynx, resulting in life-threatening airway obstruction. About 50 % of patients also manifest urticaria and pruritis. Involvement of the abdominal viscera is often associated with severe pain.

Diagnosis The abrupt onset of AE affecting an observable area is easily recognized and diagnosed.

Treatment The initial treatment often focuses on providing symptomatic relief. AE presenting with urticaria usually responds well to antihistamines and corticosteroids. Efforts to

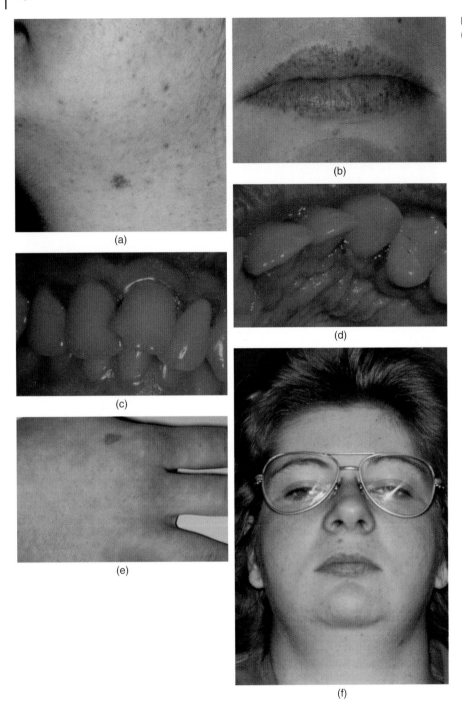

Figure 5.2 (a)–(f) HHT.

(a)

(b)

(c)

(d)

(e)

(f)

identify the cause of the AE should be undertaken, and patients with recurrent AE should be referred to an allergist or dermatologist for a comprehensive evaluation.

Erythema Multiforme

EM is an acute, typically self-limiting, and potentially recurrent mucocutaneous vesiculoerosive disorder. Severity varies from mild (EM

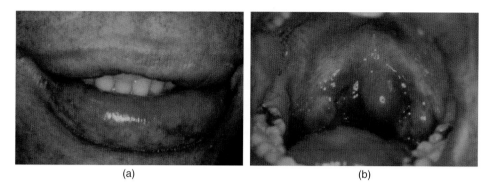

(a)   (b)

Figure 5.3 (a) and (b) Angioedema.

Table 5.2 Spectrum of erythema multiforme.

Type	Cutaneous involvement	Mucosal involvement	Outcome
EM minor	Target lesion, acral distribution, negative Nikolsky's sign	Often absent	Recovery; possible recurrence
EM major	As above	Prominent oral involvement; vesiculoerosive erosions with fibrinous pseudomembrane; characteristic hemorrhagic lip involvement	Recovery; possible recurrence; rare mortality
SJS	Widespread small blisters, macules, atypical target lesions predominate on torso; epidermal detachment <10 % body surface area; positive Nikolsky's sign	As above, possibly more extensive; ocular and genital involvement common	Fatal in 5–10% of cases; possible scarring; possible recurrence
TEN	Widespread small blisters, macules, atypical target lesions predominate on torso; epidermal detachment in >30% body surface area; positive Nikolsky's sign	As above	Fatal in up to 50% of cases; possible scarring; possible recurrence
Oral EM	Typical target lesions frequently absent	Oral lesions predominate clinical picture	Recovery; possible recurrent and chronic forms

minor) to moderate (EM major) to potentially fatal (Stevens–Johnson syndrome [SJS] and toxic epidermal necrolysis [TEN]) (Table 5.2). Some authorities consider oral EM minor/EM major and SJS/TEN to be two distinct disease processes.

The etiology of EM is most likely due to a genetically predisposed allergic host response to antigenic challenge (Table 5.3). Most cases of EM minor and EM major are related to an infectious agent, typically herpes simplex virus (HSV), while most cases of SJS and TEN are caused by exposure to a triggering drug. The incidence of EM minor and EM major is unknown, while the incidence of SJS and TEN is estimated to be two to three cases per million.

Table 5.3 Some causes of erythema multiforme.

Infectious agents	Drugs
β-Hemolytic streptococci	Allopurinol
Coccidiomycosis	Carbamazepine
Coxsackie virus	Cotrimazole
Diptheria	Lamotragine
Epstein–Barr virus	Nevirapine
Herpes simplex 1 and 2	NSAIDs (oxicam-type)
Herpes zoster	Phenobarbitol
Influenza, type A	Phenytoin
Mumps	
Mycoplasma pneumoniae	
Vaccinia	

Clinical Features Cutaneous lesions usually begin as erythematous papules that progress to form the more characteristic iris or target lesions. These lesions typically arise in an acral distribution (Figure 5.4a). In more severe forms of EM, the cutaneous lesions may present as more widespread erythematous or purpuric macules and blisters. Such patients may demonstrate a positive Nikolsky's sign. Hemorrhagic crusting of the lips is highly characteristic and virtually pathognomonic (Figure 5.4b). Intraorally, lesions on the unattached mucosal tissues predominate (Figure 5.4c and d). In the vast majority of cases, mucosal lesions tend to appear abruptly and manifest as painful vesicles, ulcerations, and erosions. Mucocutaneous lesions tend to heal completely in two to six weeks.

Diagnosis The typical abrupt onset, combined with the presence of the characteristic mucocutaneous lesions (i.e. target lesions, crusted lips, and vesiculoulcerative oral lesions) is diagnostic. Historical evidence of prior occurrence and/or exposure to a possible causative drug or infectious agent reinforces the diagnosis. For equivocal cases, a biopsy and immunofluorescence studies may be useful to rule out other conditions in the differential

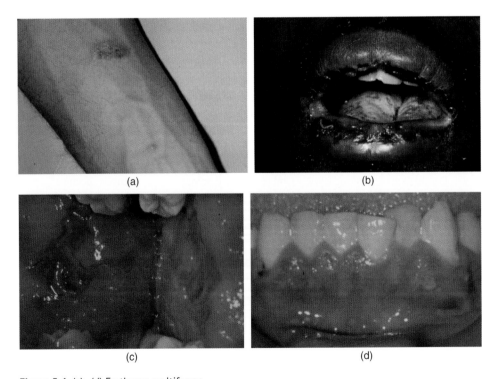

(a)　　　　　　　(b)

(c)　　　　　　　(d)

Figure 5.4 (a)–(d) Erythema multiforme.

diagnosis. Conditions that may mimic EM include erosive lichen planus (LP), pemphigus, mucous membrane pemphigoid (MMP), lupus erythematosus, herpetic gingivostomatitis, major aphthous, and hand-foot-and-mouth disease.

Treatment Most cases of EM resolve in two to six weeks, and treatment is generally palliative and supportive. Efforts to ensure adequate hydration and nutrition are mandatory, as is close monitoring. Anesthetic mouth rinses such as diphenhydramine hydrochloride and viscous lidocaine may be prescribed for oral pain, along with a bland soft nutritious diet. Antibiotic therapy may be indicated if secondary infection becomes evident. The withdrawal of any suspected causative medication should be undertaken and a careful history should be obtained to identify other possible underlying causes. Suspected cases of SJS or TEN mandate immediate referral to a physician.

Actinic Cheilosis

Actinic cheilosis is essentially actinic keratosis affecting the lip vermilion. Etiologic factors include cumulative ultraviolet radiation (UVR) exposure, skin phenotype, age, male sex, outdoor occupation, tobacco habits, and host immunological status. It represents the early clinical stage of a continuum that ultimately may progress to squamous cell carcinoma of the lip. Cumulative exposure to UVR in sunlight is the most important cause of actinic cheilosis. The true incidence of actinic cheilosis is unknown.

Clinical Features Actinic cheilosis typically develops over several years and primarily affects the lower lip. Initially, the patient may manifest a dry, unobtrusive chapped lip (Figure 5.5a). More advanced cases manifest marked parallel folds, isolated hyperkeratotic plaques, and a loss of the definition of the vermilion-cutaneous border (Figure 5.5b). In later stages, actinic cheilosis may appear mottled or opalescent in color, with a slightly elevated white or gray plaque (Figure 5.5c). The waxing and waning of erythematous or hemorrhagic areas over a prolonged period of time may represent an ominous sign.

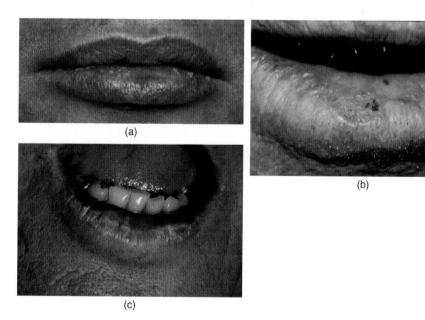

(a)

(b)

(c)

Figure 5.5 (a)–(c) Actinic cheilosis.

Diagnosis The working diagnosis of actinic cheilosis usually is straightforward and is derived by correlating the history with clinical findings in an at-risk patient. The presence of concurrent actinic keratoses on sun-exposed areas (i.e. face, neck, bald scalp, and ears) reinforces the diagnosis. Lesions that persist or do not respond to preventive measures should be biopsied. Unfortunately, the clinical appearance of actinic cheilosis does not always correlate directly with the underlying histological changes. Suspicious-looking lesions may prove to be remarkably benign, while a small area of actinic cheilosis may in fact represent severe dysplasia or even squamous cell carcinoma.

Treatment Commonly attempted ablative therapies to remove actinic cheiloses include cryotherapy with liquid nitrogen, topical 5-fluorouracil (5-FU), excision, laser ablation, and chemical peel. However, the only therapy which allows for histopathological review is vermillionectomy. Given the strong etiologic link between UVR and actinic cheilosis, reducing exposure to sunlight (or other forms of UVR) is the single most important measure for preventing actinic cheilosis. Avoiding peak sun exposure; covering up exposed skin; wearing a hat that shades the neck, face, and ears; wearing sunglasses; and using a sunscreen with a sun protection factor (SPF) of 15 or higher is recommended for all patients.

Angular Cheilitis

Angular cheilitis (perlèche) is an erythematous fissuring of the commissures of the mouth and adjacent skin. The lesions are typically infected with *Candida albicans* and staphylococci or streptococci. Factors that predispose to the development of angular cheilitis include insufficient vertical dimension of occlusion, nutritional deficiencies, endocrinopathies, medications, poor oral hygiene, dental prostheses, and conditions of altered immunity. While angular cheilitis may be an isolated occurrence, it is often

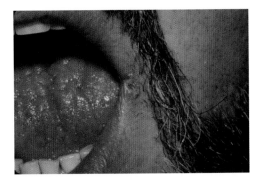

Figure 5.6 Angular cheilitis.

associated with intraoral candidiasis. The true incidence of angular cheilitis is unknown, but the number of patients who harbor *C. albicans* as a commensal organism in the oral cavity varies from 25 to 75%.

Clinical Features Angular cheilitis presents as unilateral (Figure 5.6) or bilateral (Figure 5.7) erythematous fissures of the commissures of the lips and adjacent skin. The lesion often has a glistening or moist appearance, but variable crusting may also occur.

Diagnosis The characteristic site-specific presentation of angular cheilitis makes for a straightforward diagnosis.

Treatment Mild cases of angular cheilitis are often transient and resolve uneventfully. More persistent cases typically respond to the use of a topical antifungal/steroid formulation and

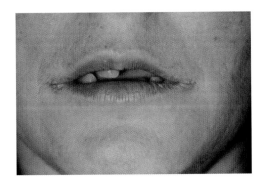

Figure 5.7 Angular cheilitis.

proper hygiene. For all cases, it is prudent to identify and, when possible, correct any predisposing factors.

5.2 Examine the Labial and Buccal Mucosa

To expose the labial mucosa, retract the upper and lower lips. Numerous minor salivary glands are located in this area. Using bidigital palpation, these glands are often apparent as small nodules. Minor salivary glands express saliva through pinpoint ducts. The function of these glands may be evaluated by everting the lips and drying the labial surfaces. Within several seconds, small beads of saliva should be expressed from these ducts. Mucoceles, extravasations of mucous-type saliva (mucin) into the connective tissue, occur frequently in the lower lip.

Still using the fingers as retractors, extend the examination to the buccal and vestibular mucosa. Observe color and other tissue characteristics. Find the parotid duct (Stensen's duct) located on the buccal mucosa adjacent to the maxillary first and second molar teeth. Assess parotid function. Firmly massaging the gland toward Stensen's duct should yield a clear fluid. Expression of casts, pus, or blood may indicate the presence of an infection, a sialolith, or a malignancy. Reduced salivary flow, dry mouth or xerostomia, is most often noted secondary to the use of anticholinergic agents, or in association with diabetes mellitus, Sjögren's syndrome, or head-and-neck radiotherapy.

A common and totally benign finding, linea alba typically presents bilaterally as a grayish-white keratotic linear plaque on the buccal mucosa that runs parallel to the adjacent occlusal plane. It is thought to represent mild occlusal trauma to the buccal mucosa characterized by hyperorthokeratosis (hyperkeratosis without retention of nuclei). More pronounced lesions may exhibit a shredded or shaggy appearance. Such pronounced cases likely indicate that a factitial habit (e.g. habitual cheek chewing) has contributed to the development of the lesion. Treatment is neither required nor recommended for linea alba. In leukoedema, a normal mucosal variation, the mucosa appears wrinkled and opalescent. Traumatic lesions and recurrent aphthous stomatitis (RAS) are commonly observed on the labial and buccal mucosa. The buccal mucosa is also a common site for the lacy linear Wickham striae of LP and the diffuse thickened white lesions of white sponge nevus, a congenital condition. Snuff keratosis is most commonly observed in the mucobuccal fold.

Pigmented lesions affecting the oral tissues are rare. Fordyce granules (ectopic sebaceous glands) appear as clusters of small yellow nodules and are frequently observed in the labial and buccal mucosa. An amalgam tattoo and a hematoma may be observed as an isolated bluish or grayish pigmentation affecting almost any area of the mouth. Examination of the buccal mucosa may also reveal commonly occurring raised or nodular lesions such as a fibroma and a papilloma, or less commonly occurring lesions such as a neuroma, hemangioma, or malignant neoplasm. Other conditions that may affect the labial and buccal mucosa include EM and pemphigus vulgaris.

Mucocele

A mucocele (mucous retention phenomenon, mucous extravasation phenomenon) represents a collection of salivary mucin entrapped within the connective tissue. It is thought that microtrauma to a minor salivary gland causes ductal disruption followed by mucin extravasation into the surrounding soft tissue. They are quite common, demonstrate no sex predilection, and occur more frequently in children, adolescents, and young adults. Mucoceles are most frequently located in the lower lip (60–70 %), but may develop at any location where minor salivary glands are present, including the soft palate, retromolar region, and buccal mucosa. Their occurrence in the maxillary lip is uncommon.

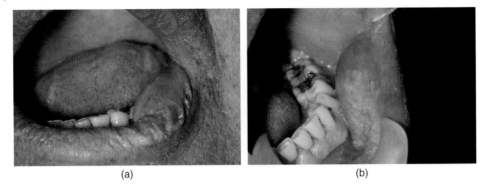

(a)   (b)

Figure 5.8 (a) and (b) Mucocele.

Clinical Features While some mucoceles may become large enough to cause a visible lip swelling (Figure 5.8a and b), typically they appear as a discrete, small, translucent, soft, painless swelling of the mucosa (Figure 5.9). Their color may range from normal pink to deep blue. A deep blue color reflects tissue cyanosis as a result of vascular congestion associated with the stretched overlying tissue and the translucent character of the accumulated fluid beneath. A more deep-seated lesion may appear as a normal colored submucosal nodule.

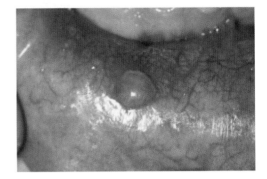

Figure 5.9 Mucocele.

Diagnosis The diagnosis of a mucocele is based principally on clinical and historical findings. The patient may or may not recall a specific inciting traumatic event. Lesions that may mimic a mucocele include a fibroma, vascular lesion, neural tumor, or salivary gland tumor.

Treatment Smaller mucoceles often undergo spontaneous involution and resolution. Lesions that persist or interfere with normal function are easily managed surgically. It is important that the surgeon remove all visible minor salivary gland tissue at the time of surgery, in order to reduce the risk of recurrence.

Dry Mouth

Dry mouth is a commonly encountered problem in dental practice. The term used to describe the patient's subjective complaint of a dry mouth is xerostomia. Numerous etiologic factors such as salivary gland disease, systemic disease, medications, head and neck irradiation, and some chemotherapy regimens contribute to dry mouth. Xerostomia is a common presenting complaint in about 30 % of patients over the age of 65 years.

Clinical Features The oral findings associated with dry mouth are variable and depend on the severity and duration of dryness. Mild acute cases may manifest no overt clinical changes. Common findings of oral dryness include a lack of saliva pooling in the floor of the mouth; inadequate wetting of the mucosal tissues (Figure 5.10a); a dry, furrowed, or fissured tongue (Figure 5.10b); patchy areas of erythema, usually indicative of candidiasis; and rampant caries (Figure 5.11a and b).

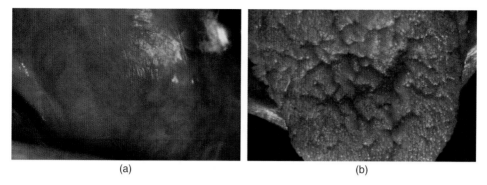

(a)   (b)

Figure 5.10 (a) and (b) Xerostomia.

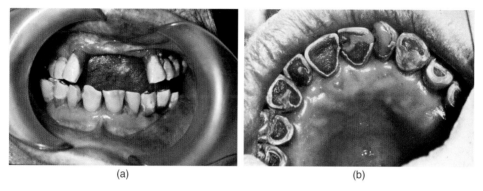

(a)   (b)

Figure 5.11 (a) and (b) Xerostomia.

Diagnosis The diagnosis of a dry mouth is relatively straightforward; the challenge is to identify the underlying cause or causes. Obtaining an exhaustive medical history is mandatory, and further medical evaluation may be necessary.

Treatment Treatment strategies for dry mouth are individually tailored and largely contingent upon the severity and duration of the dry mouth. Medication adjustment and/or underlying disease management may be all that is necessary to reestablish normal salivary production. Episodic cases, such as may occur with occasional allergy medication ingestion, may be managed with simple supportive measures such as frequent sipping of water throughout the day. In contrast, the more severe and permanent dry mouth associated with head and neck irradiation is often only minimally responsive to currently

available management protocols. These protocols consist of improved oral hygiene, saliva substitutes, fluoride therapy, and sialogogue administration.

Leukoedema

Leukoedema is a common normal variation of the buccal mucosa. The etiology is unknown, but some authorities suggest low-grade irritation contributes to an increased thickness of the epithelium, intracellular edema in the prickle cell layer, and hyperparakeratosis (hyperkeratosis with retention of nuclei). Prevalence rates vary greatly among geographic locations and among different ethnic groups. It may be present at birth, but is most often diagnosed in adolescence. Prevalence rates in black people vary from 70 to 90%, while rates in white people vary from 10 to 90%.

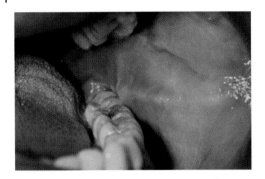

Figure 5.12 Leukoedema.

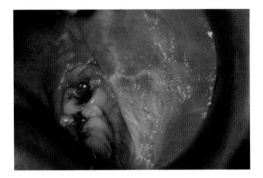

Figure 5.13 Leukoedema.

Clinical Features Leukoedema presents as a bilateral white, filmy, or milky opalescence of varying intensity affecting the buccal mucosa (Figure 5.12). The mucosa may appear folded or wrinkled (Figure 5.13). Leukoedema either disappears or undergoes significant diminution when the affected tissue is stretched. Infrequently, leukoedema affects the tongue, lips, and floor of the mouth and similar mucosal changes have been reported affecting vaginal and laryngeal mucosa.

Diagnosis The tell-tale disappearance upon stretching is diagnostic. Other white lesions that may mimic leukoedema include white sponge nevus, snuff keratosis, LP, proliferative verrucous leukoplakia, and hereditary benign intraepithelial dyskeratosis (Witkop disease).

Treatment No treatment is necessary for leukoedema. It has no malignant potential and does not change significantly after 25–30 years of age.

Recurrent Aphthous Stomatitis
"Aphthous" comes from the Greek word "aphtha," which means ulcer. RAS is a recurrent, self-limiting, noninfectious inflammatory disorder of the oral cavity characterized by painful shallow ulcerations. The actual cause of RAS remains unclear, although it is a T-cell-mediated condition and a genetic predisposition is likely. RAS is considered the most prevalent oral mucosal disease, affecting an estimated 20 % of the population, and has been associated with numerous other conditions (Table 5.4). "Aphthous stomatitis" has been used interchangeably with "aphthous ulcers" and may be more accurate terminology.

Clinical Features RAS typically presents as one or more well-circumscribed, round or oval, yellowish to white colored, shallow ulcers that are surrounded by an erythematous halo of inflamed mucosa. The lesions are typically painful and may interfere with speaking, eating, and swallowing. Some patients relate a prodromal burning sensation 24–48 hours before lesion onset. RAS characteristically affects the nonkeratinized oral mucosa, such as the labial and buccal mucosa (Figures 5.14–5.16), tongue (Figure 5.17), and soft palate. RAS may be further characterized according to its clinical appearance and severity (Table 5.5).

Table 5.4 Conditions often associated with RAS.

Local trauma (factitial or iatrogenic)	Hematological diseases (cyclic neutropenia, leukemia)
Stress	Rheumatic disorders (Behçet disease, Reiter's syndrome)
HIV infection	Allergy (food, drugs)
GI diseases (Crohn's disease, ulcerative colitis, and celiac disease)	Nutritional deficiencies (iron, folic acid, zinc, and vitamins B1, B2, B6, and B12)

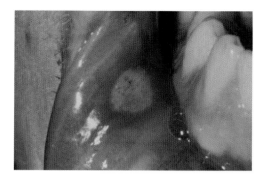

Figure 5.14 RAS.

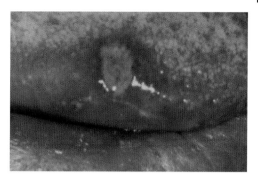

Figure 5.17 RAS.

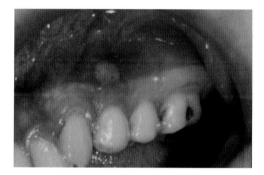

Figure 5.15 RAS.

Table 5.5 Classification of RAS.

Type	Characteristics
Minor RAS	Most common type (80%); single or multiple small ulcers (< 1.0 cm); heal without scarring in 7–10 days.
Major RAS	Less common type (10–15%); single or multiple large ulcers (> 1.0 cm); ulcers are deeper and more persistent; heal in several weeks; scarring possible.
Herpetiform RAS	Least common (5–10%), multiple small pinpoint ulcerations; clustered or cropped presentation; heal in 1–4 weeks.

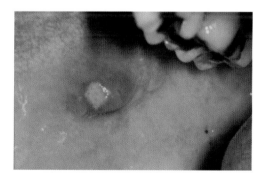

Figure 5.16 RAS.

Diagnosis The diagnosis of RAS is principally based upon the characteristic clinical presentation and history. Conditions to consider in the differential diagnosis include recurrent intraoral herpes simplex infections, primary herpetic gingivostomatitis, herpes zoster, a traumatic ulcer, EM, and ulcers associated with systemic disease.

Treatment The goals of therapy are to relieve pain, promote healing, and decrease the frequency and severity of recurrence. Although a variety of treatment modalities (topical and systemic) have been promoted to either eliminate or reduce the duration of recurrence of RAS, their clinical value remains unproven and can be controversial. On the basis of efficacy, cost, and safety, topical steroids remain the treatment of choice for patients with minor RAS. Finally, a comprehensive medical evaluation may be warranted to identify underlying systemic conditions potentially associated with RAS.

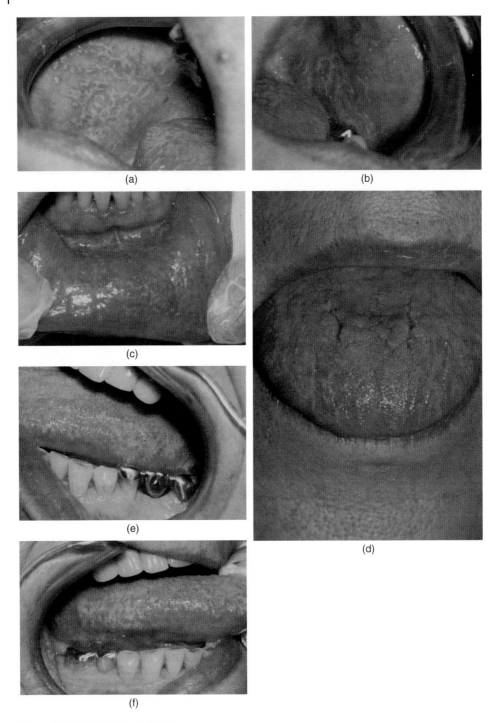

Figure 5.18 (a)–(f) Lichen planus.

Lichen Planus

LP is a cell-mediated chronic inflammatory disease involving mucous membranes and skin. It is thought to arise as a result of an immune response to certain unknown antigens within the basal cell layer of the epithelium. LP primarily occurs in middle-aged individuals, although all ages are at risk. The disease has a predilection for women (2 : 1). Up to 65 % of patients with cutaneous LP will manifest concurrent oral lichen planus (OLP), and oral lesions comprise the sole manifestation of LP in approximately 15–35 % of cases. OLP affects an estimated 0.1–4 % of the population.

Clinical Features There are at least three recognized forms of OLP: reticular, atrophic, and erosive. The reticular variant is thought to be the most common form and is characterized by mucosal keratotic lines, plaques, or papules arranged in a characteristic lacy pattern of Wickham striae (Figure 5.18a–f). The atrophic form is a combination of the reticular form and erythematous component (Figure 5.19), while the erosive form is a combination of the reticular form and a shallow ulcerative component (Figure 5.20a). All forms of LP may be accompanied by skin lesions (Figure 5.20b). Reticular lesions tend to be asymptomatic, while atrophic and erosive forms are likely to be painful. The most commonly affected sites are the buccal mucosa, tongue, lips, floor of the mouth, palate, and gingivae. OLP typically presents in a bilateral and symmetrical fashion. Patients often present with a variable mix of all three forms, and in some cases the characteristic striae may be absent. OLP may wax and wane, but seldom undergoes total remission.

Diagnosis A working diagnosis of LP is usually established when the characteristic striae are present. A confirmatory biopsy is usually recommended and is essential in order to diagnose equivocal cases. The variable appearance of OLP results in an extensive differential diagnosis including oral candidiasis, lichenoid drug reactions, EM, epithelial dysplasia, MMP,

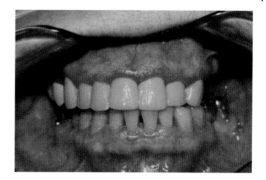

Figure 5.19 Lichen planus.

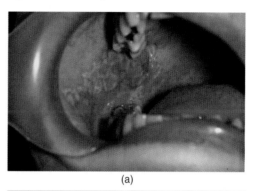

(a)

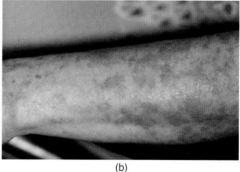

(b)

Figure 5.20 (a) and (b) Lichen planus.

pemphigus vulgaris, oral cancer, periodontal disease, graft-versus-host disease, lupus erythematosus, gastrointestinal disease, anemia, leukoplakia, erythroplakia, and linear IgA disease.

Treatment There is no cure for OLP, and treatment is based on the extent of symptoms. Asymptomatic reticular OLP requires no treatment. Symptomatic atrophic or erosive forms of OLP often respond well to topical steroids, while more severe disease may require systemic therapy. In all cases, OLP should be routinely monitored, as patients with OLP appear to be at a slightly increased risk of developing oral cancer.

White Sponge Nevus

White sponge nevus is an uncommon benign hereditary disorder that affects the mucous membranes.

Clinical Features White sponge nevus is characterized by the presence of folded or corrugated white plaques. Symmetrical involvement of the buccal mucosa is invariably observed (Figure 5.21a–d), but other oral mucosal sites, along with the nasal, vaginal, and rectal mucosa, may be affected.

Diagnosis The clinical appearance, combined with a family history of disease, makes for an easy diagnosis.

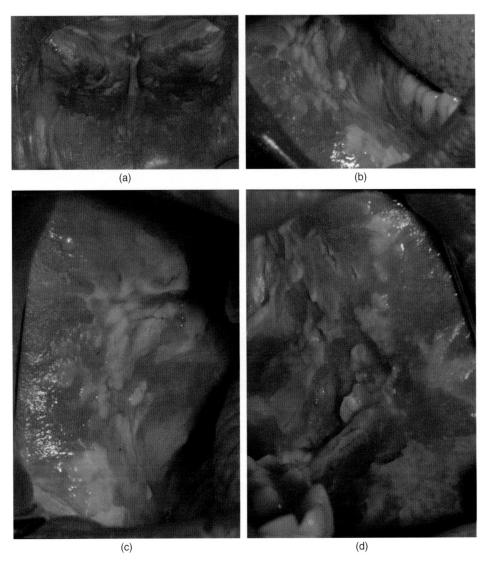

(a)

(b)

(c)

(d)

Figure 5.21 (a)–(d) White sponge nevus.

Treatment No treatment is necessary for this benign condition.

Snuff Keratosis

Snuff keratosis represents the reactive mucosal response to the placement of smokeless tobacco products. The smokeless tobacco, along with numerous other ingredients within the smokeless tobacco, acts to irritate the oral mucosal membranes. While there is a tangible risk of dysplasia occurring in snuff keratosis, recent epidemiological data suggests the prevalence of oral epithelial dysplasia in such lesions is generally low. While the rate of malignant transformation is low and the process is slow, the relative risk for carcinoma of the buccal/labial mucosa and gingivae among female chronic users is 50 times greater than among nonusers. It is estimated that 8.2 million people used smokeless tobacco products in 2011.

Clinical Features Snuff keratosis presents as a fairly characteristic corrugated or folded grayish-white plaque affecting the labial and vestibular mucosa (Figures 5.22–5.25). These lesions develop in those areas where the smokeless product is routinely placed. Most lesions are fairly well-localized, but those associated with extensive smokeless tobacco use may be widespread.

Diagnosis The clear association between smokeless tobacco placement and lesion

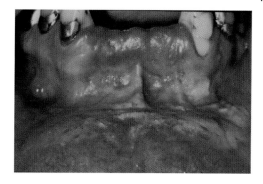

Figure 5.23 Snuff keratosis.

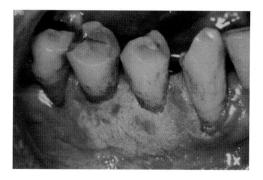

Figure 5.24 Snuff keratosis.

development makes for a straightforward diagnosis.

Treatment Any patient with snuff keratosis should be encouraged to quit using smokeless tobacco and should be advised of available cessation resources. Discontinuation of the smokeless tobacco usually results in lesion resolution. A biopsy is rarely necessary, but is indicated to assess any area of snuff keratosis that is clinically suspicious or unusual looking.

Amalgam Tattoo

An amalgam tattoo is a well-circumscribed, flat pigmented oral lesion. They arise when small particles of dental amalgam, composed primarily of silver (Ag) and mercury (Hg), are inadvertently implanted into the oral soft tissues during dental procedures. It has also been suggested that they may develop in the oral soft tissues as a result of chronic exposure

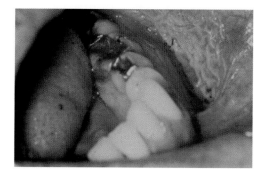

Figure 5.22 Snuff keratosis.

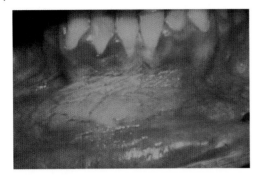

Figure 5.25 Snuff keratosis.

to restorative materials containing Hg, Ag, and sometimes copper, zinc, and tin. Amalgam tattoos are common, affecting about 8 % of the population.

Clinical Features An amalgam tattoo typically presents as an asymptomatic, solitary gray, blue, or black macule on the oral mucosa. They most commonly occur on the gingivae, alveolar ridge (Figure 5.26a), cheek, floor of the mouth, palate, and tongue. Most lesions are less than 1 cm in size. In some cases, evidence of small radiopaque amalgam flecks may be observed on a routine radiograph (Figure 5.26b).

Diagnosis The diagnosis of an amalgam tattoo is typically based on the characteristic clinical findings combined with the history of prior dental work. A biopsy is recommended for equivocal cases. Other lesions to consider in

the differential diagnosis include physiologic pigmentation, an oral melanotic macule, nevi, melanoma, Kaposi's sarcoma (KS), pigmentation associated with systemic disease (e.g. Addison's disease, Cushing's syndrome), and disorders related to blood or blood vessels.

Treatment An amalgam tattoo does not require treatment. However, all pigmented oral lesions should be viewed with suspicion and if the diagnosis is questionable, a biopsy should be performed. For lesions deemed cosmetically unacceptable, surgical or laser ablation may be accomplished.

Fibroma

A fibroma is best considered a reactive hyperplasia of fibrous connective tissue in response to local irritation. The most common sites of occurrence correspond well with areas prone to intraoral trauma. The fibroma is accepted as the most common soft-tissue tumor affecting the oral cavity.

Clinical Features A fibroma typically presents as a well-defined, smooth-surfaced nodule on the buccal and labial mucosa, gingivae, and tongue (Figures 5.27 and 5.28). The color ranges from pink to white. It is a slow-growing lesion that rarely exceeds 2 cm in size. Most examples have a sessile base, but some are pedunculated. A fibroma may demonstrate evidence of secondary trauma, such as surface ulceration or maceration.

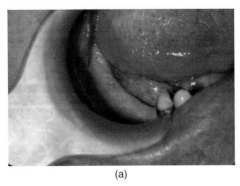

(a)

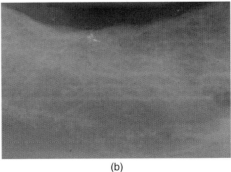

(b)

Figure 5.26 (a) and (b) Amalgam tattoo.

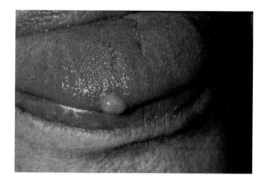

Figure 5.27 Fibroma.

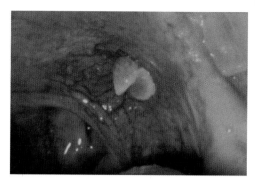

Figure 5.29 Papilloma.

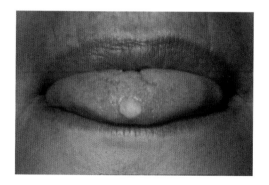

Figure 5.28 Fibroma.

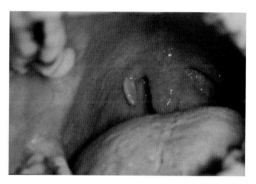

Figure 5.30 Papilloma

Diagnosis A recent episode of trauma to a pre-existing fibroma often prompts the patient to seek care. The rather banal appearance, combined with a history of trauma, makes for a straightforward initial diagnosis. A biopsy is required to establish the definitive diagnosis. Lesions to consider in the differential diagnosis include a neural tumor and a lipoma.

Treatment Simple surgical excision is the treatment of choice and recurrence is rare.

Papilloma
A papilloma is a benign exophytic growth of the epithelium caused by the human papillomavirus (HPV). There are over 100 subtypes of HPV, which can be broadly broken down into high-risk and low-risk categories. Low risk HPVs (e.g. 6, 11) are responsible for numerous benign conditions ranging from the common wart or papilloma to more serious conditions such as genital warts. High risk HPVs (e.g. 16, 18) are associated with diseases such cervical cancer and oropharyngeal cancer. Approximately 79 million Americans are currently infected with HPV and an estimated 14 million people become newly infected each year. HPV is so common that nearly all sexually-active men and women will experience at least one HPV infection during their lifetime. For HPV affecting the oral cavity, the estimated prevalence rate is 6.9%.

Clinical Features The papilloma typically presents as a solitary smooth, papillomatous, or cauliflower-like projection of the epithelium (Figures 5.29–5.32). Oral papillomas most commonly affect the palate, uvula, tongue, gingivae, and buccal mucosa. The color ranges from pink to white and pedunculation is frequently observed.

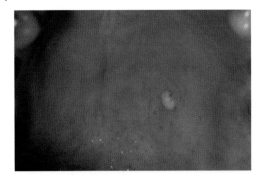

Figure 5.31 Papilloma.

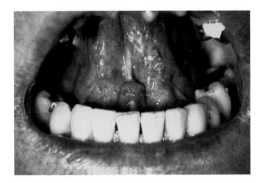

Figure 5.32 Papilloma.

Diagnosis The characteristic clinical appearance usually allows for a straightforward diagnosis. However, a biopsy is recommended to confirm the diagnosis. HPV subtyping is available but is rarely used for establishing a diagnosis. A new onset of multiple papillomas should alert the clinician to the possibility of underlying immune compromise. Conditions to consider in the differential diagnosis for papillomas include genital warts, focal epithelial hyperplasia, molluscum contagiosum, giant cell fibroma, and verruciform xanthoma.

Treatment Simple excision of a solitary papilloma is the treatment of choice.

Pemphigus Vulgaris

Pemphigus vulgaris is a rare autoimmune disorder that affects the mucocutaneous tissues. Affected patients produce IgG autoantibodies that target the desmosomal adhesion molecules (i.e. desmoglein 1 and desmoglein 3) of the squamous epithelium. This destruction results in the development of an intraepithelial split. The mean age of onset is between 40 and 60 years of age and there is no sex predilection. An increased risk has been noted in persons of Mediterranean and Jewish descent.

Clinical Features Pemphigus vulgaris typically presents as painful oral bullae, erosions, or ulcers (Figure 5.33a and b). These lesions usually develop insidiously and tend to persist. Often, a blister may be deliberately induced by rubbing an unaffected area (Nikolsky's sign). The most commonly affected sites are the palate, buccal mucosa, and gingivae.

Diagnosis The clinical appearance of pemphigus vulgaris is not specific. A biopsy and immunofluorescent studies are required to establish the presence of intraepithelial slits (Figure 5.33c) and the presence of autoantibodies (Figure 5.33d) associated with the disease. Numerous conditions may mimic pemphigus vulgaris and include MMP, EM, linear IgA disease, drug-induced reactions, and paraneoplastic pemphigus.

Treatment Pemphigus vulgaris is a potentially fatal disease for which there is no cure and a medical referral is warranted, usually to a dermatologist. Long-term disease control may be obtained with immunosuppressive therapy. For lesions restricted to the oral cavity, topical corticosteroid therapy may suffice for local control.

5.3 Examine the Hard Palate

With the patient's mouth wide open and the head tilted back, the palatal vault can be easily examined, both visually and tactilely. The incisive papilla overlies the incisive canal, and the palatal rugae present as transversely oriented palatal folds that converge toward the incisive papilla. An incisive canal cyst may present as

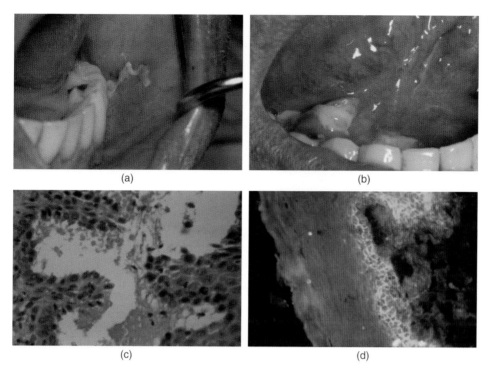

(a)

(b)

(c)

(d)

Figure 5.33 (a)–(d) Pemphigus vulgaris.

a fluctuant, midline, anterior palatal swelling. A spongy palatal swelling lateral to the midline likely indicates the presence of a periapical or periodontal abscess, or more rarely an expansile lesion such as a minor salivary gland tumor. The palatine raphe divides the palate down the midline and may be slightly elevated. A palatal torus presents as a hard, midline "swelling."

Nicotine stomatitis imparts a whitish-gray color to the mucosal tissues. The presence of diffuse palatal erythema or papillary hyperplasia affecting the denture-bearing mucosa is suggestive of atrophic candidiasis. Recurrent intraoral herpes (see "Herpetic Infections") most frequently occurs on the hard palate and is characterized by multiple small vesicles, which coalesce, then rupture to form painful shallow ulcerations. Pigmented palatal lesions such as oral melanotic macules and nevi occur with some frequency, as do amalgam tattoos. Less commonly observed but far more serious lesions include malignant melanoma and verrucous carcinoma. In patients with immunosuppression (acquired or therapeutic), KS may be observed.

Palatal Torus

A palatal torus is a common, benign, localized bony protuberance arising on the hard palate. It consists of mature dense cancellous bone covered by a rim of cortical bone of variable thickness. The etiology is unknown. A prevalence rate of 8.5 per 1000 has been reported, with a predilection for females. Palatal tori are most frequently observed in young adults and middle-aged persons, and the occurrence increases with age, achieving a plateau by the third decade. Similar lesions arising on the lingual alveolar process of the mandible are termed mandibular tori. Exophytic bone growth on the facial or buccal surfaces of the alveolar processes is known as exostosis.

Clinical Features The palatal torus presents as a bony hard exophytic mass on the palate (Figures 5.34–5.36). The shape is variable

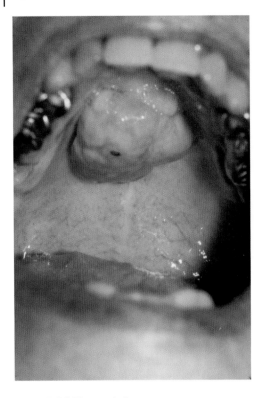

Figure 5.34 Torus palatinus.

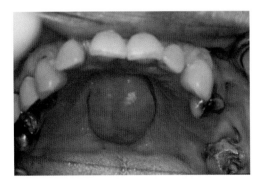

Figure 5.35 Torus palatinus.

and may be dome-shaped, spindle-shaped, nodular, or lobular. The size varies from barely discernible to very large (1.5–4 cm in diameter). If a periapical radiograph of the affected area is taken, a focal area of increased density may be noted.

Diagnosis The characteristic appearance of the palatal torus is pathognomonic. In some cases,

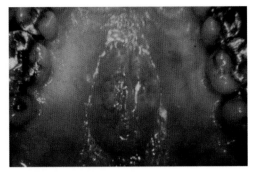

Figure 5.36 Torus palatinus.

the patient's first awareness of a torus occurs when the thin overlying mucosa becomes traumatized, prompting a visit to the dentist.

Treatment A palatal torus rarely requires treatment. However, if it interferes with function, denture placement, or is repeatedly traumatized, the torus may be surgically removed.

Nicotine Stomatitis

Nicotine stomatitis is a specific red/white lesion attributable to smoking with relatively quick resolution after smoking cessation. Although it manifests no increase in malignant transformation, if the tobacco habit involves reverse smoking (i.e. placement of the lighted end in the mouth), then the palatal lesion should be deemed as precancerous.

Clinical Features Nicotine stomatitis most frequently affects the hard and soft palate, followed by the retromolar pad and buccal mucosa. It produces a generalized thickening of the affected oral mucosa varying in appearance from a faint white-gray translucence to a distinct whitish-gray plaque (Figures 5.37 and 5.38). Palatal cases typically exhibit interspersed reddish puncta, which represent the dilated opening of minor salivary glands (Figures 5.39 and 5.40).

Diagnosis The characteristic appearance, combined with a history of tobacco exposure, makes for a straightforward diagnosis.

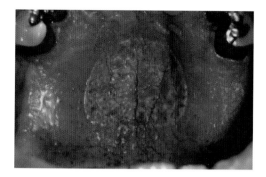

Figure 5.37 Nicotine stomatitis.

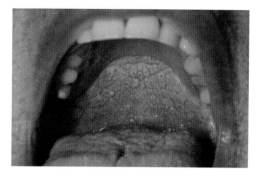

Figure 5.40 Nicotine stomatitis.

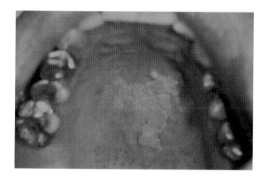

Figure 5.38 Nicotine stomatitis.

Table 5.6 Predisposing factors for candidiasis.

Endocrinopathies (diabetes mellitus, hypoparathyroidism, hypoadrenalism, pregnancy)	Acquired and therapeutic immunosuppression (HIV infection, cytotoxic drugs, corticosteroids)
Nutritional deficiencies	Qualitative and quantitative changes in salivary flow (drug-induced, radiotherapy, Sjögren's syndrome)
High carbohydrate diet	Poor oral hygiene
Antibacterial agents	Dental prostheses
Age	Smoking

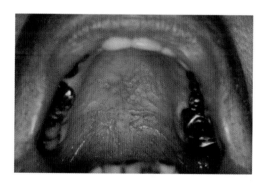

Figure 5.39 Nicotine stomatitis.

Unusual appearing cases should be biopsied to establish a definitive diagnosis.

Treatment Patients with nicotine stomatitis should be encouraged to stop using tobacco products, in which case the lesions may resolve significantly. Following discontinuation of tobacco products, the mucosa will eventually return to normal.

Candidiasis

Candidiasis is an infectious disease primarily caused by the mycelial form of *C. albicans*. A normal inhabitant of the oral cavity, *C. albicans* maintains a symbiotic relationship with *Lactobacillus acidophilus*. An alteration in host immune response likely precedes the metamorphosis from a state of commensalism to parasitism. Predisposing factors are summarized in Table 5.6.

Considering the fact that carriage rates as high as 75 % have been reported in healthy individuals, it is not surprising that candidiasis is a frequently encountered problem in clinical practice.

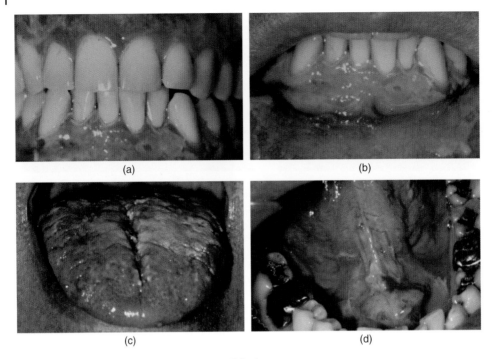

(a)

(b)

(c)

(d)

Figure 5.41 (a)–(d) Pseudomembraneous candidiasis.

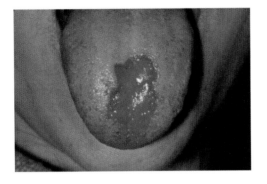

Figure 5.42 Erythematous candidiasis.

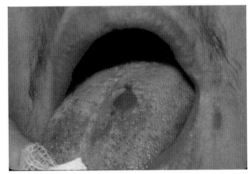

Figure 5.43 Erythematous candidiasis.

Clinical Features Patients may be asymptomatic or may complain of burning, dysgeusia, and/or dysphagia. A variety of clinical forms have been proposed and described. Pseudomembraneous candidiasis is characterized by the presence of a "cottage cheese-like" pseudomembrane, which may be wiped away, leaving a painful, bleeding mucosal surface (Figure 5.41a–d). This form is frequently observed in neonates and immunosuppressed patients. Erythematous candidiasis appears as red patches, most frequently affecting the palate or dorsum of the tongue (Figures 5.42–5.44). This form may be associated with a dry mouth, an immunosuppressive state, or exposure to antibiotics. The least common form is hyperplastic candidiasis, which is characterized by the presence of persistent, white plaques that do not wipe off (Figures 5.45–5.47). This form is usually associated with immunosuppression. Denture stomatitis

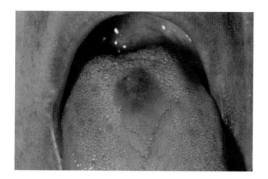

Figure 5.44 Erythematous candidiasis.

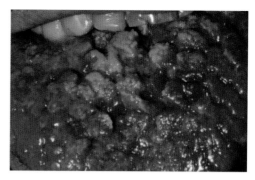

Figure 5.46 Hyperplastic candidiasis.

presents as an erythematous area beneath a denture-bearing surface (Figure 5.48). This form is frequently asymptomatic and associated with poor oral hygiene and/or continual wearing of a dental prosthesis. Median rhomboid glossitis is a candidal infection that affects the midline of the dorsum of the tongue and alters the normal appearance of the papilla in this location (Figures 5.49 and 5.50). Finally, candidiasis may also present as angular cheilitis, which has been previously described.

Diagnosis The diagnosis of candidiasis is established by correlating the typical signs and symptoms with the medical history. When doubt exists, exfoliative cytology, culture, or tissue biopsy may be used to confirm the diagnosis.

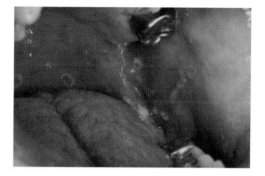

Figure 5.47 Hyperplastic candidiasis.

Treatment Measures to address any predisposing factors should be accomplished. When necessary, anti-fungal agents, both topical and systemic, are available and should be individualized based on the patient's health status and the clinical presentation and severity of infection.

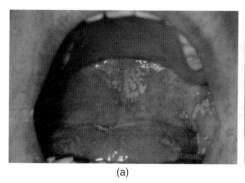

(a)

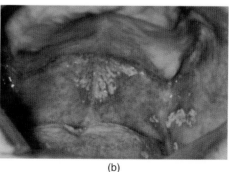

(b)

Figure 5.45 (a) and (b) Hyperplastic candidiasis.

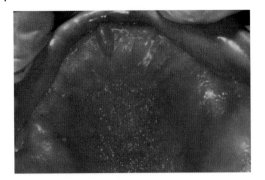

Figure 5.48 Denture stomatitis.

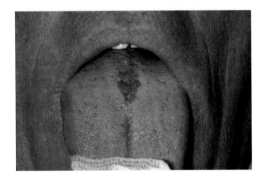

Figure 5.49 Median rhomboid glossitis.

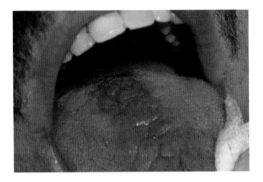

Figure 5.50 Median rhomboid glossitis.

Melanoma

Melanoma is a rare entity. Compared with its cutaneous counterpart, oral melanoma tends to follow a more rapid clinical course, and the overall prognosis is very poor. An estimated 33–50 % of all oral melanomas are believed to arise in an area of pre-existing pigmentation.

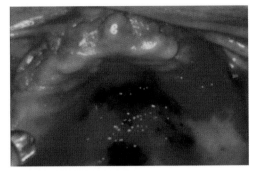

Figure 5.51 Melanoma.

Clinical Features The most common oral presentation is that of an expansile pigmented lesion most commonly affecting the palate and gingival mucosa (Figure 5.51). The color of the lesion may be pink, or it may contain any combination of blue, black, red, yellow, brown, and purple. Tooth mobility, spontaneous hemorrhage, satellite lesions, and pain may also be present.

Diagnosis A biopsy is required for the diagnosis. The grave nature of oral melanoma, and its frequent association with a pre-existing area of pigmentation, dictates that all intraoral pigmented lesions be carefully assessed.

Treatment Radical surgical resection is the treatment of choice. Additional chemotherapy, radiotherapy, and immunotherapy may be attempted, but the prognosis is very poor.

Verrucous Carcinoma

Verrucous carcinoma is an uncommon variant of squamous cell carcinoma that has a distinct predilection for the oral cavity. Compared with a typical squamous cell carcinoma, it tends to occur later in life (seventh to eight decade), is locally aggressive, and infrequently undergoes metastasis. Predisposing factors include oral tobacco use, smoking, alcohol, and poor oral hygiene.

Clinical Features Verrucous carcinoma appears clinically as a prolific warty or fungating

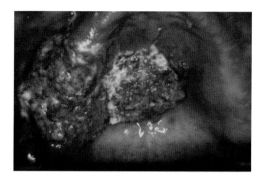

Figure 5.52 Verrucous carcinoma.

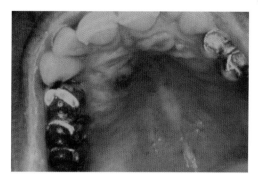

Figure 5.53 Kaposi's sarcoma.

superficial growth (Figure 5.52). The most commonly affected sites are the buccal mucosa, gingivae, palate, and larynx. Areas of ulceration may be present.

Diagnosis The characteristic clinical appearance should raise suspicion. A biopsy is warranted and should include ample sampling of the base of the lesion.

Treatment Surgical excision is the treatment of choice, but is complicated by the tendency of the tumor to extend locally and to recur.

Kaposi's Sarcoma

KS is an angioproliferative malignancy. It is the most common AIDS-associated malignancy, and its occurrence is closely associated with the sexual transmission of human herpesvirus type 8. While KS may occur anywhere in the body, up to 70 % of initially observed lesions occur in the oral cavity.

Clinical Features The most common sites of occurrence are the hard palate, gingival mucosa, and tongue (Figures 5.53 and 5.54a–c). Initial lesions present as small red to blue macules, which progress to bluish expansile nodular masses of varying size. Advanced lesions may be painful and interfere with normal function.

Diagnosis Advanced lesions observed in an HIV positive patient are difficult to miss

clinically. However, early macular lesions occurring in patients unaware of their immune status are more problematic. In all cases a biopsy is necessary to confirm the diagnosis. Other conditions to consider in the differential include benign vascular lesions, trauma, and melanocytic lesions.

Treatment Treatment of KS is palliative and targeted to alleviate pain and restore normal function. Potential therapeutic interventions include surgical excision or debulking, radiotherapy, and antineoplastic chemotherapy.

5.4 Examine the Soft Palate and Tonsillar Area

By gently depressing the base of the tongue, the soft palate and uvula can be directly examined. The soft palate functions to separate the oral cavity from the nasal pharynx and to close the nasal pharynx during swallowing and speaking. In contrast to the thick attached mucosa of the hard palate, which overlies bone, the mucosa of the soft palate is much thinner. Thus, it often appears pinker than the mucosa of the hard palate. In some patients, the underlying fat in the soft palate may impart a yellowish cast to the mucosa.

Petechiae, purpura, and ecchymosis represent extravasations of blood into the connective tissue. Such lesions frequently occur in the soft palate, usually as a consequence of intense

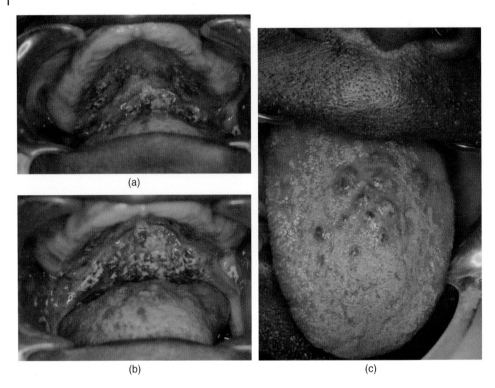

Figure 5.54 (a)–(c) Kaposi's sarcoma.

coughing, sneezing, or vomiting; a bleeding diatheses; infectious mononucleosis (IM); or fellatio. Palatal lesions may also reflect trauma (i.e. physical, chemical, thermal), infection (i.e. bacterial, viral, and fungal), salivary gland neoplasm, KS, squamous cell carcinoma, or lymphoma.

By depressing the tongue and asking the patient to say "ah," the oropharynx can be visualized. It is critical to inspect both fauces (tonsillar areas), the anterior pillars (glossopalatine arches), and the posterior pillars (pharyngopalatine arches). These areas are replete with lymphoid tissue and any abnormality should be documented and investigated.

Infectious Mononucleosis

IM is an acute viral illness associated with mild respiratory symptoms and prolonged malaise and fatigue. The Epstein–Barr virus (EBV) is the main causative agent of IM. EBV is a human herpesvirus that is present in over 90 % of the population. Most exposures occur during adolescence, and the risk of developing IM increases with age of exposure. EBV has also been linked to the development of several malignant tumors, including B-cell neoplasms such as Burkitt's lymphoma and Hodgkin's disease, certain forms of T-cell lymphoma, and undifferentiated nasopharyngeal carcinoma.

Clinical Features Most EBV infections in infants and children are asymptomatic. However, infection in adolescents or adults often results in symptomatic IM. Classic clinical features include fever, pharyngitis, and lymphadenopathy (Figure 5.55a). Petechiae affecting the soft palate may be present (Figure 5.55b). IM usually resolves over a period of weeks or months without complications.

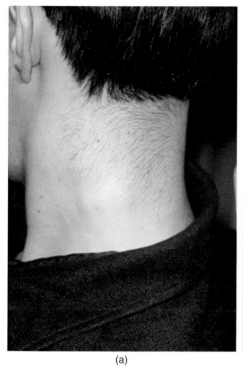

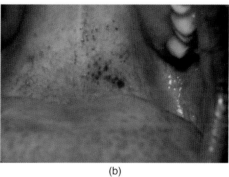

(a)   (b)

Figure 5.55 (a) and (b) Infectious mononucleosis.

Diagnosis The diagnosis of IM is attained by correlating the characteristic clinical and laboratory findings. The most diagnostic laboratory test is the serologic test for heterophil antibodies. Differential diagnosis should include group A β-hemolytic streptococcal pharyngitis or other viral infections.

Treatment Treatment of uncomplicated IM is supportive and should include nutritional supplementation, hydration, and rest. Acetaminophen may be prescribed for pain and to reduce fever. Aspirin should be avoided, since it has been associated with rare cases of Reye's syndrome during acute EBV infection.

Minor Salivary Gland Neoplasm

Minor salivary gland neoplasms constitute a heterogeneous group of both benign and malignant tumors arising in the oral cavity. The most common benign minor salivary gland neoplasms are the pleomorphic adenoma and the canalicular adenoma. The most common malignant minor salivary gland neoplasms are mucoepidermoid carcinoma, adenoid cystic carcinoma, and the polymorphous low-grade adenocarcinoma. Collectively, minor salivary neoplasms account for less than one-quarter of all salivary neoplasms.

Clinical Features Minor salivary gland neoplasms typically present as expansile well-defined submucosal nodules or tumors (Figures 5.56 and 5.57). The most common site of occurrence is the palate, but these neoplasms may arise in any area containing minor salivary gland tissue. Advanced lesions may exhibit surface ulceration and local fixation increases the concern of malignancy.

Diagnosis A biopsy is required to diagnose a minor salivary neoplasm. Small lesions should be excised at the time of biopsy.

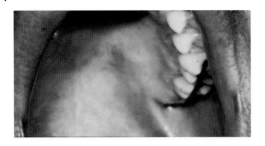

Figure 5.56 Mucoepidermoid carcinoma.

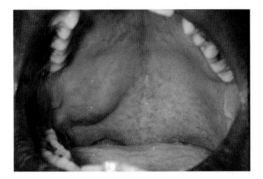

Figure 5.57 Adenoid cystic carcinoma.

Treatment Surgical removal remains the treatment of choice. The prognosis for a benign minor salivary neoplasm is excellent. For malignant salivary gland lesions, the prognosis is greatly influenced by the tumor type and stage at the time of surgery.

5.5 Examine the Tongue

The color, size, and shape of the tongue should be assessed and any variations from normal documented. The dorsal surface of the tongue is characterized by the presence of specialized papillae, which can be divided into four groups: filiform, fungiform, circumvallate, and foliate. A history of irregular and shifting areas of shortened filiform papillae, giving the tongue a "geographic" appearance, is characteristic of erythema migrans (stomatitis migrans). Excessive lengthening of the filiform papillae on the dorsal tongue is known as hairy tongue (HT). The papillae may absorb exogenous

stains or harbor chromogenic organisms, often causing a white, yellow, brown, or black discoloration. An atrophic bald erythematous patch affecting the posterior dorsal of the tongue is characteristic of median rhomboid glossitis (see "Candidiasis"). Numerous nutritional deficiencies may result in the tongue becoming beefy red, ulcerated or pale, and atrophic. A tongue that appears edematous and cyanotic may be observed in polycythemia vera, a condition of excess bone marrow activity.

Grasping the tongue with dry gauze and gently pulling it from side to side allows the clinician to inspect the lateral, ventral, and posterior aspects of the tongue. Scalloping or indentations along the lateral border may indicate the presence of a tongue sucking habit, a clenching habit, or macroglossia. Common causes of macroglossia include normal variation, vascular lesions (e.g. hemangioma, lymphangioma), acromegaly, and myxedema (hypothyroidism).

Traumatic ulcers, papillomas, and fibromas frequently occur on the tongue. The tongue is the most common location for a granular cell tumor (GCT) and hairy leukoplakia (HL). The ventral surface of the tongue often reveals pronounced varicosities, usually as a function of age. The incidence of squamous cell carcinoma of the tongue is second only to squamous cell carcinoma of the lips. Because of the tendency for carcinoma of the tongue to undergo early metastasis, the clinician must evaluate all erythroplakic, leukoplakic, and ulcerative lesions of the tongue with a high degree of suspicion.

Erythema Migrans
Erythema migrans is a poorly understood benign condition characterized by focal areas of erythema or atrophy. Putative associations with several conditions such as psoriasis, allergies, diabetes mellitus, hormonal disturbances, nutritional disturbances, psychological disorders, LP, Down syndrome, and Reiter's syndrome remain largely unproven. Erythema

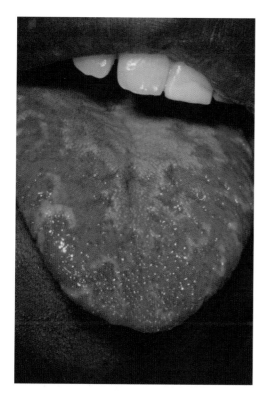

Figure 5.58 Erythema migrans.

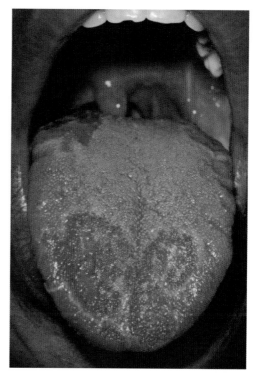

Figure 5.59 Erythema migrans.

migrans affects approximately 1–2.5 % of the population.

Clinical Features Erythema migrans typically presents as multiple circinate or irregular erythematous patches, which are marginated by whitish to yellowish keratotic lines (Figures 5.58–5.60). By far the most common site of occurrence is the dorsal tongue, in which case the erythematous patches correspond to a loss of the filiform papillae. Pain is rarely observed, but some patients complain of burning or itching of the affected sites.

Diagnosis The characteristic appearance is pathognomonic and biopsy should be reserved for equivocal cases. The differential diagnosis should include the putatively associated conditions mentioned above.

Treatment Simple recognition and patient reassurance will usually suffice. For patients

with symptomatic erythema migrans, a topical antihistamine solution, such as diphenhydramine elixir, or a steroid rinse may be prescribed to reduce symptoms.

Hairy Tongue

HT is a commonly observed benign condition associated with reduced desquamation or excess formation of the filiform papillae. Normal filiform papillae are approximately 1 mm in length, whereas filiform papillae in HT may exceed 1.5 mm in length. The specific underlying cause of HT is unclear. Predisposing factors include poor oral hygiene, smoking, alcohol, mouthwash use, numerous medications, and therapeutic radiation to the head and the neck. The prevalence varies widely among population groups, but overall it is quite common.

Clinical Features HT is characterized by a hypertrophy and elongation of the filiform

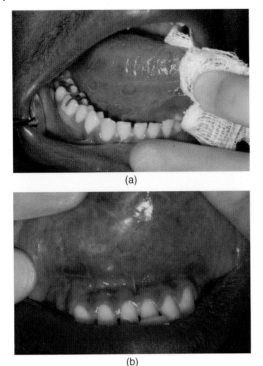

Figure 5.60 (a) and (b) Erythema migrans.

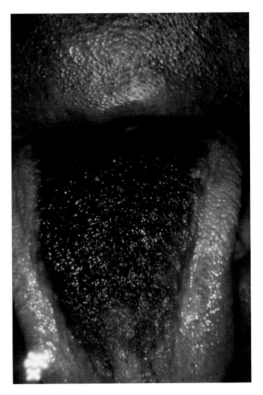

Figure 5.61 Hairy tongue.

papillae. The most frequently observed form is referred to as black HT; however, HT may also appear brown, white, green, or any of a variety of hues (Figures 5.61–5.63). It is rarely symptomatic, but interspersed deepened furrows may harbor candidal overgrowth. Patients may also develop halitosis as a result of retention of oral debris between the elongated papillae.

Diagnosis The diagnosis of HT is straightforward and is based principally on the clinical presentation. The perception of halitosis may prompt the patient to report to the dental office for an evaluation.

Treatment Management of HT consists of removing known predisposing factors and improving oral hygiene. Simple tongue brushing is often sufficient to reduce HT. In rare cases, physical removal of the elongated filiform papilla may be accomplished with electrodessication, carbon dioxide laser,

or even clipping. If a candidal infection is present, topical antifungal medications should be prescribed.

Nutritional Deficiencies

Numerous nutritional deficiencies may induce a variety of changes affecting the oral mucosa. The rate of oral mucosal cell turnover is much more rapid than that of the cutaneous tissues (3–7 days vs. up to 28 days). As a result, the oral mucosa often manifest early signs and symptoms of metabolic alteration resulting from systemic diseases, medications, or nutritional deficiencies. Commonly implicated nutrients include B vitamins (B_{12}, niacin, riboflavin, pyridoxine), iron, folic acid, and vitamin C. Underlying conditions associated with inadequate or impaired absorption, such as alcoholism, malabsorptive disorders, and eating disorders, further add to the risk.

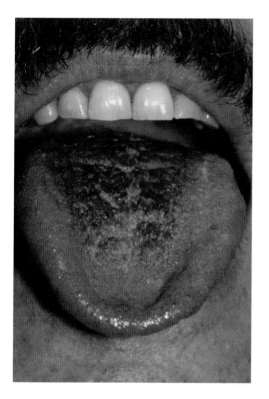

Figure 5.62 Hairy tongue.

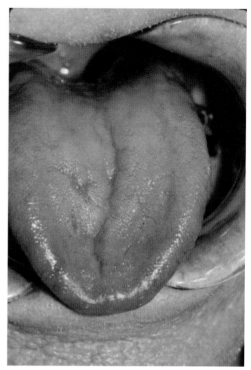

Figure 5.64 Nutritional deficiency.

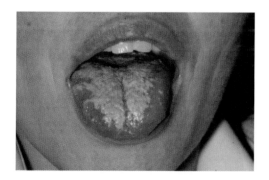

Figure 5.63 Hairy tongue.

Clinical Features The oral presentation of a patient suffering from a nutritional deficiency is variable and rarely specific. The tongue is the most frequently affected oral site. Two common descriptive entities are "beefy red tongue" and "pale tongue with papillary atrophy." The presence of pallor is suggestive of iron deficiency (Figures 5.64 and 5.65), while beefy red tongue is more typically associated

with vitamin B_{12} or folic acid deficiency (Figure 5.66a). The concomitant occurrence of angular cheilitis with either of these conditions is frequently observed (Figure 5.66b). The patient may also complain of a burning or tingling pain.

Diagnosis The diagnosis of a nutritional deficiency is established via appropriate laboratory tests.

Treatment Medical therapy to address any underlying systemic factors, combined with necessary nutritional supplementation, is usually sufficient to correct the deficiency.

Granular Cell Tumor

The GCT is an uncommon neoplasm believed to arise from either the Schwann cell or an undifferentiated mesenchymal cell. Women are affected more often than men (3 : 1), and most tumors are discovered between the fourth and sixth decades.

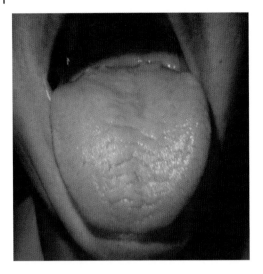

Figure 5.65 Nutritional deficiency.

Clinical Features Most GCTs occur in the head and neck region, and there is a predilection for the tongue. A GCT typically presents as a solitary, slow-growing, painless, nonulcerated, submucosal nodule or tumor (Figures 5.67 and 5.68). The surface mucosa is either normal or slightly pinkish in color.

Diagnosis A biopsy is required to confirm the diagnosis. Other lesions to consider in a differential diagnosis include a fibroma, lipoma, neural tumor, hemangioma, and lymphangioma. The GCT may exhibit histological evidence of pseudoepitheliomatous hyperplasia, and thus should be evaluated by an experienced oral pathologist.

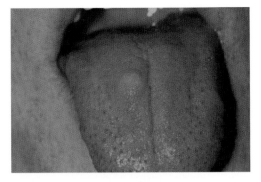

Figure 5.67 Granular cell tumor.

Treatment Surgical excision is the treatment of choice, and recurrence is rare.

Hairy Leukoplakia

HL is a unique type of leukoplakia that is almost always associated with immunosuppression. While the exact pathogenic mechanism remains to be determined, it is accepted that the presence of EBV is necessary for the development of HL.

Clinical Features HL almost always affects the lateral and dorsolateral aspects of the tongue (Figure 5.69a and b). It presents as multiple white vertical folds or corrugations that cannot be wiped off. Lesions vary in size from almost imperceptible to large plaques that may interfere with normal eating and speaking.

Diagnosis The rather characteristic clinical appearance, combined with a history of

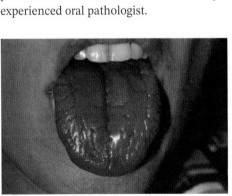

(a)

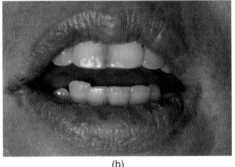

(b)

Figure 5.66 (a) and (b) Nutritional deficiency.

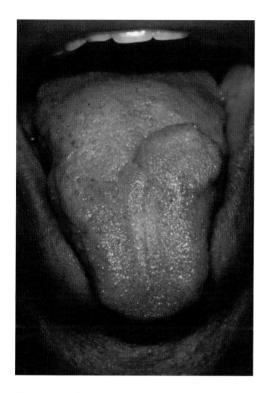

Figure 5.68 Granular cell tumor.

immunosuppression, allows for a straight-forward clinical diagnosis. A biopsy is rarely necessary. If performed, immunohistochemical staining for EBV should be used to confirm the diagnosis.

Treatment HL is generally asymptomatic and rarely requires treatment. HL will generally regress following treatment of the underlying cause of immunosuppression.

5.6 Examine the Glossopharyngeal (IX) and Vagus (X) Nerves

The glossopharyngeal nerve provides sensory function to the posterior one-third of the tongue, soft palate, and pharynx; special sense of taste to the posterior one-third of the tongue and soft palate; motor function to the stylopharyngeus muscle; secretory and motor function to the parotid glands; and it initiates the gag reflex. The vagus nerve provides overlapping motor function with the glossopharyngeal nerve for the gag reflex; sole motor innervation to the laryngeal muscles (voice); sensory innervation to the pinna of the ear; and parasympathetic innervation to the thoracic and abdominal viscera. Vagal nerve paralysis, possibly caused by diphtheria, may result in the patient having a nasal voice and food regurgitation through the nose. Clinically, the uvula may be deflected to the unaffected side.

Assess Sensory and Motor Function

The gag reflex varies among patients, but can usually be stimulated and assessed by gently stroking the pharyngeal tissue with an

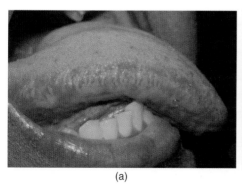

(a)

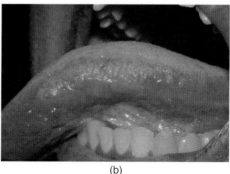

(b)

Figure 5.69 (a) and (b) Hairy leukoplakia.

applicator stick. Likewise, stroking the left and right side of the uvula is used to test the palatal reflex, whereupon the stroked side should rise. When the patient is instructed to say "ah," the entire soft palate should rise.

The hypoglossal nerve provides motor function to the tongue. Injury to the nerve, often as a consequence of surgery or trauma, results in paralysis of the tongue on the affected side. When the tongue is protruded, it will deviate to the affected side and, in time, show evidence of muscle atrophy. Additional signs of hypoglossal nerve damage are slurred speech, difficulty masticating, and an inability of the patient to resist contralateral pressure applied to the tongue.

5.7 Examine the Floor of the Mouth

The mylohyoid muscles support the floor of the mouth. Inspection and bimanual palpation of the area permit the identification of lesions arising within the supporting tissues of the region, in the major salivary glands and their ducts, and in the submandibular and submental lymph nodes. Anatomically, the sublingual glands and the superior portion of the submandibular glands lie superior to the mylohyoid muscles. The sublingual glands and the superior lobes of the submandibular glands are palpable orally. Salivary flow may be assessed by blotting dry the area of the lingual caruncle (Wharton's duct). Pressure may be applied to the submandibular area to express saliva, which will usually pool in the floor of the mouth. Anticholinergic drugs, sialoliths, infection, Sjögren's syndrome, or neoplasia may restrict salivary flow. A ranula is a variant of a mucocele affecting the sublingual or submandibular glands. Squamous cell carcinoma of the floor of the mouth typically appears as an area of erythroplakia, leukoplakia, and/or a painless ulceration with rolled indurated borders.

Ranula

The ranula is a relatively uncommon phenomenon caused by blockage of the sublingual or submandibular glands. It is generally accepted that most cases result from extravasation of saliva into the connective tissue adjacent to the sublingual gland. The prevalence of a ranula is unknown, but it appears to be more frequently observed in individuals infected with HIV.

Clinical Features The ranula usually presents as a blue-domed, translucent swelling in the floor of the mouth, resembling the "belly of a frog" (Figure 5.70). If the ranula extends down through the mylohyoid muscle, it is called a plunging ranula. This lesion manifests as a painless, nonmobile swelling in the neck.

Diagnosis A classic ranula is easily recognized; however, the plunging ranula may occur without any concurrent intraoral involvement, necessitating further assessment for confirmation. Advanced imaging techniques, particularly magnetic resonance imaging (MRI), combined with fine needle aspiration may be useful to assess these lesions. Other lesions to consider in the differential diagnosis include a hemangioma, lymphangioma, and salivary gland neoplasm.

Treatment Treatment options for the ranula include excision of the lesion with or without excision of the ipsilateral sublingual

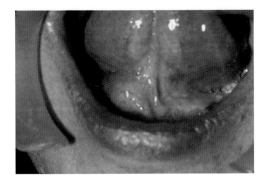

Figure 5.70 Ranula.

or submandibular gland, marsupialization, cryosurgery, and CO_2 laser excision. The choice of treatment is dependent upon the location and the size of the ranula, and the skill and experience of the surgeon.

Erythroplakia

Erythroplakia is a descriptive clinical term for any red macular lesion affecting the oral mucosa that cannot be given a specific clinical diagnosis. Erythroplakia is usually diagnosed in the sixth to seventh decade, and most patients relate a positive history of long-term tobacco use and alcohol consumption. The prevalence of erythroplakia in the United States is unknown, but estimates of up to 0.83 % have been reported in South and Southeast Asia. Histological assessment of erythroplakia reveals the presence of dysplasia, carcinoma-in-situ, or invasive squamous cell carcinoma in over 90 % of cases.

Clinical Features Erythroplakia may manifest as a homogenous red macule, a mixed macular red- and-white lesion, or as a red lesion with superimposed white granular spots (speckled leukoplakia) (Figures 5.71–5.74). Lesions are most prevalent in the ventral and lateral aspects of the tongue, the retromolar-trigone-soft palate complex, the floor of the mouth, and buccal mucosa. Although often asymptomatic, some patients may complain of discomfort, especially when eating hot or spicy food.

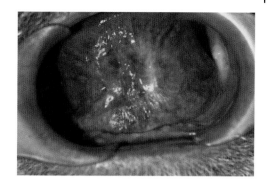

Figure 5.72 Erythroplakia.

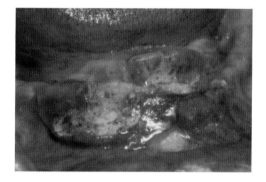

Figure 5.73 Erythroplakia.

Diagnosis Erythroplakia is strictly a clinical diagnosis, and it infers a high degree of suspicion for malignancy. Any suspicious lesion that persists for two weeks should be biopsied. The importance of recognizing and evaluating any persistent (over two weeks) erythroplakia cannot be overemphasized, as evidenced by the fact that dysplasia, carcinoma-in-situ, or invasive SCC is diagnosed microscopically in well over 90 % of the lesions characterized clinically as erythroplakia.

Treatment Ablative therapies used to treat erythroplakia include surgical excision, electrocoagulation, cryosurgery, and laser surgery. The choice of therapy is based upon clinician experience and patient desires. Counseling about tobacco and alcohol use and close long-term monitoring are indicated.

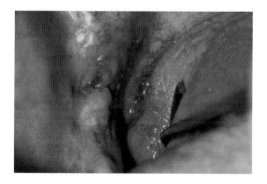

Figure 5.71 Erythroplakia.

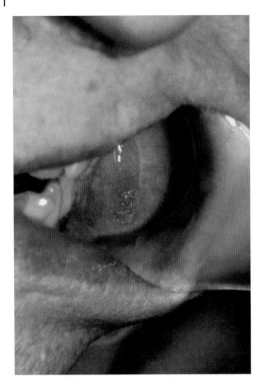

Figure 5.74 Erythroplakia.

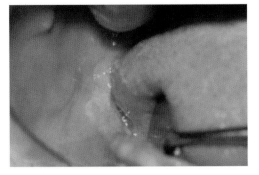

Figure 5.75 Leukoplakia

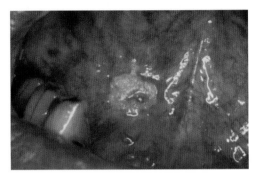

Figure 5.76 Leukoplakia.

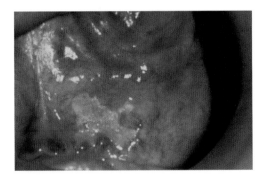

Figure 5.77 Leukoplakia.

Leukoplakia

Leukoplakia is a descriptive term for a white lesion of the oral mucosa that cannot be attributed to any other clinically definable lesion. The prevalence of leukoplakia in the United States is unknown, but it is estimated to approach 3 %. The rate of malignant transformation of leukoplakia cannot be predicted accurately, but it is important to acknowledge that up to 85 % of all precancerous lesions are leukoplakic.

Clinical Features Leukoplakia may present as a homogeneous white lesion or as a nonhomogeneous speckled, ulcerated, or papillary white-and-red lesion (Figures 5.75–5.78). It is most prevalent in the buccal mucosa and mandibular sulcular/alveolar ridge areas, the floor of the mouth, the ventral and lateral aspects of the tongue, the palate, and gingivae.

Diagnosis Similar to erythroplakia, leukoplakia is strictly a clinical term. As a rule, any lesion that persists beyond two weeks should be biopsied. Conditions to consider in a differential diagnosis include frictional keratosis, factitial injury, LP, lupus erythematosus, white sponge nevus, leukoedema, and hyperplastic candidiasis.

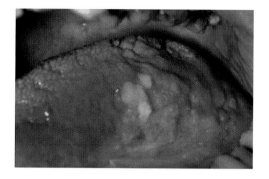

Figure 5.78 Leukoplakia.

Treatment Ablative therapies used to treat leukoplakia include surgical excision, electrocoagulation, cryosurgery, and laser surgery. The choice of therapy is based upon clinician experience and patient desires. Counseling about tobacco and alcohol use and close long-term monitoring are indicated.

5.8 Examine the Gingivae

The gingiva is a keratinized band of tissue that surrounds and attaches to the root surface of each tooth. The attachment extends onto the periosteum of the supporting alveolar bone. Visual and tactile examination allows for an assessment of gingival color, consistency, texture, architecture, and relationship to adjacent structures. Gingival pigmentation is most common in dark-skinned individuals and is usually physiologic. Discolored or dark marginal gingivae may occur as a consequence of excess exposure to lead, mercury, and bismuth. Gingival inflammation or gingivitis is characterized by gingival erythema and edema, and is usually due to local factors such as poor oral hygiene and plaque accumulation. However, gingivitis may be associated with numerous systemic conditions.

Necrotizing ulcerative gingivitis (NUG) is a painful inflammation of the gingivae with an unmistakable fetid odor. Gingival enlargement presents as enlarged, variably inflamed, firm, or edematous gingivae. Desquamative gingivitis is a descriptive term used to describe sloughing gingival tissues and may be the early presenting sign of a mucocutaneous disease (e.g. LP, pemphigus, and MMP). A common clinical presentation of herpetic infections is primary herpetic gingivostomatitis. Spontaneous gingival bleeding may be seen in association with gingivitis, thrombocytopenia, polycythemia vera, aplastic anemia, hemophilia, and drug therapy (e.g. antithrombotic agents, warfarin, and heparin). Some of the more common exophytic lesions that occur on the gingivae are a pyogenic granuloma, peripheral giant cell granuloma (PGCG), and peripheral ossifying fibroma (POF). Less frequently occurring lesions include carcinomas and sarcomas.

Necrotizing Ulcerative Gingivitis

NUG is a bacterial infection of the gingivae associated with elevated levels of *Prevotella intermedia* and other pathogenic spirochetes. Predisposing factors include poor oral hygiene, smoking, poor nutrition, stress, and immunosuppression. Most cases occur in young to middle-aged adults, and the exact prevalence is unknown.

Clinical Features The hallmark features of NUG are pain, gingival ulceration with necrosis, and bleeding (Figures 5.79 and 5.80). The interdental papillae frequently demonstrate a "punched out" appearance with loss of vertical height. Other common signs and symptoms include fetid breath, sialorrhea, metallic taste, fever, and lymphadenopathy. Extension of the disease to include the underlying alveolar osseous tissues can lead to necrotizing ulcerative periodontitis (NUP).

Diagnosis The abrupt onset of the characteristic presentation of NUG makes for an easy clinical diagnosis. Bacterial culturing is not indicated in the routine clinical setting.

Treatment The treatment of NUG consists of simple debridement and the institution

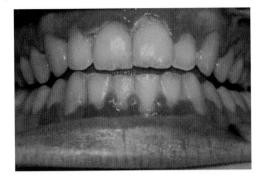

Figure 5.79 Necrotizing ulcerative gingivitis.

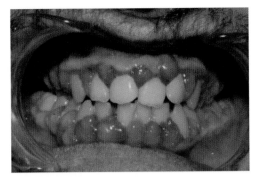

Figure 5.81 Gingival hyperplasia.

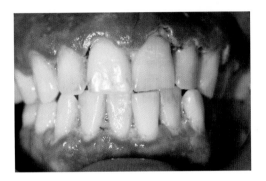

Figure 5.80 Necrotizing ulcerative gingivitis.

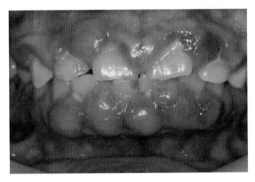

Figure 5.82 Gingival hyperplasia.

of improved oral hygiene. Antibiotic therapy may be considered for cases presenting with fever and lymphadenopathy. Nonresponsive cases must be evaluated further to rule out the presence of more serious systemic conditions such as immunosuppression or leukemia.

Gingival Enlargement

Potential causes of gingival enlargement include inflammation, hereditary predisposition, certain syndromes, and drug exposure. The most frequently implicated medications are the anticonvulsant drugs phenytoin and valproic acid, the immunosuppressant drug cyclosporine, and numerous calcium channel blocking agents. The prevalence of gingival enlargement in the normal population is estimated to vary between 4.0 and 7.5%.

Clinical Features Gingival enlargement initially manifests as generalized enlargement

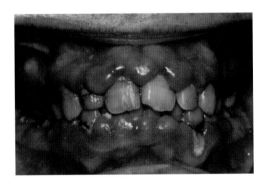

Figure 5.83 Gingival hyperplasia.

involving the interproximal papillae (Figures 5.81–5.84). Progression results in more widespread involvement and extension of the gingival tissues around the teeth. Severe cases may eventually spread to cover the clinical crowns of the dentition. In many cases, the edentulous areas will be spared.

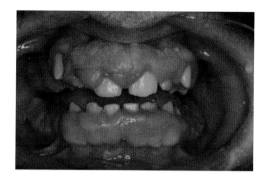

Figure 5.84 Gingival hyperplasia.

Diagnosis The diagnosis is straightforward. A thorough medical history is necessary to identify any contributing factors such as medication exposure or genetic predisposition.

Treatment Drug-induced gingival enlargement may improve if the offending drug can be identified and discontinued. However, most cases of gingival enlargement require surgical therapy to remove redundant

tissue. If contributing factors are not removed, recurrence is likely.

Mucous Membrane Pemphigoid
MMP, a form of autoimmune vesiculoulcerative disease, has a predilection for involving the oral and conjunctival mucosa. Affected patients develop autoantibodies that target the basement membrane zone of the epithelium. The typical patient is a woman between the ages of 60 and 80 years.

Clinical Features The onset of MMP is insidious, and the most commonly affected oral site is the gingivae (Figure 5.85a–d). The gingivae often demonstrate erythema and desquamation. Signs of ocular involvement include conjunctivitis, burning, and photophobia.

Diagnosis A biopsy and immunofluorescent studies are required to establish a definitive diagnosis. Other conditions to consider in a differential diagnosis include pemphigus

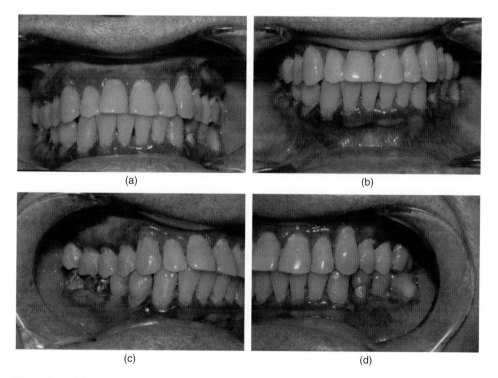

(a)

(b)

(c)

(d)

Figure 5.85 (a)–(d) Mucous membrane pemphigoid.

vulgaris, EM, herpetic simplex infection, LP, and lupus erythematosus.

Treatment There is no cure for MMP. Topical or systemic immunosuppressive agents may be useful to manage oral lesions. Systemic therapies should be accomplished in close consultation with the patient's physician. All MMP patients should receive an ophthalmologic examination to rule out ocular involvement.

Herpetic Infections

The HSV is a ubiquitous virus that is spread through contact with infected secretions. Two strains are acknowledged: HSV-1, which is associated with oral infections, and HSV-2, which is associated with genital infections. However, this site specificity is not absolute. Most cases of HSV-1 occur in children. Exposure rates as high as 90 % have been reported, and age-specific prevalence rates appear to be decreasing in industrialized countries.

A unique feature of all herpes viruses is their ability to establish latency in an infected host. The most frequent site of latency for HSV-1 is the trigeminal ganglion. Reactivation of the latent virus may occur following ultraviolet light exposure, mechanical trauma, fever, immunosuppression, decompression of the trigeminal nerve, and dietary factors. About 40 % of patients with prior exposure experience recurrent infection and approximately 100 million cases of recurrent infections occur each year in the United States.

Clinical Features Two stages of infection are recognized, primary, and recurrent. In reality, over 90 % of primary infections result in either asymptomatic or mildly symptomatic illness. The classical clinical illness is primary herpetic gingivostomatitis. After a prodromal period characterized by malaise, irritability, headache, and fever, patients

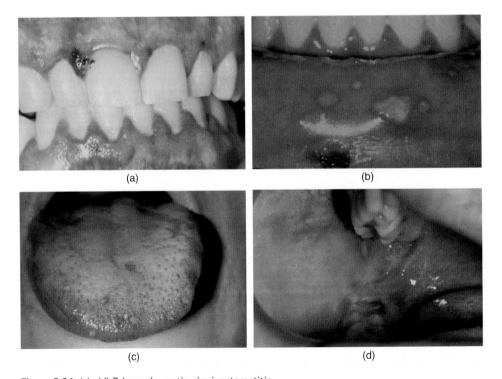

(a)

(b)

(c)

(d)

Figure 5.86 (a)–(d) Primary herpetic gingivostomatitis.

develop gingivitis, but painful vesicular eruptions may arise on any oral mucosal surface (Figure 5.86a–d). Within 24–48 hours, the vesicles rupture producing small, round, shallow, and painful erosions. Vesicles and erosions often coalesce to form large irregular lesions that heal within 7–14 days. Associated pain may be so severe as to adversely affect the patient's ability to eat, swallow, and speak.

Over 90 % of recurrent herpetic infections occur on the lips (RHL) unaccompanied by systemic illness (Figure 5.87a–d). The patient may relate a prodromal period of hyperesthesia or altered sensation, erythema, and edema at the site of involvement. Within hours, a localized vesicular eruption develops, which subsequently coalesces and crusts over during the next few days. Total resolution is noted in about 10–14 days.

Recurrent herpetic infections may also occur intraorally, where they tend to affect

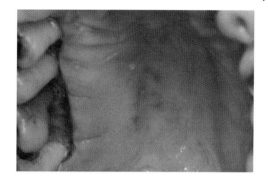

Figure 5.88 Recurrent intraoral herpes.

the keratinized mucosa of the hard palate or gingivae (Figures 5.88–5.91).

While most cases of primary and recurrent HSV infections resolve uneventfully, immunocompromised patients are at risk for developing severe complications, for example, encephalitis and blindness.

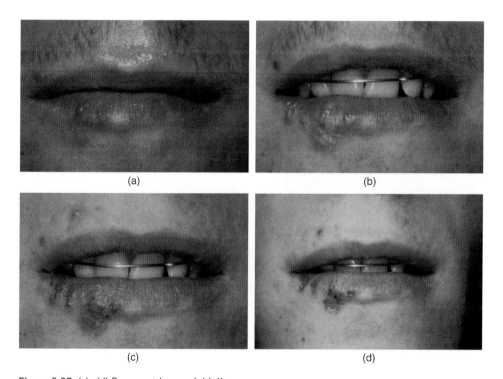

(a)

(b)

(c)

(d)

Figure 5.87 (a)–(d) Recurrent herpes labialis.

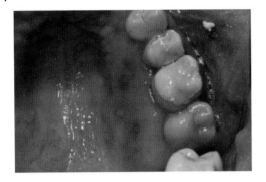

Figure 5.89 Recurrent intraoral herpes.

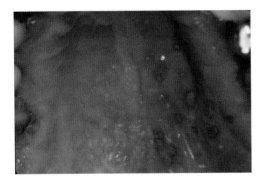

Figure 5.90 Recurrent intraoral herpes.

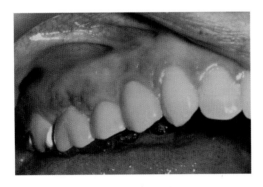

Figure 5.91 Recurrent intraoral herpes.

Diagnosis The diagnosis of primary or recurrent HSV-1 infections is typically made based upon history and the characteristic clinical presentation. Specific laboratory tests are available but are rarely necessary to establish a diagnosis. Conditions to consider in a differential diagnosis include herpetiform

RAS, herpangina, pemphigus, EM, NUG, and hand-foot-and-mouth disease.

Treatment For primary infections, the goal of therapy is to provide palliative and supportive care. Successful management consists of controlling fever and pain, preventing dehydration, shortening the duration of lesions, and monitoring for systemic viremia. RHL often does not require treatment. Several over-the-counter and prescription products are marketed to relieve pain and promote healing. The use of lip balms and lotions with an SPF of at least 15 may prevent sun-induced recurrent infections. In all cases, proper hygiene to reduce the risk of transmission and autoinoculation should be enforced. Antiviral chemotherapy should be considered for patients at an increased risk of developing systemic dissemination.

Pyogenic Granuloma
The pyogenic granuloma is a commonly observed reactive inflammatory response to local irritation. The exact etiology is often unknown but most cases occur as a response to an irritant such as plaque, calculus, or foreign material. Hormonal alterations likely modulate the development of a pyogenic granuloma, as evidenced by a distinct female predilection and an increased risk of occurrence during pregnancy (pregnancy tumor). The exact prevalence is unknown.

Clinical Features The pyogenic granuloma presents as a bright red pedunculated or sessile mass of variable size (Figures 5.92 and 5.93). These lesions are highly vascular, bleed easily, and often exhibit exuberant growth. The most common location is the gingivae.

Diagnosis While the clinical appearance is highly suggestive, particularly during pregnancy, a biopsy is recommended for persistent lesions. A differential diagnosis should include a fibroma, POF, the PGCG, and a benign neural tumor.

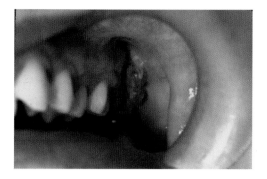

Figure 5.92 Pyogenic granuloma.

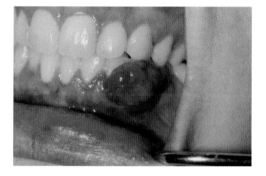

Figure 5.93 Pyogenic granuloma.

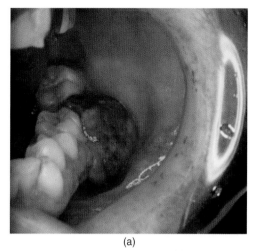

(a)

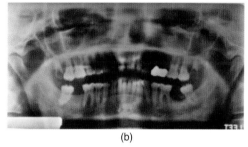

(b)

Figure 5.94 (a) and (b) Peripheral giant cell granuloma.

Treatment A small pyogenic granuloma may undergo spontaneous involution after the implementation of improved oral hygiene or after delivery. Persistent or large lesions should be excised and the adjacent teeth should be thoroughly scaled and curetted.

Peripheral Giant Cell Granuloma
The PGCG is best considered as the soft-tissue counterpart of the central giant cell granuloma. The etiology and prevalence are unknown. Most lesions occur in young adult females, and there is a predilection for the mandible.

Clinical Features A PGCG is clinically indistinguishable from a pyogenic granuloma. Compared with the pyogenic granuloma, the color may appear more deeply purple, and the PGCG only arises on gingivae or edentulous alveolar ridge (Figure 5.94a). Superficial osseous erosion or cupping of the underlying bone may be noted on a radiograph (Figure 5.94b).

Diagnosis A biopsy is required to establish a definitive diagnosis. Conditions that may mimic the PGCG include a fibroma, a pyogenic granuloma, POF, and benign neural tumor.

Treatment Surgical excision is the treatment of choice, followed by thorough scaling and curettage of the affected teeth.

Peripheral Ossifying Fibroma
The POF is a reactive hyperplastic inflammatory lesion. It is considered to arise from the periosteum or from periodontal ligament mesenchymal cells in response to local irritants such as plaque, calculus, and foreign material. Females are affected more often than males,

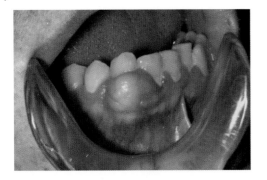

Figure 5.95 Peripheral ossifying fibroma.

and most patients are between the ages of 5 and 25 years of age.

Clinical Features A POF usually presents as a well-circumscribed nodular mass usually arising from the anterior gingival mucosa (Figure 5.95). The surface may be smooth or ulcerated. Like the PCGC, POF only arises on the gingiva or edentulous alveolar ridge. POF frequently causes separation and/or divergence of the adjacent teeth (Figure 5.96a and b). Occasionally, it may be associated with minimal underlying osseous resorption.

Diagnosis A biopsy is necessary in order to establish a definitive diagnosis. Other conditions to consider in a differential diagnosis include a pyogenic granuloma, PGCG, fibroma, or an odontogenic tumor.

Treatment Treatment consists of surgical excision down to the periosteum and the elimination of any local irritants. Tooth extraction is seldom necessary, and the prognosis is quite good. Recurrence rates as high as 16 % have been reported.

5.9 Examine the Teeth

Note the Number of Teeth

Developmental disturbances affecting the number of teeth may manifest as partial or total anodontia or hypodontia and supernumerary teeth (hyperdontia). Hypodontia is a relatively common finding in the permanent dentition, and the most common missing teeth are third molars, mandibular second premolars, maxillary second premolars, and maxillary lateral incisors, respectively. If several teeth are missing, the possibility of ectodermal dysplasia, Reiter's syndrome, or incontinentia pigmenti should be considered. Hyperdontia or supernumerary teeth are commonly found in the anterior maxilla as mesiodens and in the molar area, usually as fourth molars. Hyperdontia may also be a manifestation of cleidocranial dysplasia and Gardner's syndrome.

Note the Size of Teeth

Developmental disturbances affecting the size of teeth may manifest as microdontia,

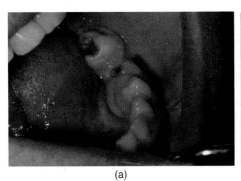

(a)

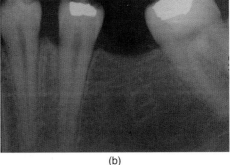

(b)

Figure 5.96 (a) and (b) Peripheral ossifying fibroma.

macrodontia, and taurodontism. Microdontia is characterized by smaller than normal teeth and may be secondary to pituitary hypofunction during childhood. Macrodontia is characterized by larger than normal teeth and may be secondary to pituitary hyperfunction during childhood. Taurodontism is characterized by radiographic evidence of abnormally large pulp chambers extending apically.

Note the Shape of Teeth

Developmental disturbances affecting the shape of teeth may manifest as germination, fusion, concrescence, and dens invaginatus. Germination usually affects permanent incisors and is believed to be the result of a tooth germ attempting to divide, resulting in a double crown or a double root. Fusion, more common in the primary dentition, is the result of two adjacent tooth germs joined by enamel and/or dentin. Concrescence is characterized by radiographic evidence of the roots of two adjacent teeth joined by cementum. Dens invaginatus commonly affects maxillary lateral incisors and manifests as invagination (sometimes into the pulp) on the palatal surfaces of affected teeth.

Note the Color of Teeth

Inherited disturbances affecting the color of teeth include amelogenesis imperfecta (AI) and dentinogenesis imperfecta. In AI, the enamel is often absent and the exposed dentin has a yellowish to brown discoloration. The color of the teeth in dentinogenesis imperfecta and osteogenesis imperfecta is opalescent, ranging from a slightly golden brown to a bluish tinge.

Reactive disturbances affecting the color of teeth may be secondary to inflammation, vitamin deficiencies, trauma, and exposure to tetracycline or excess fluoride. An isolated tooth with a grayish-blue hue may indicate the presence of a necrotic pulp, often due to prior trauma. A tooth that appears pink (pink tooth of Mummery) invariably signals the presence of internal resorption. Yellow to violet staining that fluoresces under ultraviolet light characterizes tetracycline staining. Fluorosis or "mottled enamel" is caused by ingestion of fluoride in the drinking water in excess of 1.5 ppm The extent of discoloration may vary from mild chalky white blotching to yellow and even brown staining and is dependent on the extent of fluoride exposure.

Amelogenesis Imperfecta

AI is a heterogeneous inherited disorder with defective tooth enamel formation caused by various gene mutations in the absence of any generalized or systemic disease. AI has an estimated prevalence of 1 in 718 to 1 in 14 000, depending on the population studied.

Clinical Features The clinical presentation of AI may include a reduction in the amount of enamel produced (hypoplasia) and/or a defect in mineralization of the enamel (hypomineralization). The teeth may have fine enamel or grooves and pits scattered across the surface of the teeth arranged in rows or columns; exhibit a mottled, opaque white-brown yellow discoloration; or show enamel that has a very low mineralization, manifested clinically by pigmented, softened, and easily detachable enamel (Figure 5.97a–c).

Diagnosis The diagnosis of defects in dental enamel must be based on clinical, radiographic, and, when possible, laboratory data. Although molecular and biochemical methods have shown differences in the composition of the enamel with some types of AI, other AI-associated gene defects remain unknown, making routine clinical and radiographic observations extremely important. In the differential diagnosis, the clinician should consider acquired defects (chemical insult, nutritional deficiencies, infections,

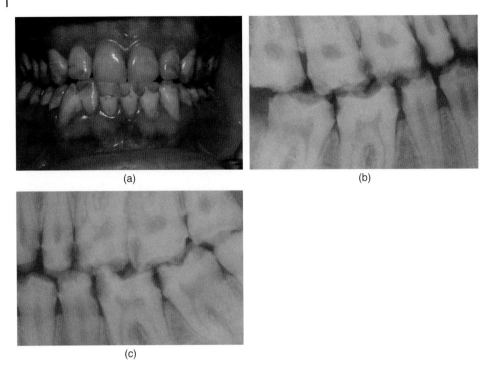

(a)

(b)

(c)

Figure 5.97 (a)–(c) Amelogenesis imperfecta.

and trauma), dentinogensis imperfecta, and tricho-dento-osseous syndrome.

Treatment The management depends on the severity of the problem. Treatment strategies include composite resin veneers and jacket crowns for anterior teeth, as well as steel crowns for posterior teeth. Full crowns will improve cosmetic appearance and protect the teeth from damage.

Fluorosis

Dental fluorosis (DF) is a permanent hypomineralization of enamel resulting from the ingestion of excessive amounts of fluoride (chronic exposure) during tooth formation. Fluoride only causes fluorosis in concentrations of greater than 1 ppm The main documented risk factors for fluorosis are use of fluoridated drinking water, fluoride supplements, fluoride toothpaste, and infant formulas reconstituted with fluoridated water used before the age of six years. It is now believed that fluorosis occurs when fluoride interacts with mineralizing tissues, causing alterations in the mineralization process.

Clinical Features Fluorosis varies in appearance from white striations to stained pitting of enamel (Figure 5.98a–c). The very mild and mild forms of enamel fluorosis appear as small, barely visible, white flecks found primarily on cusp tips and on facial surfaces of a tooth's enamel surface that are not readily apparent to the affected person or casual observer. In the moderate form, more than 50 % of the enamel surface is opaque white. The rare, severe form manifests as pitted and brittle enamel. After eruption, teeth with moderate or severe fluorosis might develop areas of brown stain. In the severe form, the compromised enamel might break away, resulting in excessive wear of the teeth. Fluorosis of the primary teeth occurs less often and is milder than that of the permanent teeth.

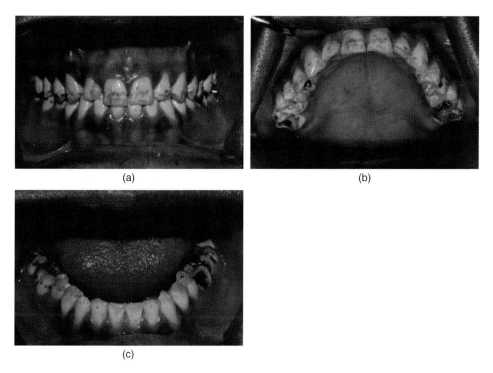

(a)

(b)

(c)

Figure 5.98 (a)–(c) Fluorosis.

Diagnosis Diagnosis of DF is based on clinical presentation and history of excessive fluoride intake. Definitive diagnosis requires that the defect is present bilaterally in a symmetric pattern, and evidence of prior excessive fluoride intake or elevated levels of fluoride in the enamel or other tissues should be found.

Treatment Preventive management of DF includes de-fluoridation of drinking water in endemic areas, water low in fluoride for dilution of infant formulas, cautious use of fluoride supplements and supervision of the use of fluoride toothpaste by children aged below five years. Aesthetically objectionable discoloration may be managed by bleaching, micro-abrasion, veneering, or crowning. The choice between these treatments depends on the severity of the fluorosis.

Note Acquired Dental Defects

Acquired dental defects include dental caries, attrition, abrasion, and erosion. Dental caries is an infectious process. Attrition is the wearing away of tooth structure due to tooth-to-tooth contact. Abrasion is the wearing away of tooth structure through an abnormal mechanical process. Erosion refers to the loss of tooth structure due to chemical action.

5.10 Summary

The clinical manifestations of many diseases, either local or systemic, characteristically affect the lips, labial, or buccal mucosa, hard palate, soft palate and tonsillar areas, tongue, floor of the mouth, gingivae, and teeth. Knowledge of the more common presentation patterns of a given disease assists the practitioner in determining a diagnosis. It must be remembered, however, that no diagnostic index or outline can fully account for the capriciousness of a disease or the different reactions of an individual host to a disease.

Therefore, the evaluation and integration of the clinical appearance and characteristics of a disease, along with the history of development and other appropriate diagnostic findings, are often necessary to determine the final diagnosis.

Suggested Reading

Akintoye, S.O. and Greenberg, M.S. (2014). Recurrent aphthous stomatitis. *Dent. Clin. North Am.* 58 (2): 281–297.

Al Quran, F.A. and Al-Dwairi, Z.N. (2006). Torus palatinus and torus mandibularis in edentulous patients. *J. Contemp. Dent. Pract.* 7: 112–119.

Baccaglini, L., Atkinson, J.C., Patton, L.L. et al. (2007). Management of oral lesions in HIV-positive patients. *Oral Surg. Oral Med. Oral Pathol. Oral Radiol. Endod.* S50 (103 Suppl): e1–e23.

Baurmash, H. (2003). Mucoceles and ranulas. *J. Oral Maxillofac. Surg.* 61: 369–368.

Black, M., Mignogna, M.D., and Scully, C. (2005). Number II. Pemphigus vulgaris. *Oral Dis.* 11: 119–130.

Brunet, L., Miranda, J., Roset, P. et al. (2001). Prevalence and risk of gingival enlargement in patients treated with anticonvulsant drugs. *Eur. J. Clin. Invest.* 31: 781–788.

Cabay, R.J., Morton, T.H. Jr., and Epstein, J.B. (2007). Proliferative verrucous leukoplakia and its progression to oral carcinoma: a review of the literature. *J. Oral Pathol. Med.* 36 (5): 255–261.

Centers for Disease Control and Prevention (CDC) (2012). Current tobacco use among middle and high school students – United States, 2011. *MMWR* 61: 581–585.

Centers for Disease Control and Prevention (CDC). 2017. Genital HPV Infection – Fact Sheet. Available at: www.cdc.gov/std/HPV/STDFact-HPV.htm (accessed 16 December 2020).

Cicardi, M. and Zingale, L.C. (2007). The deficiency of C1 inhibitor and its treatment. *Immunobiology* 212: 325–331.

Cohen-Brown, G. and Ship, J.A. (2004). Diagnosis and treatment of salivary gland disorders. *Quintessence Int.* 35: 108–123.

Corbet, E.F. (2004). Diagnosis of acute periodontal lesions. *Periodontol.* 34: 204–216.

Cornacchio, A.L., Burneo, J.G., and Aragon, C.E. (2011). The effects of antiepileptic drugs on oral health. *J. Can. Dent. Assoc.* 77: b140.

Cozad, J. (1996). Infectious mononucleosis. *Nurse Pract.* 21: 14–16, 23, 27–28.

Cuisia, Z.E. and Branon, R.B. (2001). Peripheral ossifying fibroma – a clinical evaluation of 134 pediatric cases. *Pediatr. Dent.* 23: 245–248.

Denbesten, P. and Li, W. (2011). Chronic fluoride toxicity: dental fluorosis. *Monogr. Oral Sci.* 22: 81–96.

Ebell, M.H. (2004). Epstein-Barr virus infectious mononucleosis. *Am. Fam. Physician* 70: 1279–1287.

Epstein, J.B., Cabay, R.J., and Glick, M. (2005). Oral malignancies in HIV disease: changes in disease presentation, increasing understanding of molecular pathogenesis, and current management. *Oral Surg. Oral Med. Oral Pathol. Oral Radiol. Endod.* 100: 571–578.

Esmeili, T., Lozada-Nur, F., and Epstein, J. (2005). Common benign oral soft tissue masses. *Dent. Clin. N. Am.* 49: 223–240.

Farthing, P., Bagan, J.-V., and Scully, C. (2005). Erythema multiforme. *Oral Dis.* 11: 261–267.

Foloyan, M.O. (2004). The epidemiology, etiology, and pathophysiology of acute necrotizing ulcerative gingivitis associated with malnutrition. *J. Contemp. Dent. Pract.* 5: 28–41.

Frigas, E. and Park, M. (2006). Idiopathic recurrent angioedema. *Immunol. Allergy Clin. North Am.* 26: 739–751.

Gadhia, K., McDonald, S., Arkutu, N., and Malik, K. (2012). Amelogenesis imperfecta: an introduction. *Br. Dent. J.* 212: 377–379.

Gillison, M.L., Broutian, T., Pickard, R.K. et al. (2012). Prevalence of oral HPV infection in the United States, 2009-2010. *JAMA* 307: 693–703.

Gonsalves, W.C., Chi, A.C., and Neville, B.W. (2007). Common oral lesions: Part I. Superficial mucosal lesions. *Am. Fam. Physician* 75: 501–507.

Govani, F.S. and Shovlin, C.L. (2009). Hereditary haemorrhagic telangiectasia: a clinical and scientific review. *Eur. J. Hum. Genet.* 17: 860–871.

Gryfe, R. (2009). Inherited colorectal cancer syndromes. *Clin. Colon Rectal Surg.* 22: 198–208.

Gurvits, G.E. and Tan, A. (2014). Black hairy tongue syndrome. *World J Gastroenterol.* 20 (31): 10845–10850.

Hayashida, A.M., Zerbinatti, D.C., Balducci, I. et al. (2010). Mucus extravasation and retention phenomena: a 24-year study. *BMC Oral Health* 10: 15. https://doi.org/10.1186/1472-6831-10-15.

Huber, M.A. (2003). Herpes simplex type-1 virus infection. *Quintessence Int.* 34: 453–467.

Huber, M.A. (2004). Oral lichen planus. *Quintessence Int.* 35: 731–752.

Huber, M.A. and Tantiwongkosi, B. (2014). Oral and oropharyngeal cancer. *Med. Clin. N Am.* 98: 1299–1321.

Huber, M.A. and Terézhalmy, G.T. (2006). The patient with actinic cheilosis. *Gen. Dent.* 54 (4): 274–282.

Jafarzade, H., Sanatkhani, M., and Mohtasham, N. (2006). Oral pyogenic granuloma: a review. *J. Oral Sci.* 48: 167–175.

Lalla, R.V., Patton, L.L., and Dongari-Bagtzoglou, A. (2013). Oral candidiasis: pathogenesis, clinical presentation, diagnosis and treatment strategies. *J. Calif. Dent. Assoc.* 41: 263–268.

Lavanya, N., Jayanthi, P., Rao, U.K., and Ranganathan, K. (2011). Oral lichen planus:

an update on pathogenesis and treatment. *J Oral Maxillofac Pathol* 15: 127–132.

Lopez, J.P. (2008). White sponge nevus: presentation of a new family. *Pediatr. Dermatol.* 25: 116–117.

Madani, F.M. and Kuperstein, A.S. (2014). Normal variations of oral anatomy and common oral soft tissue lesions: evaluation and management. *Med. Clin. North Am.* 98 (6): 1281–1298.

Markopoulos, A., Albanidou-Farmaki, E., and Kayavis, I. (2004). Actinic cheilitis: clinical and pathologic characteristics in 65 cases. *Oral Dis.* 10: 212–216.

Martelli, H. Jr., Pereira, A.M., Rocha, T.M. et al. (2007). White sponge nevus: Report of a three-generation family. *Oral Surg. Oral Med. Oral Pathol. Oral Radiol. Endod.* 103: 43–47.

Meleti, M., Rene Leemans, C., Mooi, W.J. et al. (2007). Oral malignant melanoma: a review of the literature. *Oral Oncol.* 43: 116–121.

Meleti, M., Vescovi, P., Moori, W.J., and van der Waal, I. (2008). Pigmented lesions of the oral mucosa and perioral tissues: a flow-chart for the diagnosis and some recommendations for the management. *Oral Surg. Oral Med. Oral Pathol. Oral Radiol. Endod.* 105: 606–616.

Mockenhaupt, M. (2011). The current understanding of Stevens-Johnson syndrome and toxic epidermal necrolysis. *Expert Rev. Clin. Immunol.* 7: 803–813. quiz 814–815.

Moynihan, P.J. (2007). The relationship between nutrition and systemic and oral well-being in older people. *J. Am. Dent. Assoc.* 138: 493–497.

Munde, A. and Karle, R. (2016). Proliferative verrucous leukoplakia: an update. *J. Cancer Res. Ther.* 12 (2): 469–473.

Olson, M.A., Rogers, R.S. 3rd, and Bruce, A.J. (2016). Oral lichen planus. *Clin. Dermatol.* 34 (4): 495–504.

Peñarrocha-Diago, M.A., Cervera-Ballester, J., Maestre-Ferrín, L., and Peñarrocha-Oltra, D. (2012). Peripheral giant cell granuloma associated with dental implants: clinical case and literature review. *J. Oral Implantol.* 38 Spec No: 527–532.

Porter, S.R., Scully, C., and Hegarty, A.M. (2004). An update of the etiology and management of xerostomia. *Oral Surg. Oral Med. Oral Pathol. Oral Radiol. Endod.* 97: 28–46.

Preeti, L., Magesh, K., Rajkumar, K., and Karthik, R. (2011). Recurrent aphthous stomatitis. *J Oral Maxillofac Pathol* 15: 252–256.

Rye Rasmussen, E.H., Bindslev-Jensen, C., and Bygum, A. (2012). Angioedema--assessment and treatment. *Tidsskr. Nor. Laegeforen.* 132: 2391–2395.

Sabba, C., Pasculli, G., Lenato, G.M. et al. (2007). Hereditary hemorrhagic telangiectasia: clinical features in ENG and ALK1 mutation carriers. *J. Thromb. Haemost.* 12: 1149–1157.

Schlosser, B.J., Pirigyi, M., and Mirowski, G.W. (2011). Oral manifestations of hematologic and nutritional diseases. *Otolaryngol. Clin. North Am.* 44: 183–203.

Sherman, R.G., Prusinski, L., Ravenel, M.C., and Joralmon, R.A. (2002). Oral candidosis. *Quintessence Int.* 33: 521–532.

Silva, S.C., Nasser, R., Payne, A.S., and Stoopler, E.T. (2019). Pemphigus Vulgaris. *J. Emerg. Med.* 56 (1): 102–104.

Slots, J., Saygun, I., Sabeti, M., and Kubar, A. (2006). Epstein-Barr virus in oral diseases. *J. Periodontal Res.* 41: 235–244.

Stoopler, E.T. and Alawi, F. (2008). Clinicopathologic challenge: a solitary submucosal mass of the oral cavity. *Int. J. Dermatol.* 47: 329–333.

Stoopler, E.T. and Balasubramaniam, R. (2013). Topical and systemic therapies for oral and perioral herpes simplex virus infections. *J. Calif. Dent. Assoc.* 41: 259–262.

Stoopler, E.T. and Sollecito, T.P. (2014). Oral mucosal diseases: evaluation and management. *Med. Clin. North Am.* 98 (6): 1323–1352.

Terézhalmy, G.T. and Bergfeld, W.F. (1998). Cicatricial pemphigoid (benign mucous membrane pemphigoid). *Quintessence Int.* 29: 429–437.

Terézhalmy, G.T. and Moore, W.S. (2004). Mucocele. *Quintessence Int.* 35: 766–767.

Terézhalmy, G.T. and Moore, W.S. (2004). Amelogenesis imperfecta. *Quintessence Int.* 35: 338–339.

Terézhalmy, G.T., Riley, C.K., and Moore, W.S. (2000). Pyogenic granuloma (pregnancy tumor). *Quintessence Int.* 31: 440–441.

Terézhalmy, G.T., Riley, C.K., and Moore, W.S. (2002). Oral verruca vulgaris. *Quintessence Int.* 33: 162–163.

Thompson, G.R. 3rd, Patel, P.K., Kirkpatrick, W.R. et al. (2010). Oropharyngeal candidiasis in the era of antiretroviral therapy. *Oral Surg. Oral Med. Oral Pathol. Oral Radiol. Endod.* 109: 488–495.

Touger-Decker, R. (1998). Oral manifestations of nutrient deficiencies. *Mt. Sinai J. Med.* 65: 355–361.

Tredwin, C.J., Scully, C., and Bagan-Sebastian, J.V. (2005). Drug-induced disorders of teeth. *J. Dent. Res.* 84: 596–602.

Triantafillidou, K., Dimitrakopoulos, J., Iordanidis, F., and Koufogiannis, D. (2006). Mucoepidermoid carcinoma of minor salivary glands: a clinical study of 16 cases and review of the literature. *Oral Dis.* 12: 364–370.

Vieira, R.A., Minicucci, E.M., Marques, M.E., and Marques, S.A. (2012). Actinic cheilitis and squamous cell carcinoma of the lip: clinical, histopathological and immunogenetic aspects. *An. Bras. Dermatol.* 87: 105–114.

Warnakulasuriya, K.A. and Ralhan, R. (2007). Clinical, pathological, cellular and molecular lesions caused by oral smokeless tobacco – a review. *J. Oral Pathol. Med.* 36: 63–77.

Warnakulasuriya, S., Johnson, N.W., and van der Waal, I. (2007). Nomenclature and classification of potentially malignant disorders of the oral mucosa. *J. Oral Pathol. Med.* 36: 575–580.

Weindl, G., Wagener, J., and Schaller, M. (2010). Epithelial cells and innate antifungal defense. *J. Dent. Res.* 89: 666–675.

Wroblewski, M.E., Washing, D.J., and Zaher, A. (2004). Pathologic quiz case. A 29-year-old man with a tongue lesion. Granular cell tumor. *Arch. Pathol. Lab. Med.* 128: 1059–1060.

Yih, W.-Y., Kratochvil, F.J., and Stewart, J.C.B. (2005). Intraoral minor salivary gland neoplasms: review of 213 cases. *J. Oral Maxillofac. Surg.* 63: 805–810.

6

Radiographic Examination

Diagnostic radiography is an integral part of the clinical process. It is predicated on a careful correlation of patient history, vulnerability to oral disease, and clinical findings. Radiographs should be ordered in those instances in which the clinician anticipates that the expected information obtained will contribute materially to the proper diagnosis, treatment, and prevention of disease. Consequently, the clinician's responsibility in obtaining radiographs involves two major considerations: (i) the clinical decision to order radiographic studies;

and (ii) the selection of an appropriate number and type of radiographic views necessary to conduct the examination.

In order to maximize diagnostic yield yet minimize the risk of unnecessary exposure, clinicians are responsible for assuring that all radiographs are obtained in accordance with the current standard of care. Periodically, the American Dental Association and the Food and Drug Administration publish joint guidelines addressing the use of radiography in dentistry to serve as a decision making

Physical Evaluation and Treatment Planning in Dental Practice, Second Edition.
Géza T. Terézhalmy, Michaell A. Huber, Lily T. García and Ronald L. Occhionero.
© 2021 John Wiley & Sons, Inc. Published 2021 by John Wiley & Sons, Inc.
Companion Website: www.wiley.com/go/terezhalmy/physical

resource for the practitioner. These guidelines categorize five specific patient categories: (i) child with primary dentition (prior to eruption of the first permanent tooth); (ii) child with transitional dentition (after eruption of the first permanent tooth); (iii) adolescent with permanent dentition (prior to eruption of third molars); (iv) adult who is dentate or partially edentulous; and (v) adult who is edentulous. The clinician must remember that disease and risk status may change over time and that an individual's radiographic recall interval may need to be changed accordingly.

The type of radiographs, the number of films taken, the date on which they were taken, and the diagnostic data obtained should be documented in the progress notes. Furthermore, since radiographs often represent the only evidence of past dental treatment or disease and serve as the basis for future treatment decisions, they must be retained as part of the patient's permanent record.

Before initiating any radiographic procedures, the clinician is further responsible for obtaining the patient's consent. The consent given by the patient may be implied or expressed. An implied consent is sufficient for commonly performed procedures that have few known risks. When a procedure has perceived or potential risks associated with it, such as the use of ionizing radiation on a child or a pregnant woman, the clinician should receive the guardian's or the pregnant patient's expressed consent (Table 6.1).

6.1 Radiographic Examination of the New Patient

Child with Primary Dentition

Open contacts in the primary dentition will often allow the clinician to visually inspect the proximal surfaces of posterior teeth. However if proximal surfaces cannot be visualized or probed, an individualized radiographic exam consisting of selected periapical/occlusal views and/or posterior bitewings is recommended.

Child with Transitional Dentition

The incidence of dental caries tends to increase in children with a transitional or mixed dentition as a result of socialization, dietary modifications, and changes in daily oral hygiene procedures. Thus, an individualized radiographic exam consisting of posterior bitewings with panoramic exam or posterior bitewings and selected periapical images is recommended.

Adolescent with Permanent Dentition

Increased independence and socialization, changing dietary patterns, and decreased attention to daily oral hygiene characterize this age group. Each of these factors may result in an increased risk for dental caries. Although proximal surfaces continue to show caries development, there is a tendency for caries activity to shift from proximal surfaces to surfaces with pits and fissures. An individualized radiographic examination should consist of posterior bitewing radiographs with a panoramic exam or posterior bitewings and selected periapical images. If the patient has clinical evidence of generalized oral disease or a history of extensive dental treatment, the attainment of a full mouth intraoral radiographic exam is preferred.

Adult Dentate or Partially Edentulous Patient

Although the incidence of proximal caries in the adult patient population is declining, it is important to assess proximal surfaces in

Table 6.1 Elements of an expressed consent in diagnostic dental radiography.

Why are the radiographs necessary?

What alternate diagnostic aids are available?

What risks are inherent in the use of ionizing radiation?

What radiation protection measures will be taken?

What effect the lack of quality dental radiographs may have on the diagnosis, treatment, and prognosis?

new adult patients for primary and recurrent disease activity (the incidence of root surface caries increases with age, but the usual method of detecting such lesions is by clinical examination). In addition, adult patients may have signs and symptoms of periodontal and/or pulpal disease, or have missing teeth requiring replacement. Therefore, the protocol for the Adolescent with Permanent Dentition above is recommended.

Adult Edentulous Patient

Radiographic examination for occult disease in this patient population cannot be justified on the basis of disease prevalence, morbidity, mortality, radiation dose, and cost. Thus, the recommendation is for an individualized radiographic exam, based on clinical signs and symptoms.

6.2 Radiographic Examination of the Recall Patient

No Clinical Caries and No Evidence of High-Risk Factors for Caries

Child with Primary and Transitional Dentition
In spite of the general decline in the incidence of dental caries, subgroups of children have a higher caries experience than the general population. The identification of patients in these subgroups may be difficult on an individual basis. Consequently, children with primary dentition with closed posterior contacts that show no clinical caries and that are not at risk for the development of caries benefit from an examination consisting of posterior bitewing radiographs, performed at intervals of 12–24 months if proximal surfaces cannot be examined visually or with a probe. This recommendation is based on evidence that dental caries progress more rapidly in primary teeth (thinner enamel with higher organic components) than in permanent teeth.

Adolescent Patient
The caries process in the permanent dentition typically takes more than 36 months

to progress from initial involvement of the enamel surface to the dentin. Consequently, it is recommended that in adolescents who show no clinical caries and are not at high risk for the development of caries, an examination consisting of posterior bitewing radiographs be performed at intervals of 18–36 months.

Adult Dentate or Partially Edentulous Patient
Advancing age, changes in the diet, and periodontal and systemic disease in adult dentate patients may increase the risk of dental caries. Consequently, dentate adults who show no evidence of clinical caries and are not at high risk for the development of caries still benefit from an examination consisting of posterior bitewing radiographs performed at intervals of 24–36 months.

Clinical Caries and Evidence of High-Risk Factors for Caries

Child with Primary and Dentition Transitional Dentition and Adolescent Patient
Children and adolescents who are at increased risk for developing dental caries because of such factors as poor oral hygiene, high frequency of exposure to sucrose-containing food, and deficient fluoride intake are more likely to have proximal caries. Therefore, the recommendation is to perform a bitewing examination at 6–12 month intervals if the proximal surfaces cannot be examined visually or with a probe.

Adult Dentate or Partially Edentulous Patient
Adult patients who manifest clinical dental caries or other risk factors for dental caries should be monitored carefully for any new or recurrent lesions that are detectable only by radiographic examination. The frequency of recommended radiographic recall should be determined on the basis of caries risk assessment. As a consequence the interval can vary from 6 to 18 months.

Radiographic Examination of the Recall Patient with Periodontal Disease

The frequency and type of radiographic examinations for these patients should be based on a clinical examination of the periodontium and documented signs and symptoms of periodontal disease. Structures or conditions to be assessed should include the level of supporting alveolar bone, condition of the interproximal bony crest, length and shape of roots, bone loss in furcations, and calculus deposits. Therefore, it is recommended that clinical judgment be used in determining the need for, and type of radiographic images necessary for, evaluation of periodontal disease. Imaging may consist of, but is not limited to, selected bitewing and/or periapical images of areas where periodontal disease (other than nonspecific gingivitis) can be identified clinically.

Patient (New and Recall) for Monitoring of Dentofacial Growth and Development, and/or Assessment of Dental/Skeletal Relationships

A child with primary and transitional dentition prior to the eruption of the first permanent tooth, radiographic examination to assess growth and development, in the absence of clinical signs and symptoms, is unlikely to yield productive information. Consequently, any abnormality of growth and development suggested by clinical findings should be evaluated radiographically on an individual basis.

In the adolescent patient, there is often a need to assess the growth status and/or the dental and skeletal relationships of patients in order to diagnose and treat their malocclusion. Appropriate radiographic assessment of the malocclusion should be determined on an individual basis. Another major concern for patients in this age group is to determine the presence, position, and development of third molars. This can best be accomplished through a radiographic examination consisting of selected periapical films or a panoramic view on a single occasion once the patient is in late adolescence (16–19 years of age).

Adult Dentate, Partially Edentulous, or Edentulous Patient

In the absence of any clinical signs or symptoms suggesting abnormalities of growth

and development in adults, no radiographic examinations are indicated for this purpose. Patients may present with other circumstances including but not limited to proposed placement of dental implants or the presence of existing implants, other dental and craniofacial pathoses, restorative or endodontic treatment needs, treated periodontal disease and caries remineralization. Clinical judgment for the individual patient should be exercised in determining the need for, and type of radiographic images necessary for evaluation and/or monitoring of these other circumstances.

6.3 Introduction to Radiographic Interpretation

In approaching radiographic diagnosis, the first step is to recognize the presence of an abnormality. This is best accomplished by systematically scanning the radiograph. Once an abnormality is encountered, it should be described in general terms and categorized based on location and radiographic appearance. It must, however, be emphasized that in no instance should a clinician arrive at a definitive diagnosis on the basis of radiographic findings alone. The radiographic diagnosis must correlate with the historical profile, physical examination, and, when indicated, with the clinical laboratory data and microscopic analysis.

Radiolucent Versus Radiopaque

As a general rule, lesions in osseous tissue may be divided into three categories: radiolucent, radiopaque, or mixed. Radiolucency indicates some measure of bone destruction. Conversely, radiopacity is more frequently associated with slow-growing lesions that although cause osseous alteration can be regarded as relatively nondestructive. There are exceptions to this concept, especially when the radiopacity is directly associated with a radiolucent area.

A mixed radiolucent/radiopaque appearance is often associated with fibro-osseous lesions, which both resorb and produce bone.

In radiopaque and mixed lesions, it is very important to notice the degree of radiopacity. Enamel is the most radiopaque and homogeneous tissue in the human body. Dentin and cementum are as homogeneous as enamel but less radiopaque. Bone, while similar to dentin and cementum in terms of radiopacity, is usually less homogeneous and is characterized by the presence of loose or dense trabeculation.

Unilocular Versus Multilocular

Multiloculation in a single radiolucent area suggests the presence of a slow-growing neoplasm. Round locules presenting a soap bubble appearance are usually noted in well-circumscribed yet locally aggressive tumors like the ameloblastoma or myxoma.

Peripheral Outline

The lesion, whether it is radiolucent or radiopaque, may have a distinct border, or its margins may be rough, irregular, or indistinct. A distinctive opaque lamina or sclerotic border around a radiolucent area suggests a slowly growing noninvasive lesion, as seen in "typical" cystic lesions. A definite, relatively smooth, easily identifiable margin between a radiolucent area and the surrounding bone may be observed when solid granulation tissue develops in bone.

Rough, irregular, or indistinct peripheral margins suggest tissue growth or the spread of infection beyond the present capacity of the body to wall off or circumscribe. A radiolucent line around a radiopaque area is characteristic of odontomas, particularly the cementomas and the compound composite and complex composite odontomas. A rather easily observed differentiation between an opaque mass and the surrounding bone, even though these tissues blend together, is often associated with a sclerotic bone lesion such as an enostosis.

Trabecular Pattern

Maxillary trabecular pattern is usually quite fine and without any particular directional arrangement. Trabecular bone in the mandible tends to run horizontally and the pattern is larger and more elliptical than those in the maxilla. The normal trabecular pattern, particularly in the mandible, may be altered to show fewer, coarser trabeculae arranged in a horizontal fashion. This gives a so-called "stepladder" appearance to the trabeculae and suggests a disturbance of the hematopoietic system.

The normal pattern may also be replaced by a fine, almost web-like network of bone trabeculae that look like ground glass, as in fibrous dysplasia and various stages of Paget's disease. When the web-like, reticulated, or ground-glass appearance is associated with a reduction in opacity, one must suspect calcium depletion, as may be seen with hyperparathyroidism. Following recalcification, these areas may present a cotton-wool appearance.

Dimensional Changes

Changes in bone size or shape are usually manifest clinically. Expansion of bone apparently takes place as a compensatory mechanism resulting from bone resorption in a directly adjacent area, which may be associated with pressure, chronic infection, or a slow-growing neoplastic lesion. Soft-tissue tumors that have metastasized to bone expand bone inversely to the rapidity of tumor growth. Bone tumors that are true neoplastic osteogenic lesions are inherently expansile. Here the bone growth is due to normal bone formation in an abnormal location at an abnormal rate.

Many expansile lesions cause a characteristic response in the periosteum of the overlying bone; this is called "periosteal reaction." Various appearances have been described such as "onion skin," "sunburst," or "Codman's triangles." Each appearance can be associated with a particular disease entity.

6.4 Radiographic Manifestations of Common Conditions

In this chapter, radiographic lesions are introduced as they present in the clinical setting: (i) coronal and pericoronal radiolucent, radiopaque, or mixed lesions (Table 6.2);

Table 6.2 Coronal and pericoronal lesions.

	Condition	Predominant gender	Predominant age	Predominant jaw	Predominant region	Other features
Radiolucent	Caries (Figure 6.1)	M ≈ F	>15 years	Maxilla ≈ mandible	Premolar/molar	Many variants of this disease exist
	Periodontal disease (Figures 6.2 and 6.3)	M > F	Adults	Maxilla	Posterior	
	External resorption (Figures 6.4 and 6.5)	M ≈ F	Adolescents	Maxilla	Anterior	May be iatrogenic (orthodontic)
	Follicular space (Figures 6.6 and 6.7)	M ≈ F	18–25 years	Mandible ≈ maxilla	3rd molar Cuspid	Considered normal if <2.5 mm on periapical radiographs and 3 mm on panoramic radiographs
	Dentigerous cyst (Figures 6.8 and 6.9)	M > F (2 : 1)	20+ years	Mandible	3rd molar	Often encompasses crown from CEJ to CEJ
Radiopaque	Ameloblastic fibroma (Figure 6.10)	M > F (1.5 : 1)	10–15 years	Mandible	Posterior	May extend beyond CEJ
	Compound odontoma (Figure 6.11)	M ≈ F	Second decade	Maxilla	Anterior	Multiple small tooth-like formations
	Complex odontoma (Figures 6.12 and 6.13)	M ≈ F	Second decade	Mandible	Posterior	Homogeneous mass
	Enamel pearl (Figure 6.14)	M ≈ F	Younger patients	Maxilla	Molar	1–3 mm radiopacity in the furcation area
	Pulp stone (Figure 6.15)	M ≈ F	Increases with age	Maxilla ≈ mandible	Premolar/molar	May be solitary or multiple
Mixed	Ameloblastic fibro-odontoma	M ≈ F	Second decade	Maxilla ≈ mandible	Anterior Posterior	Often associated with a missing tooth
	Adenomatoid odontogenic tumor (Figure 6.16a–c)	M < F (1 : 2)	10–20 years	Maxilla	Canine	Often associated with impacted tooth
	Calcifying odontogenic tumor (Gorlin cyst)	M ≈ F	30–50 years	Maxilla ≈ mandible	Premolar/molar	Usually multilocular
	Calcifying epithelial odontogenic tumor (Pindborg tumor)	M ≈ F	10–20 years	Maxilla ≈ mandible	Anterior Posterior	Exists in multiple subtypes

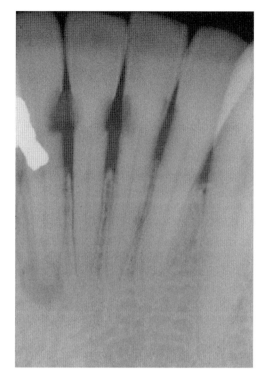

Figure 6.1 Caries.

Figure 6.2 Periodontal disease.

Figure 6.3 Periodontal disease.

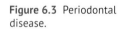

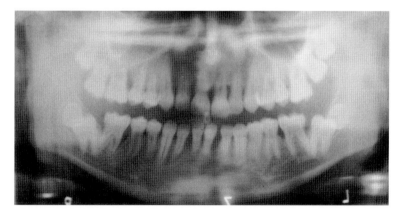

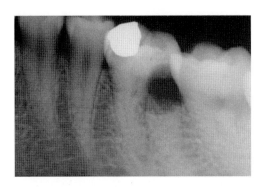

Figure 6.4 External resorption.

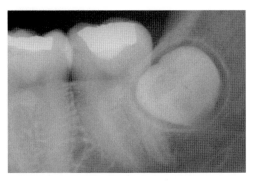

Figure 6.6 Follicular space.

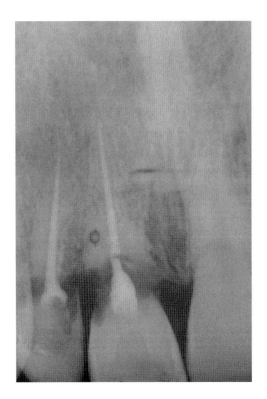

Figure 6.5 External resorption.

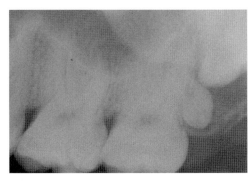

Figure 6.7 Follicular space.

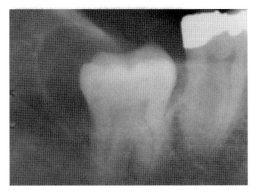

Figure 6.8 Dentigerous cyst.

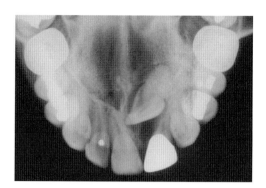

Figure 6.9 Dentigerous cyst.

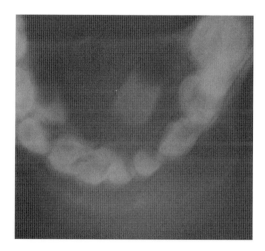

Figure 6.10 Ameloblastic fibroma.

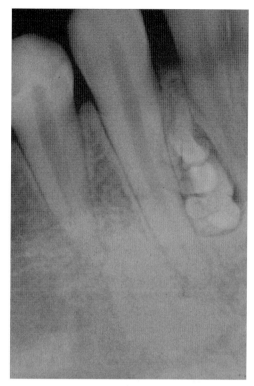

Figure 6.11 Compound odontoma.

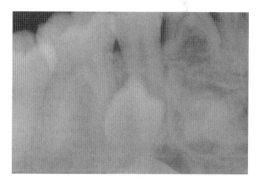

Figure 6.12 Complex odontoma.

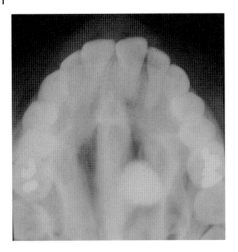

Figure 6.13 Complex odontoma.

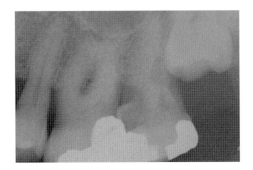

Figure 6.14 Enamel pearl.

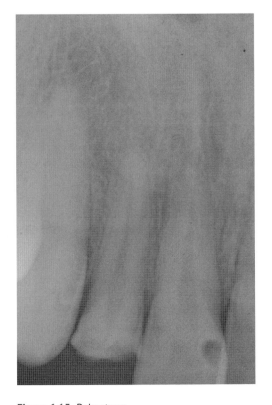

Figure 6.15 Pulp stone.

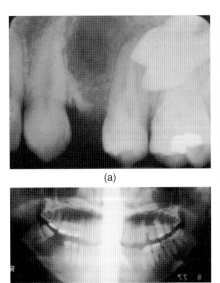

(a)

(b)

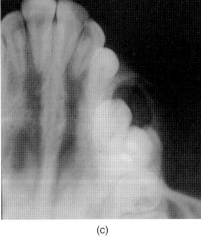

(c)

Figure 6.16 (a)–(c) Adenomatoid odontogenic tumor.

Table 6.3 Periapical, intraradicular, or interradicular lesions.

	Condition	Predominant gender	Predominant age	Predominant jaw	Predominant region	Other features
Radiolucent	Internal resorption (Figures 6.17–6.20)	M > F	Fourth–fifth decades	Maxilla ≈ mandible	Cuspids, 1st and 2nd molars	
	Periapical periodontitis (Figure 6.21), abscess (Figure 6.22), cyst (Figure 6.23), granuloma (Figure 6.24a), scar (Figure 6.24b)	M > F	Third–sixth decades	Maxilla (60%)	Incisors/cuspids	The apex is usually the epicenter of the lesion
	Lateral periodontal cysts	M > F	Fifth–sixth decades	Mandible	Cuspid/premolar	Teeth are usually vital
	Incisive canal cyst (Figure 6.25)	M > F (2.3 : 1)	<20 years of age	Maxilla	Anterior (midline)	Median-palatine cyst is the same lesion located posteriorly
Radiopaque	Traumatic bone cyst (Figure 6.26)	M > F (2 : 1)	Second decade	Mandible	Premolar/molar	Pseudo-cyst, no epithelial lining
	Osteosclerosis	M ≈ F	All ages	Mandible	Canine/premolar	Normal anatomic variant
	Pulp obliteration (Figure 6.27)	M ≈ F	Adults	Maxilla ≈ mandible	Anterior	Consider systemic conditions
	Hypercementosis	M ≈ F	Third–fourth decades	Mandible	Molar	Unknown etiology
	Condensing osteitis	M ≈ F	All ages	Mandible	Molar/premolar	
Mixed	Periapical cemental dysplasia (Figure 6.28)	M < F	Fourth decade	Mandible	Anterior	Three stages; often misdiagnosed as a periapical radiolucency
	Cementoblastoma (Figures 6.29 and 6.30)	M > F	Second–third decades	Mandible	1st molars	Lesion is fused to the roots
	Florid cemento-osseous dysplasia	M < F	Fourth decade	Maxilla ≈ mandible	Found in all regions	Usually multiple lesions

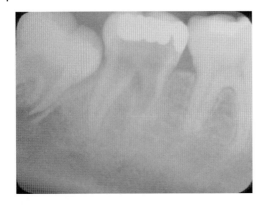

Figure 6.17 Internal resorption.

(ii) periapical, intraradicular, or interradicular radiolucent, radiopaque, or mixed lesions (Table 6.3); (iii) unilocular and multilocular radiolucent lesions of the jaw bones with distinct borders (Table 6.4); (iv) solitary radiopaque or mixed lesions within jaw bones with distinct border (Table 6.5); and (v) multiple or generalized radiolucent lesions with distinct borders, radiolucent lesions with indistinct borders, radiopaque lesions, or mixed lesions within jaw bones (Table 6.6).

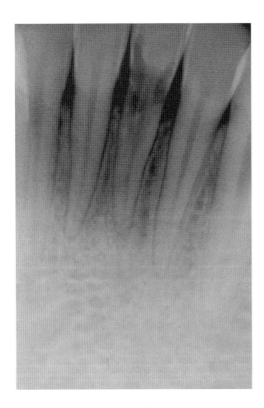

Figure 6.18 Internal resorption.

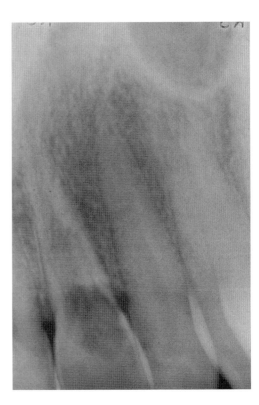

Figure 6.19 Internal resorption.

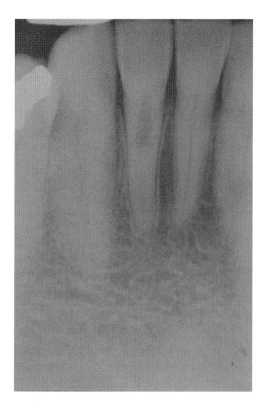

Figure 6.20 Internal resorption.

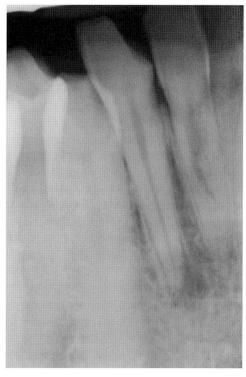

Figure 6.22 Periapical abscess.

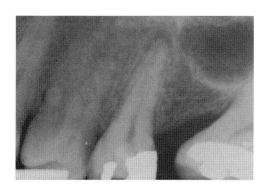

Figure 6.21 Periapical periodontitis.

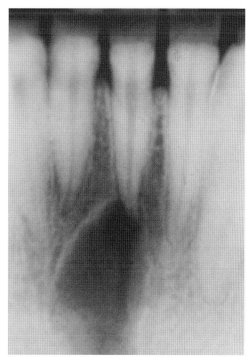

Figure 6.23 Periapical cyst.

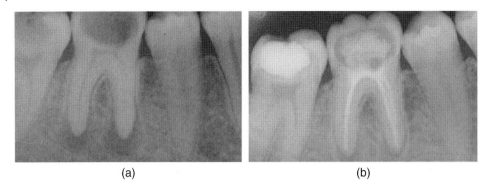

(a)   (b)

Figure 6.24 (a) Periapical granuloma. (b) Periapical scar.

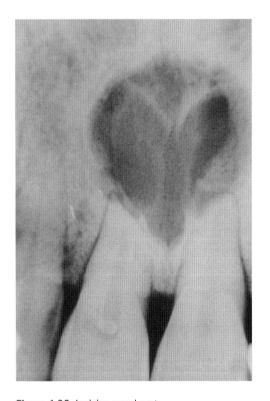

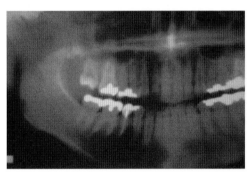

Figure 6.26 Traumatic bone cyst.

Figure 6.25 Incisive canal cyst.

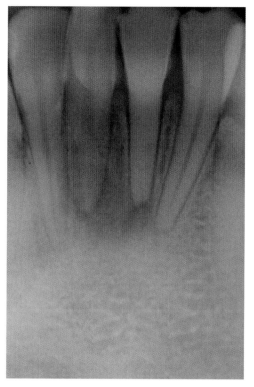

Figure 6.27 Pulp obliteration.

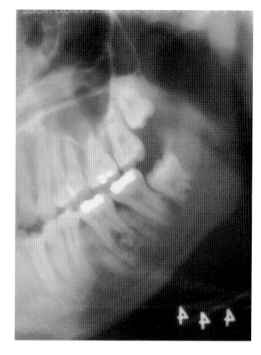

Figure 6.29 Cementoblastoma.

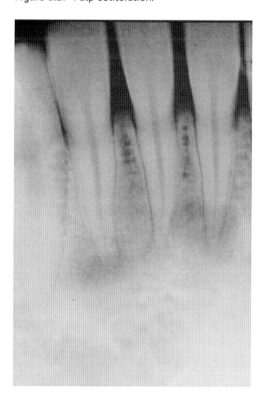

Figure 6.28 Periapical cemental dyslasia.

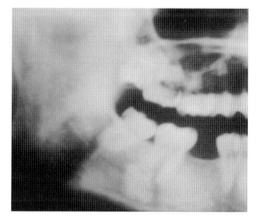

Figure 6.30 Cementoblastoma.

Table 6.4 Unilocular and multilocular radiolucent lesions within the jaw bones.

	Condition	Predominant gender	Predominant age	Predominant jaw	Predominant region	Other features
Unilocular	Salivary gland depression	M ≈ F		Mandible	Posterior	Inferior to the mandibular canal
	Fibrous healing defects (Figures 6.31 and 6.32)	M ≈ F	>30 years	Maxilla	Anterior	
	Hematopoietic bone marrow defect	M < F	Fourth decade and up	Mandible	Posterior	
	Residual cyst (Figure 6.33)	M > F	Older patients	Slightly more in the mandible	All areas	Prior surgical history often noted
	Langerhans cell disease (Histiocytosis-X)	M > F (2 : 1)	Children and adolescents	Mandible	Posterior areas bilaterally	May be isolated or part of a syndrome
	Odontogenic keratocyst	M > F (1.5 : 1)	Third–fourth decades	Mandible	Posterior	High recurrence rate
Multilocular	Ameloblastoma (Figures 6.34 and 6.35)	M > F	Third–fourth decades	Mandible	Posterior	Typical soap bubble appearance
	Central giant cell granuloma (Figures 6.36 and 6.37)	M < F (1 : 2)	<20 years of age	Mandible	Anterior	Generally anterior to 1st molars
	Aneurismal bone cyst (Figure 6.38a–c)	M < F (2 : 3)	<30 years of age	Mandible	Posterior	
	Odontogenic myxoma	M < F	10–30 years of age	Mandible	Posterior	Typical geometric septation
	Central hemangioma (Figure 6.39a–c)	M < F (1 : 2)	Children and toddlers	Mandible	All areas	Auscultation may reveal pulse, bruit

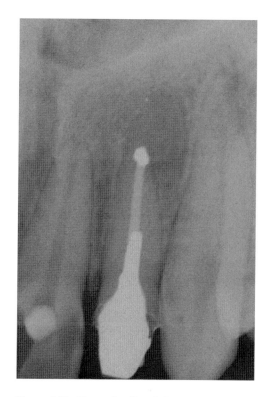

Figure 6.31 Fibrous healing defect.

Figure 6.32 Fibrous healing defect.

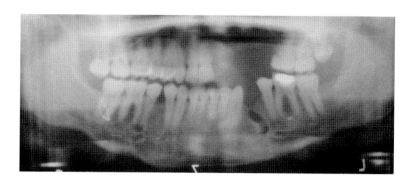

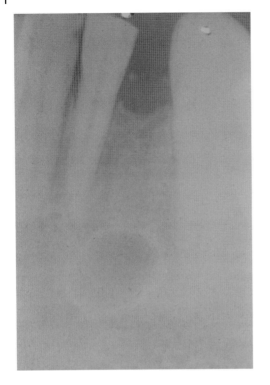

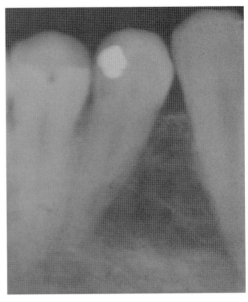

Figure 6.34 Ameloblastoma.

Figure 6.33 Residual cyst.

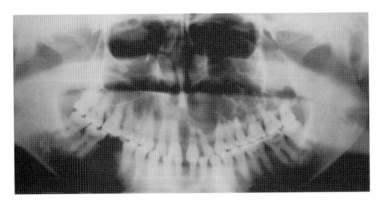

Figure 6.35 Ameloblastoma left maxillary sinus.

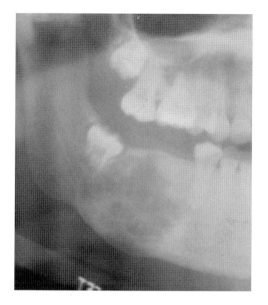

Figure 6.36 Central giant cell granuloma.

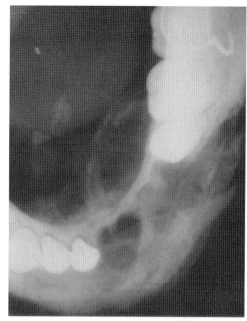

Figure 6.37 Central giant cell granuloma.

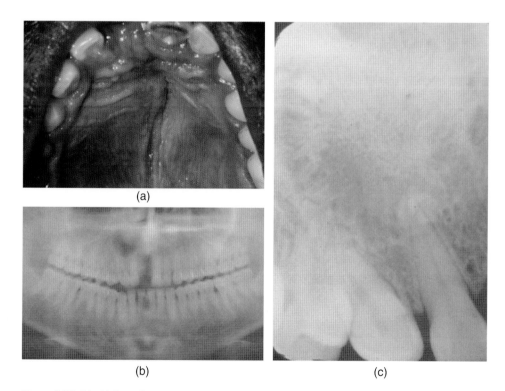

(a)

(b)

(c)

Figure 6.38 (a)–(c) Aneurismal bone cyst.

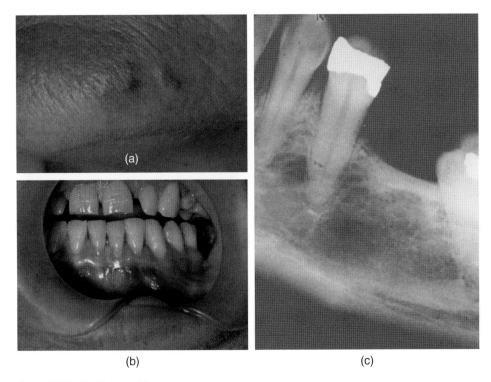

Figure 6.39 (a)–(c) Central hemangioma.

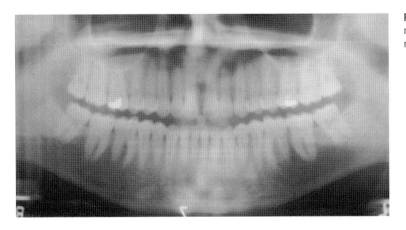

Figure 6.40 Mucous retention phenomenon right maxillary sinus.

Table 6.5 Solitary radiopaque lesions within the jaw bones.

	Condition	Predominant gender	Predominant age	Predominant jaw	Predominant region	Other features
Radiopaque	Exostosis	M ≈ F		Maxilla	Buccal aspect of canines and molars	
	Root fragments	M ≈ F				
	Socket sclerosis	M < F (1 : 2)	Middle-age adults	Maxilla ≈ mandible	Premolar/molar	
	Torus		Middle age	Both	Midpalate	
	Enostosis	M ≈ F	All ages	Mandible	Premolar/molar	Attached to the endosteal surface of the cortex, not detected clinically
	Osteoma	M > F	Older than 40 years of age	Mandible	Posterior/ramus	
	Osteoblastoma	M > F (2 : 1)	Second and third decades	Maxilla ≈ mandible	Posterior/ramus	
	Chondrosarcoma (Figure 4.16a–g)	M ≈ F	Adults	Maxilla ≈ mandible	Maxilla: anterior regions Mandible: condylar head/neck	
	Osteosarcoma (Figure 4.15a–d)	M > F (2 : 1)	Fourth decade and older	Mandible	Mandible: angle and ramus	
	Cementifying and osseous fibroma	M < F	Adolescents and young adults	Mandible	Molar/premolar	
Mixed	Mucous retention phenomenon (maxillary sinus) (Figure 6.40)	M > F	All ages	Sinus		Incidental finding

Table 6.6 Generalized or multiple lesions within the jaw bones.

	Condition	Predominant gender	Predominant age	Predominant jaw	Predominant region	Other features
Radiolucent (distinct borders)	Multiple myeloma (Figure 6.41a–d)	M > F	35–70 years	Mandible	Posterior/ramus	Multiple punched out lesions
	Cherubism (Figure 6.42)	M ≈ F	2–6 years	Mandible	Always bilateral	Regresses with age
	Nevoid basal cell carcinoma (Gorlin syndrome)	M ≈ F	5–30 years	Maxilla	Posterior	Jaw manifestation is one of many symptoms
	Osteomyelitis	M > F (5 : 1)	>30 years	Mandible (95%)	Posterior	Frequently seen with immunosuppression
	Osteo-radionecrosis (Figure 6.43)	M > F	Elderly	Mandible		History of head and neck irradiation
	Osteopetrosis	M ≈ F	Childhood	Maxilla	Bilateral	Hereditary disorder
Radiolucent (indistinct borders)	Rickets	M ≈ F	Children	Generalized		
	Hyperparathyroidism (Figure 6.44a–c)	M < F	40–50 years	Generalized		
	Sickle cell anemia	M ≈ F	Children and adolescents	Generalized	Autosomal dominant disease	
	Gardner's syndrome (Figure 4.19a–g)	M ≈ F	Younger patients	Maxilla ≈ mandible	All regions	Hereditary
	Paget's disease (Figure 6.45)	M > F (1.8 : 1)	>40 years	Enlargement of both the maxilla and mandible		
Radiopaque	Fibrous dysplasia (Figure 4.13a–d)	M ≈ F (Albright only female)	Monostatic: second decade; Polyostotic: <10 years	Maxilla	Posterior	
	Metastatic tumors	M ≈ F	>60 years	Mandible	Posterior	
Mixed	Florid cemento-osseous dysplasia	M < F	Fourth decade	Maxilla ≈ mandible	Bilateral	

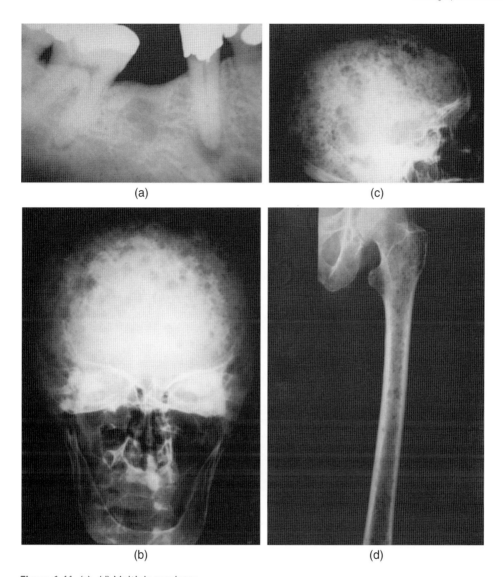

Figure 6.41 (a)–(d) Multiple myeloma.

Figure 6.42 Cherubism.

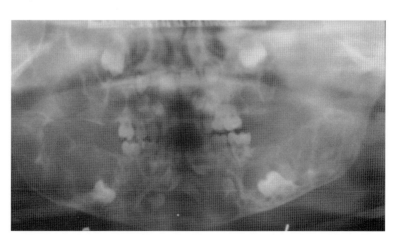

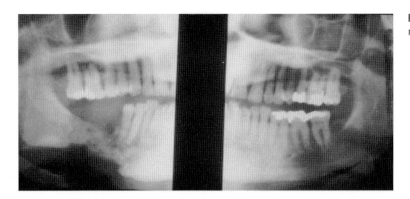

Figure 6.43 Osteo-radionecrosis.

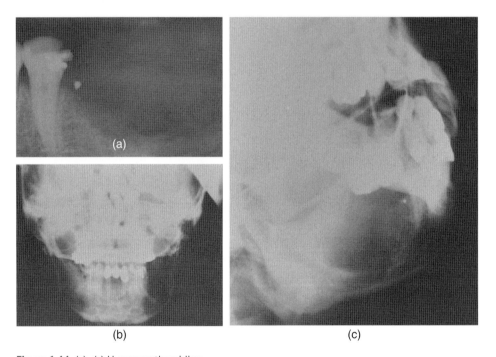

Figure 6.44 (a)–(c) Hyperparathyroidism.

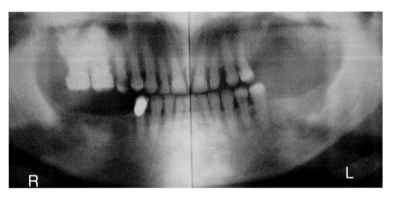

Figure 6.45 Paget's disease.

6.5 Conclusion

Oral healthcare providers must use clinical judgment to determine the type, frequency, and extent of each radiographic examination. Radiographic imaging should be individualized for each patient and should never be based on administrative or arbitrary requirements such as insurance needs or a fixed time schedule. The goal is to eliminate unnecessary or capricious exposures; that is, follow the dictum of ALARA (As Low As Reasonably Achievable), yet maximize diagnostic yield.

Suggested Reading

American Dental Association and the U.S. Department of Health and Human Services. (2012). The selection of patients for dental radiographic examinations. http://www.fda.gov/radiation-emittingproducts/radiationemittingproductsandprocedures/medicalimaging/medicalx-rays/ucm116504.htm (accessed 16 December 2020).

Coleman, G. and Nelson, J.F. (1989). Review of dental radiographic interpretation, part II: differential diagnosis of radiopacities, mixed radiolucent-radiopaque lesions, maxillary sinus disease, and soft tissue calcifications. *Compendium* 10 (8): 434–437, 440.

Langlais, R.P., Langland, O.E., and Nortjé, C.J. (1995). *Diagnostic Imaging of the Jaws*. Malvern, PA: Williams & Wilkins.

Mileman, P.A. and Van den Hout, W.B. (2003). Preferences for oral health states: effect on prescribing periapical radiographs. *Dentomaxillofac. Radiol.* 32 (6): 401–407.

Rushton, M.N. and Rushton, V.E. (2012). A study to determine the added value of 740 screening panoramic radiographs compared to intraoral radiography in the management of adult (>18 years) dentate patients in a primary care setting. *J. Dent.* 40 (8): 661–669.

Stuart, S.C. and Pharoah, M.J. (2014). *Oral Radiology Principles and Interpretation*, 7e. St. Louis, MO: Elsevier Mosby.

White, S.C. and Pharoah, M.J. (eds.) (2004). Principles of radiographic interpretation. In: *Oral Radiology: Principles and Interpretation*, 5e, 281–296. C.V. Mosby.

7

Laboratory Methods

In physical evaluation, clinical laboratory procedures may provide the final clue essential to confirm a diagnosis. They may also lead to the early detection of disorders with vague signs and symptoms, contribute to the discovery of significant, unexpected conditions, or provide a baseline against which response to or the safety of a therapeutic intervention

Physical Evaluation and Treatment Planning in Dental Practice, Second Edition.
Géza T. Terézhalmy, Michaell A. Huber, Lily T. García and Ronald L. Occhionero.
© 2021 John Wiley & Sons, Inc. Published 2021 by John Wiley & Sons, Inc.
Companion Website: www.wiley.com/go/terezhalmy/physical

may be measured. Consequently, in some situations, clinical laboratory information may be essential prior to the initiation of therapy. In other instances, it may be an important component of a diagnostic or therapeutic follow-up evaluation. Prior to ordering laboratory procedures, the clinician should elicit a careful medical history, perform a thorough physical examination, evaluate radiographic studies, and then request the tests from the laboratory that are most likely to either confirm or exclude the provisional diagnosis. A primary organic abnormality may be reflected in specific laboratory findings that may suggest a specific diagnosis or group of diagnoses, prompting the clinician to initiate appropriate therapy, consultation, or referral. This chapter briefly reviews some of the more frequently ordered tests or procedures utilized in medicine and dentistry.

7.1 Hematology Screening

The complete blood count (CBC) is an automated test that yields valuable information about red blood cells (RBCs), white blood cells (WBCs), and platelets. It is actually a broad screening panel consisting of several tests utilized to identify numerous disorders such as anemia, leukemia, infection, and other disorders (Table 7.1). To understand fully the relevance of these tests, it is necessary to examine the clinical significance of elevated or diminished values for the various determinants included in a CBC. However, it should be emphasized that the various blood elements are closely interrelated and individual values must be interpreted in the context of the entire hematological examination.

Red Blood Cell (RBC) Count

Erythrocytes transport oxygen to all tissues and carbon dioxide to the lungs. Their production is stimulated by hypoxia or anoxia and mediated by erythropoietin. The RBC count expresses

Table 7.1 Components of CBC.

Red blood cell count	Male: 4.7–6.1 million cells/mcl
	Female: 4.2–5.4 million cells/mcl
Platelet count	150 000–400 000/mcl
White blood cell count	4500–10 000 cells/mcl
Hemoglobin	Male: 13.8–17.2 g/dl
	Female: 12.1–15.1 g/dl
Hematoctrit	Male: 40.7–50.3%
	Female: 36.1–44.3%
RBC Indices	
MCV	80–100 fentoliter
MCH	27–31 picograms/cell
MCHC	32–36 g/dl

the number of RBCs per microliter of whole blood. Erythrocytosis polycythemia refers to an abnormal increase of RBCs and hemoglobin. An absolute or primary increase in the total number of circulating RBCs is referred to as polycythemia. It can be caused by chronic hypoxia, myeloproliferative syndromes, and other bone marrow abnormalities or it can be congenital. Polycythemia can also be relative (secondary). This is often caused by a decrease in plasma volume caused by dehydration or can be a result of acute hypoxia.

Hematocrit (Hct)

The hematocrit (Hct) is the percent volume of packed RBCs in a unit volume of whole blood and provides information about the number and size of RBCs. An elevated Hct may occur with dehydration, burns, polycythemia, and other conditions associated with low oxygen tension (smoking, living at high altitudes, congenital heart disease). A low Hct may be caused by anemia, hemorrhage, bone marrow failure, hemolysis, leukemia, nutritional deficiency, multiple myeloma, and rheumatoid arthritis.

Hemoglobin (Hgb)

Hgb is the oxygen-carrying molecule in erythrocytes and its concentration is reported in

Table 7.2 Common types of anemia.

Type	Cause
Normocytic normochromic	Acute hemorrhage Hemolysis Aplastic anemia
Microcytic hypochromic	Chronic hemorrhage Iron deficiency Hemoglobinopathies
Microcytic normochromic	Erythropoietin deficiency due to kidney failure
Macrocytic normochromic	Folic acid deficiency Vitamin B_{12} deficiency

grams per deciliter of whole blood. Low Hgb values are usually indicative of either anemia or blood loss.

RBC Indices

The RBC indices consist of three parts. The mean corpuscular volume (MCV), which is a reflection of the relationship between the Hct and the RBC count, is an assessment of the average size of RBCs. RBCs with low, normal, and high MCV values are described as microcytic, normocytic, and macrocytic, respectively. The mean corpuscular hemoglobin (MCH), which is a reflection of the relationship between the Hgb and the RBC count, is an assessment of the average amount of hemoglobin per RBC. RBCs with low, normal, and high MCH values are described as hypochromic, normochromic, and spherocytic, respectively. The mean corpuscular hemoglobin concentration (MCHC), which is a reflection of the relationship between Hgb and Hct, is an assessment of the hemoglobin concentration in relation to the size of RBCs. The RBC indices provide valuable information used to characterize anemia (Table 7.2).

White Blood Cell (WBC) Count

There are several types of WBCs or leukocytes (Table 7.3) that contribute to the WBC count. Neutrophils are the body's predominant phagocytic cell. Neutrocytosis is generally seen with bacterial infections B-lymphocytes synthesize and secrete antibodies. T-lymphocytes help mediate B-lymphocyte function and have cytotoxic activity against abnormal or virus-infected cells. Monocytes serve as sentinel cells against numerous pathogens and can turn into activated macrophages. Eosinophils and basophils, seen in allergic reactions and parasitic infections, release numerous substances that modulate the immune response.

The normal WBC count may vary in a particular individual during the course of the day. Conditions of WBC excess (leukocytosis) are associated with infection, inflammatory disease, leukemia, severe emotional stress, or extensive tissue damage. Conditions of WBC deficiency may be observed with bone marrow failure, certain autoimmune disorders, exposure to cytotoxic drugs or chemicals, radiation exposure, or diseases of the liver and spleen. Minor variations outside the normal range are not significant as long as the differential count on the peripheral blood is normal. The differential count is typically performed if the WBC count is outside the normal range. In a differential count the various types of leukocytes are visually identified and counted on a peripheral blood smear.

7.2 Evaluation of Hemostasis

A physiologic mechanism by which the body controls undesirable blood loss is called hemostasis. Adequate hemostasis is dependent on the proper function of its three essential phases: the vascular phase, the platelet phase, and the coagulation phase (Figure 7.1). A discrepancy in one or more of these phases may result in a bleeding disorder, which may be either inherited or acquired.

Vascular Phase

The vascular phase of hemostasis is dependent on the integrity and function of the vasculature.

Table 7.3 WBC differential and associated abnormalities.

WBC type	Normal range (%)	Conditions of excess	Conditions of lack
Neutrophil	40–60	Acute bacterial infection, eclampsia, gout, myelocytic leukemia, rheumatoid arthritis, rheumatic fever, acute stress, thyroiditis, trauma	Aplastic anemia, chemotherapy, influenza, overwhelming bacterial infection, radiation therapy/exposure
Lymphocytes	20–40	Chronic bacterial infection, infectious hepatitis, infectious mononucleosis, lymphocytic leukemia, multiple myeloma, viral infection, recovery from bacterial infection	Chemotherapy, HIV infection, leukemia, radiation therapy/exposure, sepsis
Monocytes	2–8	Chronic inflammatory disease, parasitic infection, tuberculosis, viral infection	NA
Eosinophils	1–4	Allergic reaction, parasitic infection, Hodgkin's disease	NA
Basophils	0.5–1	Acute rheumatic fever, polycythemia vera, myeloproliferative disease	Acute allergic reaction

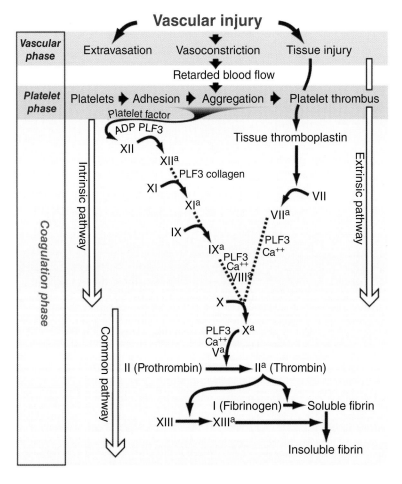

Figure 7.1 Phases of hemostasis.

When a blood vessel is damaged, it constricts to reduce blood flow. Examples of inherited disorders associated with impaired vascular function include hereditary hemorrhagic telangiectasia (HHT) and Ehlers–Danlos syndrome. The most likely acquired disorder of vascular function is allergic purpura. When necessary, a tourniquet test may be performed to clinically assess vessel integrity. In this provocative test, a blood pressure cuff is inflated to maintain pressure halfway between systolic and diastolic for five minutes. After deflating the cuff, the skin is allowed to return to its normal color, at which time the number of petechiae visible in a 1-in.-square area on the ventral surface of the forearm is determined (normal: <20/square inch).

Platelet Phase

The successful formation of a platelet plug is largely dependent on the availability of an adequate number of functioning platelets. The platelet count is a component of the CBC (Table 7.1). A high platelet count (thrombocytosis) may be associated with polycythemia vera, post-splenectomy syndrome, anemia, and certain malignancies. A low platelet count (thrombocytopenia) may be associated with cancer chemotherapy, disseminated intravascular coagulation (DIC), idiopathic thrombocytopenic purpura (ITP), leukemia, and prosthetic heart valves.

Traditional tests to assess the functional capacity of platelets, such as bleeding time (BT) are no longer used. Today, most large hospitals use an automated system, the Platelet Function Analyzer–100 (PFA–100®) to assess platelet function. Inherited disorders of platelet function include von Willebrand's disease and other rare diseases such as Bernard–Soulier syndrome, Glanzmann's thrombasthenia, and storage pool diseases. Acquired disorders of platelet function are far more common than the inherited disorders and may be caused by medications, autoimmune diseases, myeloproliferative diseases, and uremia.

Coagulation Phase

The coagulation phase of hemostasis consists of two distinct pathways, the extrinsic and intrinsic pathways of coagulation (Figure 7.1). The extrinsic pathway is activated in response to tissue damage, while the intrinsic pathway is activated in response to blood vessel wall damage.

Prothrombin Time (PT)

The prothrombin time (PT) reflects the efficacy of the extrinsic pathway (factors II, VII, X) of coagulation to induce clot formation. Normal PT results range from 11 to 16 seconds. A high PT may be associated with liver disease, bile duct obstruction, vitamin K deficiency, warfarin therapy, malabsorptive disorders, DIC, or deficiencies of factors II, VII, and X.

The PT is utilized not only to assess an undiagnosed bleeding disorder but also to monitor the therapeutic effect of oral anticoagulants (e.g. warfarin). However, testing reagents used to determine PT vary from laboratory to laboratory, which precludes direct comparisons between results. Efforts to solve the problem of variability among testing reagents culminated with the adoption, by the World Health Organization (WHO), of the International Normalized Ratio (INR) system. The INR is the PT ratio that one would have obtained if the WHO reference reagent had been used to perform the PT on the sample.

For most clinical scenarios in which an anticoagulant effect is indicated, a moderate-intensity anticoagulant effect with a targeted INR of 2.0–3.0 is appropriate. Anticoagulant therapy for patients with prosthetic heart valves is optimal when the INR is between 3.0 and 4.0. With a less intense therapeutic range (INR 2.0–3.0), the risk of bleeding is reduced significantly compared with the greater intensity protocols. Abnormal bleeding that occurs when the INR is below 3.0 is typically associated with an obvious underlying cause such as concomitant use of antithrombotic agents, or serious coexisting systemic conditions such as renal insufficiency, anemia, the presence of a structural defect (such as a polyp in the colon), or bladder tumor.

Prior to an oral surgical procedure, an assessment of the patient's level of anticoagulation is essential to ensure the INR value is within the targeted therapeutic range. Routine dental care (including simple oral surgical procedures) can be delivered with an INR of 4 or less, provided local hemostatic measures are used. For cases in which the INR exceeds 4, it is the responsibility of the patient's physician to make dosage adjustments. Warfarin has a plasma half-life of 36–42 hours; consequently, any change in the dosage will require about two days to be reflected in the INR value. Once an acceptable therapeutic range has been achieved, one may perform the procedure. Local anesthesia should be administered cautiously to minimize the risk of hematoma formation. Further measures to augment hemostasis include minimizing surgical trauma, obtaining primary closure when possible, placing sutures to stabilize the tissues, and using local hemostatic agents.

Activated Partial Thromboplastin Time (aPTT)

The activated partial thromboplastin time (aPTT) reflects the efficacy of the intrinsic pathway of coagulation to induce clot formation. Normal aPTT results range from 25 to 35 seconds. An elevated aPTT may be associated with numerous disease states, for example, cirrhosis, DIC, hypofibrinogenemia, malabsorption, von Willebrand's disease, lupus, or deficiency of coagulation factors VIII, IX, or XII. Such deficiencies are typical of hereditary coagulation disorders. The aPTT also reflects the level of anticoagulation produced by heparin therapy.

Traditional unfractionated heparin therapy is provided intravenously and thus requires hospitalization. Frequent monitoring is required to maintain the ratio of the patient's aPTT to the mean control aPTT within a defined range. For anticoagulation, an aPTT of 1.5–2.5 times normal is usually desired. When deemed necessary by the physician, heparin therapy may be discontinued approximately four hours before oral surgical procedures. Surgery is performed utilizing local anesthesia, atraumatic surgical technique, application of local hemostatic agents, and careful suturing. Heparin therapy is usually reinstated on the day of surgery if there is no active postsurgical bleeding.

The aPTT is also used to monitor the therapeutic efficacy of low molecular weight heparins (LMWHs). LMWHs have a predictable bioavailability and can be self-administered. Their use may serve as a more cost-effective approach to manage patients on warfarin for whom anticoagulation level adjustment is required prior to undergoing extensive surgery. Prior to the availability of LMWHs, the patient was admitted to the hospital, where traditional heparin therapy was substituted for warfarin therapy (the so-called heparin window). Typically on the fifth day of hospitalization, the patient would undergo the surgical procedure, at which time the warfarin would be reintroduced. Once the therapeutic level of warfarin is reestablished, the patient is released. By prescribing an LMWH in lieu of traditional heparin, the physician can now prepare the patient for the anticipated surgery on an outpatient basis.

It is important for the practitioner to remember that currently there are newer classes of anticoagulant drugs including direct thrombin inhibitors and Factor Xa inhibitors. The effect on clotting is not dependent on platelet number or function or vascular function. Nor can it be measured by the tests usually used to assess intrinsic or extrinsic arms of the coagulation cascade.

7.3 Biochemical Tests

From the analysis of large numbers of biochemical profiles, certain patterns emerge that are sufficiently characteristic to suggest a specific diagnosis or group of diagnoses. This

Table 7.4 Biochemical tests.

Test	Normal values
Liver panel	
ALT	N/A
AST	10–34 IU/l
ALT	44–147 IU/l
Bilirubin	
Total	0.3–1.9 mg/dl
Direct	0.0–0.3 mg/dl
TP	6.0–8.3 g/dl
Albumin	3.4–5.4 g/dl
A/G	1.5–2.5/1
LDH	105–333 IU/l
Fasting blood glucose	60–100 mg/dl
HbA1c	<5%
Lipid panel	
Cholesterol	<200 mg/dl
LDL	< 100 mg/dl
HDL	>60 mg/dl
Triglycerides	< 150 mg/dl
BUN	7–20 mg/dl
Uric acid	3.0–7.0 mg/dl
Creatine	0.8–1.4 mg/dl
Calcium	8.5–10.2 mg/dl
PO_4	2.4–4.1 mg/dl

IU = International unit.
l = liter.
dl = deciliter.
mg = milligram.
g = gram.

is analogous to the pathologist's recognition of tissue patterns when examining specimens and may be thought of as a "biochemical biopsy." A primary organic abnormality is typically reflected in the findings of certain tests, and abnormalities detected by other tests help to arrive at a more specific diagnosis and may signal secondary involvement of other systems. Some of the more common laboratory tests to diagnose specific abnormalities are discussed (Table 7.4). Many of these tests are ordered in groups or panels. For example a liver panel consists of alanine aminotransferase (ALT),

alkaline phosphatase (ALP), aspartate aminotransferase (AST), bilirubin, albumin, and total protein.

Alanine Aminotransferase (ALT) and Aspartate Aminotransferase (AST)

ALT is an enzyme found predominately in the liver and to a lesser degree in the kidneys, heart, and muscles. AST is an enzyme found predominantly in the liver and heart, and to a lesser extent in other organs. High ALT levels are specific for liver disease or exposure to hepatotoxic drugs. High AST levels may be associated with liver disease and other conditions such as acute pancreatitis, acute renal failure, myocardial infarction, severe burns, muscle trauma, surgery, or progressive muscular dystrophy.

Alkaline Phosphatase (ALP)

ALP is a ubiquitous enzyme found predominately in the liver, bone, and placenta. Various isoenzymes of ALP exist, each correlating with a specific tissue type. High ALP levels may be associated with liver disease, anemia, biliary obstruction, Paget's disease, bone healing, leukemia, or pregnancy. Low ALP levels may be associated with a nutritional deficiency.

Bilirubin

Bilirubin is a by-product of hemoglobin metabolism derived mainly from physiological red cell destruction in the reticuloendothelial (RE) system. The water-insoluble plasma bilirubin is transported to the liver, where it is conjugated with glucoronide and eliminated into the bile. Conjugated bilirubin is referred to as direct bilirubin and unconjugated bilirubin is referred to as indirect bilirubin. The typical bilirubin assay determines both the total bilirubin and direct bilirubin values, allowing for a deductive determination of the indirect bilirubin level. High indirect bilirubin levels are associated with hemolytic anemia, sickle cell anemia, pernicious anemia, transfusion reaction, and Gilbert's disease. High direct bilirubin levels are associated with liver disease and bile duct obstruction.

Total Protein (TP), Albumin, and Albumin/Globulin (A/G) Ratio

Dietary proteins are hydrolyzed in the alimentary canal into amino acids and transported to the liver and the RE system for the synthesis of body proteins. Blood proteins are classified as either albumins or globulins. Albumins are produced by the liver and are the predominant proteins in the plasma. They serve to transport many small molecules (e.g. hormones, vitamins, drugs, ions) in the blood and are also essential for the maintenance of the osmotic pressure of the blood. Globulins are further classified as being alpha-1, alpha-2, beta, and gamma globulins. The gamma globulins include the various antibody types (M, G, A, E) and are synthesized by the RE system.

TP is a composite of the albumin plus globulin values. An elevated albumin value may occur with dehydration, while an elevated TP may be associated with chronic infection or inflammation, multiple myeloma, and Waldenström's disease. Low albumin and/or TP values may be associated with liver disease, renal disease, malabsorptive disorders, malnutrition, and severe burns. A reversed albumin/globulin ratio may be associated with malnutrition, chronic liver disease, and hypergammaglobulinemia.

Lactate Dehydrogenase (LDH)

Lactate dehydrogenase (LDH) is an intracellular enzyme present in virtually all metabolically active cells, with its highest concentration found in erythrocytes, heart, liver, kidneys, and skeletal muscle. High levels of LDH are usually associated with destructive processes, that is, myocardial infarction, cerebrovascular accident, hemolytic anemia, hepatitis, pancreatitis, or muscle injury.

Blood Glucose and HbA1c

Most carbohydrates are metabolized into glucose and stored in the liver as glycogen. The utilization of glucose by the body is under the influence of insulin, which facilitates its transfer across cell membranes. The most accurate determination of the blood glucose level is obtained by having the patient fast for at least six hours prior to undergoing the test (fasting glucose). Elevated blood glucose (hyperglycemia) is usually associated with either impaired glucose tolerance or diabetes mellitus. Low blood glucose (hypoglycemia) is usually associated with an inadequate dietary intake of sugar, exogenous insulin overdose, or therapy with oral hypoglycemic agents.

The HbA1c is a test used to monitor blood glucose control over an extended period. It represents the percentage of hemoglobin in RBCs that become glycosylated (that is, chemically linked to glucose) during their life span. HbA1c reflects glucose levels in the blood over the previous 6–12 weeks prior to the test. An elevated HbA1c is usually indicative of poorly controlled diabetes mellitus, which is associated with an increased risk of developing eye disease, kidney disease, heart disease, stroke, and nerve damage.

Lipid Panel Testing

Lipid panel testing measures cholesterol, high density lipoproteins (HDL), low density lipoproteins (LDL), very low density lipoproteins (VLDL), and triglycerides.

Lipid panel testing is a valuable tool to assess cardiovascular risk. Cholesterol is an essential body constituent required for cell membrane formation, the synthesis of bile acids, and the synthesis of steroid hormones. Water insoluble, it is carried by various lipoproteins (VLDLs, LDLs, and HDLs). Triglycerides are compounds used to move fatty acids (formed when fats or oils are consumed) through the blood. Fatty acids may be metabolized for energy or stored (as fat) for later use.

The cholesterol value is a summation of the VLDL, LDL, and HDL and should ideally be less than 200 mg/dl. Elevated cholesterol levels may be associated with a high-cholesterol diet, hypercholesterolemia, hypothyroidism, diabetes mellitus, and nephrotic syndrome. Low cholesterol levels may be indicative of nutritional deficiency, hyperthyroidism, liver disease, and pernicious anemia. Of all the components of the lipid panel, the LDL appears to be the strongest predictor of cardiovascular risk.

Blood Urea Nitrogen (BUN)

Blood urea nitrogen (BUN) is the chief nitrogenous by-product of protein metabolism. It is produced in the liver and excreted primarily by the kidney. The BUN is commonly ordered to assess renal function. An elevated BUN may be associated with renal disease, cardiovascular disease, urinary tract obstruction, dehydration, and excess protein ingestion.

Uric Acid

Uric acid is a metabolite of nucleic acid degradation, which occurs mainly in the bone marrow and organs of high metabolic activity such as the liver. It is the end product of purine metabolism and is excreted primarily by the kidneys. High uric acid levels may be associated with gout, diabetes mellitus, alcoholism, hypoparathyroidism, lymphoproliferative or myeloproliferative disorders, and renal disease.

Creatinine

Creatine, a natural amino acid derivative, is synthesized in the liver, kidney, and pancreas and is supplied exogenously through the diet (meat, fish). Cells with high-energy requirements such as skeletal muscle use creatine in the form of phosphocreatine, which serves as a phosphate donor to generate ATP from ADP. Serum concentrations of creatinine, a waste product of creatine, reflect creatine utilization, which is proportional to the body's muscle mass, and its excretion by the kidney. Elevated levels may be associated with renal disease, muscular dystrophy, rhabdomyolysis, and acromegaly.

Calcium

Over 90 % of calcium in the body is found in the skeleton and teeth. Although the calcium concentration of the extracellular fluid is relatively small, its level is precisely regulated by parathyroid hormone, total protein, vitamin D, and calcitonin. Elevated calcium levels (hypercalcemia) may be associated with hyperparathyroidism, Paget's disease, malignancies, hyperthyroidism, drug therapy, excess calcium ingestion, or sarcoidosis. Low serum calcium levels (hypocalcemia) may be a sign of vitamin D deficiency, pregnancy, renal disease, hypoparathyroidism, or drug therapy.

Phosphorus

About 85 % of the total phosphorus is combined with calcium in the skeleton and the rest is distributed as phosphate (PO_4) ion in the blood and other tissues. PO_4 is involved in most metabolic processes. The parathyroid hormone mediates an increased rate of absorption of both calcium and phosphorus and regulates phosphate loss and calcium retention by its effect on renal tubular reabsorption. Elevated PO_4 levels (hyperphosphatemia) may be associated with renal disease, hypoparathyroidism, bone metastasis, liver disease, sarcoidosis, or hypocalcemia. Low PO_4 levels (hypophosphatemia) may be associated with hyperparathyroidism, hypercalcemia, and inadequate dietary intake of PO_4 or vitamin D.

7.4 Tissue Studies

There are striking similarities among the many lesions affecting oral tissues. It is essential in the differential diagnostic process that all possibilities are considered before making a definitive diagnosis. In some instances the history of a given lesion, combined with the characteristic clinical, radiographic, and laboratory findings, may be sufficient to confirm the clinical impression. However, at other times a biopsy may be required to arrive at a specific diagnosis. This is especially true for oral soft-tissue lesions. As a rule, a biopsy is indicated in the management of any suspicious lesion that either persists or does not respond to conventional therapy within 7–14 days.

Scalpel Biopsy

Histologic assessment of a biopsy specimen represents the gold standard for diagnosing any suspicious oral lesion. An excisional biopsy is the technique of choice when a lesion is relatively small and the surgical removal is considered curative. The lesion is excised in its entirety. An incisional biopsy is indicated when a lesion is too large for easy excision or when diagnosing oral manifestations of mucocutaneous diseases such as lichen planus, lupus, or pemphigus vulgaris. A pie-shaped wedge of lesional or perilesional tissue, depending on the suspected underlying condition, is removed. In some instances, where there might be differences in the appearance of a lesion (ulcerative in one area, hypertrophic at another portion of the lesion) several specimens may have to be obtained to allow for an adequate microscopic evaluation. In performing a biopsy, certain guidelines should be followed (Table 7.5). Finally, if the practitioner is uncomfortable performing a biopsy or believes the lesion in question is malignant, he or she must promptly refer the patient for appropriate management.

Brush Biopsy

Some authorities have expressed concern that small mucosal lesions that appear to be harmless may be overlooked and thus not

Table 7.5 Guidelines for performing a biopsy.

Do not inject anesthesia directly into the lesion.
Do not crush or macerate the tissue.
Orient the specimen properly.
Immediately place the specimen in an appropriate preservative.
Provide the pathologist with an adequate history, clinical description to include exact location, photographs, and radiographs.
If the initial biopsy fails to confirm, or is inconsistent with, the clinical impression, a repeat biopsy and close monitoring of the lesion must be performed.

undergo appropriate follow-up scrutiny (i.e. scalpel biopsy). This reality has led some to advocate the use of the brush biopsy technique to assess the malignant potential for such innocent-appearing lesions. A refinement of the technique is marketed as the OralCDx™ kit (CDx Diagnostics, Suffern, NY).

Proper utilization of the sampling instrument incurs minimal discomfort or bleeding and assures the attainment of an adequate biopsy sample of all three epithelial layers (superficial, intermediate, and basal) of the lesion. All specimens are stained in accordance with a modified Papanicolaou method prior to being scanned by a computer and positive specimens are assessed by an oral pathologist.

Since architectural integrity of the tissue layers are not maintained, all positive findings from OralCDx mandate a definitive scalpel biopsy for diagnosis, and negative results may result from inadequate sampling. The utility of the technique should be limited to that of a bridging procedure for the patient who is either averse to undergoing a biopsy or likely to not return for the two-week follow-up assessment of the initial lesion.

Exfoliative Cytology

Exfoliative cytology may be defined as the microscopic examination of cells harvested from the surface of a lesion (as opposed to

Table 7.6 Guidelines for performing exfoliative cytology.

Scrape a moist tongue depressor gently over the entire surface of the lesion.

Spread the collected cells evenly on a glass slide.

Spray the slide with an appropriate fixative.

Submit the specimen to the pathologist, along with an adequate history, a clinical description to include exact location, and any photographs.

Table 7.7 DIF desquamative autoimmune conditions.

Condition	DIF characteristics
Pemphigus	Intercellular reticulate deposits of IgG and C3
MMP	Linear deposition of IgG and C3 in area of dermo-epidermal basement membrane zone
Linear IgA dermatosis	Linear deposits of IgA at the basement membrane

the examination of tissue blocks in biopsy). The procedure is inexpensive, quick, easy, and painless (Table 7.6). Properly used, oral exfoliative cytology may be useful in determining if a lesion is due to viral infections, candidiasis, and, in rare instances, changes suggesting dysplasia or cellular atypia. Any such findings must be either biopsied or promptly referred for management.

Direct Immunofluorescence

Bullous or blistering autoimmune diseases are divided into two general groups, pemphigus and pemphigoid. Pemphigus is characterized by intraepithelial splitting leading to the development of fragile thin-walled blisters. The pemphigoid group is characterized by subepithelial splitting and the development of thicker-walled blisters. This group encompasses bullous pemphigoid, mucous membrane pemphigoid, and linear IgA dermatosis. For all of these conditions, routine histologic analysis of biopsy specimens is often insufficient to establish the diagnosis. Tissue specimen should ideally be obtained from intact, perilesional tissue.

Direct immunofluorescent (DIF) testing is useful in diagnosing a variety of the bullous or desquamative autoimmune conditions. To be diagnostic, the specimen must entail intact epithelium and should be large enough to be easily split into two separate specimens. One specimen is submitted in formalin for routine histologic interpretation. The specimen submitted for DIF must be kept moist

on saline-soaked gauze or filter paper and immediately delivered to the laboratory. If immediate delivery is not feasible, appropriate transport media (e.g. Michel's solution) is available from the biopsy service. Fluorescent tagged anti-human immunoglobins are applied to the specimen to determine the presence of specific tissue-bound autoantibodies such as immunoglobulin G (IgG), immunoglobulin M (IgM), immunoglobulin A (IgA), complement factor 3 (C3), and fibrin. Specific autoantibodies localization correlates well with specific bullous or desquamative autoimmune conditions (Table 7.7).

Indirect Immunofluorescence

Indirect immunofluorescence (IIF) is used to detect circulating serum autoantibodies. For pemphigus disease, monkey esophagus is used as the substrate to test for the presence of IgG autoantibodies. For bullous disorders, a sodium chloride split skin technique is used to define the specific diagnosis.

Gram's Staining Method

The Gram stain is a valuable and time-tested method used to assess an infected body fluid or tissue (Table 7.8). It provides preliminary information that helps in choosing the best antibacterial agent to prescribe while awaiting definitive identification by a culture. The Gram stain technique is a simple laboratory

Table 7.8 Gram's staining method.

Crystal violet wash for 1 minute.
Rinse with water.
Gram's iodine wash for 1 minute.
Rinse with water.
Decolorize with acetone and alcohol.
Rinse with water.
Counterstain for 10–30 seconds with 2.5% safranin.
Wash and dry.

procedure that produces diagnostic slides requiring only an oil emersion microscope for interpretation. It separates microorganisms into two general categories: gram-negative organisms, which appear red following discoloration by alcohol and counterstaining with safranin; and Gram-positive microorganisms, which preclude the extraction of the crystal violet-iodine complex by alcohol and appear deep purple in color. Based on their morphologic appearance, microorganisms responsible for bacterial infections may also be described as cocci or bacilli.

Culturing

Based on various culturing methods, microorganisms may also be classified an aerobic, anaerobic, or facultative. Aerobic organisms are those requiring oxygen to survive, and anaerobic organisms are those that must avoid oxygen to survive. Some organisms may be facultative and survive either with or without oxygen. Clinical clues to the presence of anaerobes include the formation of abscesses, the presence of tissue necrosis, the production of gas within the tissues, the presence of a foul odor (the absence of an odor does not rule out anaerobes), and a failure to grow bacteria on an aerobic culture media.

7.5 Summary

A primary organic abnormality is typically reflected in the findings of laboratory and tissue studies that are sufficiently characteristic to suggest a specific diagnosis or groups of diagnoses and prompt the clinician to initiate appropriate therapy, consultation, or referral.

Suggested Reading

Brennan, M.T., Hong, C., Furney, S.F. et al. (2008). Utility on an international normalized ration testing device in a hospital-based dental practice. *J. Am. Dent. Assoc.* 139 (6): 697–703.

Eming, R., Hertl, M., and Autoimmune Diagnostics Working Group (2006). Autoimmune bullous disorders. *Clin. Chem. Lab. Med.* 44: 144–149.

Fakhri, H.R., Janket, S.J., Jackson, E.A. et al. (2013). Tutorial in oral antithrombotic therapy: biology and dental implications. *Med. Oral Pathol. Oral Cir. Bucal.* 18 (3): e461–e472.

Jeske, A.H. and Suchko, G.D. (2003). Lack of a scientific basis for routine discontinuation of oral anticoagulation therapy before dental treatment. *J. Am. Dent. Assoc.* 134: 1492–1497.

Jilma, B. (2001). Platelet function analyzer (PFA-100): a tool to quantify congenital or acquired platelet dysfunction. *J. Lab. Clin. Med.* 138: 152–163.

McClelland, R. (2001). Gram's stain: key to microbiology. *Med. Lab. Obs.* 33 (4): 20–28.

McPherson, R.A. and Pincus, M.R. (eds.) (2007). *Henry's Clinical Diagnosis and Management by Laboratory Methods*, 21e. Saunders.

Oliver, R.J., Sloan, P., and Pemberton, M.N. (2004). Oral biopsies: methods and applications. *Br. Dent. J.* 196 (6): 329–333.

8

Diagnostic and Treatment Planning Considerations for Orofacial Pain

The most common complaint causing a person to seek the services of an oral healthcare provider is pain. Orofacial pain conditions may be grouped into one of three major categories: (i) neurovascular, e.g. toothache and migraines; (ii) musculoskeletal, e.g. temporomandibular disorders (TMDs); and (iii) neuropathic, e.g. peripheral and central nervous system disorders. A patient may experience multiple, overlapping pain syndromes making localization of the source and diagnosis difficult.

In order to obtain the correct diagnosis, a disciplined, and methodical approach to patient assessment should be employed. First and foremost, the practitioner should obtain a sufficient history to verify that the patient may be safely treated. However if the situation permits, it is wise to always obtain a comprehensive medical history, as information attained may prove valuable in establishing the diagnosis. The next step is to obtain and assess the patient's pain history (subjective information) and to perform a clinical examination (objective findings). Again, when possible the clinical examination should be comprehensive. A good rule of thumb is to always examine the area of concern last, not first. Occasionally, the history and/or examination will reveal classic symptoms (e.g. a 30 second excruciating electric shock-like facial pain, suggestive of trigeminal neuralgia or the sharp pain on biting associated with a visibly cracked tooth) that point to the diagnosis. In other instances, the diagnosis may be equivocal or the necessary therapy may be beyond the purview of the practitioner. For such cases, referral to a specialist for further assessment or therapy may be warranted. The purpose of this chapter is to briefly review a basic methodical approach the practitioner may use to assess the patient presenting with pain.

Physical Evaluation and Treatment Planning in Dental Practice, Second Edition.
Géza T. Terézhalmy, Michaell A. Huber, Lily T. García and Ronald L. Occhionero.
© 2021 John Wiley & Sons, Inc. Published 2021 by John Wiley & Sons, Inc.
Companion Website: www.wiley.com/go/terezhalmy/physical

8.1 Subjective Information

The chief complaint should be recorded in the patient's own words to minimize misinterpretation, e.g. "my tooth is throbbing," or "I have a burning, gnawing pain in my gum." It is best to start the conversation with an open question which (i) invites the patient to tell their story and (ii) helps establish good rapport. Generally speaking, the more information obtained the better. Determine the domain (location), character (qualities) and intensity (on a 0–10 scale, where 0 is no pain and 10 is the worst pain imaginable) of pain. Did the symptoms develop slowly or rapidly? Is the pain sharp or dull? Does pain appears spontaneously and disappears quickly or does it have a persistent quality? Is the pain localized or does it radiate (refer) to other anatomic locations? Ask the patient about aggravating and alleviating influences. What is the effect of mastication on the character and intensity of pain? Are the symptoms worse when the patient is chewing? In some instances, mastication relieves symptoms; in others, it aggravates them. Has the pain become worse or better over time? Similar insights related to swallowing, drinking, and speaking are also useful. Characteristics of orofacial pain categories are presents in Table 8.1.

Neurovascular Pain

Neurovascular pain such as dental pulpalgia or migraine headaches is characterized as throbbing, pounding, or sharp. Pulpal pain is often aggravated by thermal changes such as drinking a hot or cold beverage, postural changes such as when the patient assumes a supine position, and may occur spontaneously and awaken the patient from a sound sleep.

Musculoskeletal Pain

Pain associated with a TMD such as myalgia or temporomandibular joint (TMJ) arthralgia is characterized as aching, pressure-like, dull,

Table 8.1 Characteristics of orofacial pain categories.

Pain category	Quality	Additional symptoms
Musculoskeletal (e.g. TMD)	Ache	May have burning in background
	Pressure	Worsens with functional and/or parafunctional activities
	Dull	
	Tight	Worsens with stress
	Stiff	Improves with relaxation and/or heat
	Occasionally sharp Occasionally throbbing	
Neurovascular (e.g. toothache and migraine)	Throbbing	Tooth pain may worsen with thermal changes, laying down, may occur spontaneously, and may awaken patient
	Pounding	
	Sharp	
Neuropathic (e.g. peripheral and central nervous system disorder)	Burning	Numbness
	Shooting	Paresthesia
	Electric shock-like	Hyperalgesia
	Cutting	Allodynia
	Itching	Dysesthesia

Source: Adapted from de Leeuw and Klasser (2013).

tight, and/or stiff. Throbbing may occur when the pain is severe, a burning quality may linger in the background, and the patient may experience intermittent sharp pain. Symptoms are aggravated by functional and parafunctional activities such as eating, clenching, and stress. Relaxation and the application of heat have salutary effects.

Neuropathic Pain

Neuropathic pain is characterized as burning, shooting, electric shock-like, cutting, or itching. The patient may also report numbness, paresthesia (partial loss of sensation), hyperalgesia (exaggerated pain from a painful stimulus), allodynia (painful response to a non-painful stimulus, such as pressure from a cotton swab) and/or dysesthesia (painful, unpleasant sensations). A burning sensation accompanied by aching, pressure-like, or dull symptoms is likely to be musculoskeletal pain.

8.2 Objective Findings

Careful consideration of the attained subjective information guides the practitioner during the objective phase of data collection. For example, if the subjective information provided by the patient is suggestive of musculoskeletal pain, the practitioner should begin by determining the range of mandibular motion. The accepted minimum of normal for these movements are 40 mm on opening (including the anterior tooth overlap), 7 mm to each lateral jaw movement, and 6 mm protrusive movement.

During physical examination, the practitioner should also try to identify the source of pain by reproducing and/or temporarily eliminating the patient's pain, where practical. Reproducing the patient's pain typically requires provocation, which is often accomplished through palpation, percussion using an instrument to allow testing of a single tooth (such as a tooth sloth or similar device), thermal challenges, and by probing periodontal pockets. Localization of the pain may also be determined by selectively anesthetizing finite sites or regions.

Locating the Source of Pain

Superficial somatic tissues of the face and mouth are highly innervated, while deep somatic tissues are not as well innervated. Consequently, superficial somatic pain, e.g. pain associated with tissue damage (trauma and inflammation) involving skin and mucosa, is readily localized. On the other hand, deep somatic pain, e.g. pain associated with tissue damage (trauma and inflammation) involving muscle and bone is frequently referred to adjacent anatomical areas.

It is not uncommon for a patient to point to a specific tooth as the source of his/her pain yet physical examination provides objective evidence that another tooth is the source of the patient's pain. It is also not uncommon for a patient to localize pain to a tooth or several teeth, while in reality, the pain is actually being referred from an adjacent anatomical structure such as the masseter muscle, the TMJ, or the maxillary sinus.

Failure to properly diagnose the source of pain may result in the patient receiving inappropriate and ineffectual care, such as unnecessary endodontic procedures (Figure 8.1) and/or unnecessary extractions. It is estimated that 680,000 teeth/year receive endodontic therapy to manage pain of non-endodontic origin. When the patient complains of a toothache and/or alveolar bone pain for which there is no objective evidence of pathosis at the perceived location, it is prudent to defer irreversible treatment.

In general, it is prudent to assume that the source of pain is at the location where the patient feels the pain. If this is found not to be the case, consider the source may be in an area adjacent to where the patient feels the pain. Selectively anesthetizing a limited anatomical area may also help localize the source of pain. If the source of pain cannot be attributed in the

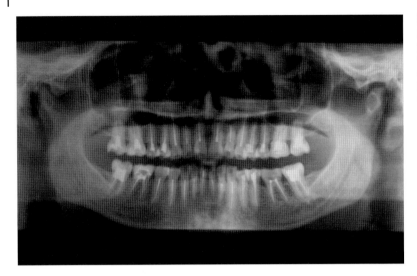

Figure 8.1 Panoramic radiograph of patient with TMD whose primary complaint was painful teeth. Wright (2014).

region, then consider that the pain is referred, leading to the possibility that the pain may have a central etiology.

Evaluating Patients with Tooth Pain

Whenever possible, it is best to accomplish an initial visual and tactile examination of the oral cavity prior to asking the patient to point out the area of pain. Procedures useful in evaluating tooth pain include palpation, percussion, thermal challenge (hot and cold), exploration, occlusal assessment, and periodontal probing to assess the periodontium. Radiographs often reveal valuable information pertaining pain etiology (e.g. periradicular abscess, fracture, periodontal disease, osseous pathology).

Percussion is a proven and simple protocol used to assess for tooth pain and the pattern of response provides valuable information. In this regard, it is beneficial to percuss all of the teeth. If a single tooth is responsive to percussion testing, the likelihood of it being the source of the pain is increased. However if multiple posterior maxillary teeth are percussion positive, the likelihood of pain due to sinusitis is increased. Furthermore, when the patient experiences percussion tenderness in multiple mandibular and maxillary teeth the possibility of significant parafunctional habits should be

considered. Such patients may benefit from wearing a diagnostic occlusal appliance to help determine if the etiology of pain is related to nighttime or daytime clenching habits.

When localization by palpation or percussion is equivocal, a protocol using step-by-step diagnostic anesthetic injections could help. In these situations a local anesthetic agent may be administered around a tooth by intraligamentary injection, regionally by inferior alveolar nerve block, or by maxillary infiltration. The technique is predicated on anesthetizing the smallest area possible that is considered to be the domain and progress to larger regions as may be necessary. For example, if a single tooth is suspected of being the source of pain, an intraligamentary injection could be administered to that specific tooth. An intraligamentary injection is preferred to rule out pain in a single tooth, because buccal or lingual infiltration or an inferior alveolar block will anesthetize more teeth, soft tissue, and masticatory muscles in the region. However, the practitioner must be cognizant that an intraligamentary injection may anesthetize as many as two teeth on each side of the injected tooth.

If the source of pain is determined not to be a tooth, the possibility of referred pain should be investigated. Pain referral patterns associated

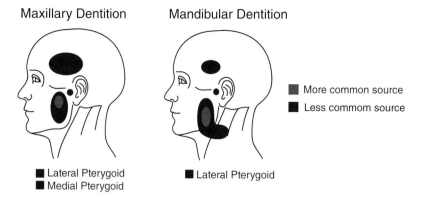

Maxillary Dentition Mandibular Dentition

■ More common source
■ Less commom source

■ Lateral Pterygoid   ■ Lateral Pterygoid
■ Medial Pterygoid

Figure 8.2 Locations responsible for producing referred pain to the teeth, gingiva, and alveolar bone. Adapted from Wright (2014). The superficial sites that caused referred pain to the labeled regions are highlighted on the drawing and the intraoral palpation locations are listed below the drawing.

with TMDs, are fairly consistent and palpable trigger points or nodules are usually present. Pain referred to maxillary posterior teeth can most often be reproduced by palpating tender nodules within the superior portion of the masseter muscle; pain referred to mandibular posterior teeth can most commonly be produced by palpating tender nodules within the inferior portion of the masseter muscle.

To reproduce referred tooth pain, the practitioner should palpate the tenderest nodule within the masseter muscle. Pressure is then applied to load the nodule, up to the patient's tolerance level (this technique requires a significant amount of force) and held for approximately five seconds or until the tooth pain is reproduced. While applying pressure on the masseter muscle, the palm of the other hand is placed on the contralateral side of the mandible to stabilize it.

If loading the first nodule did not reproduce the patient's tooth pain, the process is repeated by loading the next tender nodule. If such testing proves negative, less common sources of referred pain (Figure 8.2) should be investigated. If the tooth pain could not be reproduced from the musculoskeletal structures, but the masticatory muscles are quite tender, trial therapy with either a muscle relaxant taken

Table 8.2 Medications to temporarily reduce sinus pain.

Category	Medication	Instructions
Oral decongestant	60 mg pseudoephedrine HCl	1 tab q 4–6 hours
Nasal spray decongestant	0.05% oxymetazoline HCl	2 sprays in each nostril q 12 hours
Antibiotic	500 mg amoxicillin/ clavulanate	1 tab t.i.d. for 10 days

Source: Reproduced with permission from Wright EF (2014), Manual of Temporomandibular Disorders. 3rd ed. Wiley Blackwell Publishing Co, Ames, IA. © 2014, John Wiley & Sons.

at night or an occlusal appliance worn at night should be considered and the response assessed.

If no tooth- or TMD-related pathoses are found in the perceived area of pain, the patient should be re-queried whether he/she has a cold, flare-up of allergies, or sinus congestion. If so, it may be beneficial to prescribe the patient one or more of the medications listed in Table 8.2 to determine whether the medications temporarily relieve the patient's pain. It is of note that if the pain is of recent onset due to a cold, it is probably of viral origin and antibiotics would not be beneficial.

When there is no evidence of overt odontogenic pathoses that may explain the patient's tooth pain, when the pain cannot be reproduced and/or its intensity cannot be modulated by various manipulations, when no verifiable referral points are in play, or when pain is not significantly reduced by various selective pharmacological means, the practitioner should suspect that the pain may be due to a central disorder and the patient should be referred to a neurologist for evaluation.

Evaluating Patients with Symptoms of TMD

When evaluating patients initially suspected to have TMD pain, the aforementioned palpation assessment for referred tooth pain should be accomplished. When palpating the masticatory muscles and associated structures, a comparison should be made as to which area is most tender and most readily reproduces the pain complaint. Additionally during the clinical exam, TMJ noises, and range of motion should be evaluated.

During the initial evaluation for suspected TMD, precipitating and contributing factors (e.g. nocturnal parafunctional habits, neck pain, poor sleep, and stress) should be identified from the history. The most cost-effective therapy for TMD generally focuses on reducing identified TMD contributing factors, which then enables the body to heal itself. In evaluating pain associated with TMDs, one must also consider non-TMD-related causes.

Just as TMD pain can be referred to the teeth, a tooth can refer pain to the masticatory muscles and the TMJ. Muscles often tighten in respond to pain in the region (protective muscle splinting) and odontogenic pain commonly causes the masseter muscles to tighten. This muscle tension increases TMJ loading and, thereby, causes pain within the masticatory muscles as well as the TMJ. Hence, the pain is commonly misdiagnosed as being of TMD origin.

A study of patients whose pain was originally diagnosed by general dentists as TMD pain, but was later diagnosed to be primarily referred odontogenic pain, reported that none of the periapical radiographs revealed apical pathosis and that palpable musculoskeletal triggers points were present. The study identified four helpful characteristics of tooth pain masquerading or referring as TMD pain:

- A sensation of throbbing was a consistent finding.
- Pain often awakened the patient from sleep.
- Increased pain intensity occurred when the patient assumed a supine position.
- Increased pain intensity occurred when the patient drank hot or cold liquids.

When pain of odontogenic origin is suspected as the cause of, or contributing factor, to a patient's perceived symptoms of TMD, the practitioner must make every effort to identify the offending tooth. In attempting to identify the offending tooth, one should remember that anterior teeth – canine to contralateral canine – may refer bilaterally, while the premolars and molars may refer pain to the ipsilateral side.

Even bilateral symptoms of TMD do not exclude the possibility of referred pain from a posterior tooth. It is common to observe patients with posterior odontogenic pain contributing to their symptoms of bilateral ache, pressure, and/or dull pain in addition to unilateral throbbing pain. The offending tooth is subsequently identified as a posterior tooth on the throbbing side, and the contralateral ache, pressure, and/or dull pain is due to coexisting TMD.

If a patient reports his/her musculoskeletal pain increases when drinking hot or cold liquids, he or she should be asked to identify the offending quadrant or tooth. Appropriate provocative testing (e.g. palpation, percussion, thermal challenge, and exploration) can then be accomplished to identify the pain source. All patients in the study mentioned earlier, who were diagnosed initially with TMD pain, had tooth-related tenderness to percussion. Patients with a positive hyper-responsive thermal test also reported lingering pain within the tooth and confirmed that the pain did refer to the location of their chief complaint (e.g. masseter muscle). Finally, their practitioners confirmed that the tests reproduced the cycle or pattern of pain described by patients during their initial interviews.

When the thermal test reveals a hyper-responsive pulp, an intraligamentary injection of a local anesthetic to the suspected tooth will help determine its contribution to the perceived TMD pain. Prior to the injection, the patient should rate their current TMD pain on a 0–10 scale, where 0 is no pain and 10 is the worst pain imaginable. If the intraligamentary injection dramatically reduces or eliminates the TMD pain, odontogenic pain is significantly contributing to the pain complaint.

An intraligamentary injection technique is recommended for anesthetic testing, because traditional injections may anesthetize the ipsilateral lateral pterygoid or medial pterygoid muscles. As previously noted, an intraligamentary injection may cause pulpal anesthesia of as many as two teeth on each side of the anesthetized tooth. Therefore, traditional provocative testing should be used to identify the suspect tooth before an anesthetic challenge is performed.

Pain associated with a TMD most commonly occurs in the preauricular, masseter, and/or anterior temporalis muscle regions and cervical pain is frequently referred to these regions. Indeed, it has been shown that cervical pain is a contributing factor in about 50% of the patients diagnosed with a TMD. When cervical pain is a significant contributor to the symptoms of a TMD, the patient will not be able to obtain significant symptom relief without treating the cervical pain as well.

Referred cervical pain can usually be brought on by palpating tender trigger points at the base of the posterior skull within the splenius capitis and trapezius muscles. While placing the non-palpating hand on the patient's forehead to stabilize the head, the practitioner can identify the trigger points by placing a fingertip approximately 1 in. below the base of the posterior skull, and then pressing inward and upward. The trigger points feel like firm knots and are tenderer than the surrounding muscle. In general, several trigger points can be identified on patients with TMD and/or cervical pain. Once located, each trigger point should be loaded as previously described to determine and document the referred pain locations.

Evaluating Patients with Intraoral Neuropathic Pain

The diagnosis of neuropathic pain is essentially one of exclusion and should be considered after neurovascular and musculoskeletal sources have been exhausted. In general, patients can accurately identify the location of their intraoral neuropathic pain and practitioners can confirm the domain by light palpation. The application of a topical anesthetic over the region may provide further confirmatory information. If the topical anesthetic agent does not provide significant pain relief, local anesthesia may be administered to determine its effect. This technique will usually provide the confirmatory information necessary to substantiate the clinical impression. The final diagnosis and management of neuropathic pain is best accomplished by a practitioner experienced in the field such as a pain specialist tor a neurologist.

8.3 Plan: Treatment Options

The diagnosis will provide the rational or justification for therapeutic intervention. When there are multiple, overlapping problems, the diagnoses may have to be ordered as primary, secondary, and so on, whereby the primary source represents the most likely cause of the patient's pain. For such cases, the patient must be reminded that while the initial therapeutic intervention may alleviate their pain, more work will be necessary to restore their oral health.

If the patient's pain is determined to be of odontogenic origin (e.g. root sensitivity, caries, pulpitis, cracked tooth, etc.) appropriate restorative, endodontic, or oral surgical interventions should be accomplished. If the pain is determined to be of periodontal origin appropriate periodontal or oral surgical care should be rendered. If the patient's pain is believed to be related to a sinus problem, the patient should be referred to the patient's primary care provider or to an otolaryngologist.

A diagnosis of reversible pulpalgia not associated with dental caries may be related to a

Table 8.3 TMD self-management instructions.

1. Massage your painful muscles, as you find this beneficial. Use your index, middle, and ring fingers in a rolling motion over your skin with a pressure slightly greater than what is needed to produce your pain. Some patients find it beneficial to locate and knead the most painful portion of the muscle for approximately one minute. Be careful not to hurt yourself by too aggressively massaging your muscles.
2. Apply heat, ice or a combination of heat and ice to the painful areas. Determine and use which ever provides you with the greatest amount of relief; most patients prefer heat.
   a. Use heat for 20 minutes two or four times each day. Some patients prefer to use moist heat, whereas others find dry heat just as effective and less of a hassle. Moist heat can be obtained by wetting a thin washcloth with very warm water. The washcloth can then be kept warm by placing it against a heating pad separated by a piece of plastic wrap.
   b. Use the combination of heat and ice two to four times each day. Apply heat to the painful area for approximately 5 minutes (less if it aggravates your pain). Then apply an ice cube wrapped in a thin washcloth.
   c. Apply ice wrapped in a thin washcloth until you first feel some numbness and then remove it (this usually takes about 10 minutes).
3. Eat soft foods like casseroles, canned fruits, soups, eggs, and yogurt. Do not chew gum or eat hard foods (e.g. raw carrots) or chewy foods (e.g. caramels, steak, and bagels). Cut other foods into small pieces, evenly divide the food on both sides of your mouth, and chew on both sides.
4. Avoid caffeine because it stimulates your muscles to contract and hold tension. Caffeine or caffeine-like drugs are found in coffee, tea, most sodas, and chocolate. Decaffeinated coffee also has some caffeine, whereas Sanka has none.
5. Your teeth should never touch except lightly when you swallow. Closely monitor yourself for a clenching or grinding habit. People often clench their teeth when they are irritated, drive a car, use a computer, or concentrate. Learn to keep your jaw muscles relaxed, teeth separated, and tongue resting lightly on the roof of your mouth just behind your upper front teeth.
6. Observe for and avoid additional habits that put unnecessary strain on your jaw muscles and joints. Some habits include, but are not limited to, resting your teeth together; tapping your teeth together; resting your jaw on your hand; biting your cheeks, lips, fingernails, cuticles, or any other objects you may put in your mouth; pushing your tongue against your teeth; and holding your jaw in an uncomfortable or tense position.
7. Posture appears to play a role in TMD symptoms. Try to maintain good head, neck, and shoulder posture. You may find that a small pillow or rolled towel supporting your lower back may be helpful. Ensure you maintain good posture when using a computer and avoid poor postural habits such as cradling the telephone against your shoulder.
8. Your sleep posture is also important. Avoid positions that strain your neck or jaw, such as stomach sleeping. If you sleep on your side, keep your neck and jaw aligned.
9. Set aside time once or twice a day to relax and drain the tension from your jaw and neck. Patients often benefit from simple relaxation techniques such as sitting in a quiet room while listening to soothing music, taking a warm shower or bath, and slow deep breathing. Once you have learned to relax and drain the tension from your jaw and neck, continually monitor these. Whenever tension is observed, release it.
10. Restrain from opening your mouth wide, such as yawning, yelling, or prolonged dental procedures.
11. Use anti-inflammatory and pain-reducing medications, such as non-steriodal anti-inflammatory, ibuprofen, acetaminophen, and aspirin, to reduce joint and muscle pain. Avoid over-the-counter medications containing caffeine with aspirin.

Source: Adapted from Wright (2014).

high restoration where the offending tooth is the first closure contact. These rather common occurrences respond well to minor occlusal adjustment. For tooth pain due to heavy daytime and/or nighttime parafunctional habits, there are three therapeutic options:

- Ask the patient to observe for and break the clenching or grinding habit (some patients may be unable or unwilling to do so).
- Prudently adjust the occlusion (e.g. remove the excursive contacts on a posterior tooth). Appropriate expertise is necessary to accomplish this irreversible intervention.
- Fabricate a stabilization appliance, which while interposed between the opposing teeth will interfere with the habit.

If the perceived tooth pain is not due to local or regional factors, but is referred from a masticatory muscle or TMJ, therapies should be directed toward treating the structures that reproduce the patient's symptoms. Most symptoms of chronic TMD pain can be effectively managed by using TMD self-management techniques (Table 8.3) and by eliminating parafunctional and muscle-tensing habits. It is useful to distinguish whether the TMD pain occurs only at night, only during the day, or around the clock. Specific strategies to address nocturnal, daytime, and around the clock TMD pain are presented in Tables 8.4, 8.5, and 8.6 respectively.

Table 8.4 Primary therapies for patients who awake with TMD symptoms (recommend providing in this order).

1. Ask the patient to improve sleep posture (e.g. stop sleeping on stomach)
2. Provide a stabilization appliance for the patient to wear at night
3. Prescribe a medication that decreases nocturnal EMG activity [e.g. gabapentin 100 mg, 2–3 tabs h.s.; nortriptyline – 10 mg, 1–5 tabs, 0–3 h prior to bed; or cyclobenzaprine (Flexeril) 5 mg, 1–2 tabs h.s.]
4. Fabricate a soft appliance to oppose the patient's hard or intermediate appliance
5. Ask the patient to perform a relaxation session just prior to going to sleep, which may require a referral to a psychologist to train the patient how to perform this

Awaking headache may also be from heavy snoring or sleep apnea causing fragmented sleep and/or a decrease in oxygen levels during sleep.

Some treatment effects generally carry over to the other portion of the day, so patients with mild daytime pain may find these therapies provide them with satisfactory improvement.

Source: Adapted from Wright (2014).

Table 8.5 Primary therapies for patients with daytime TMD symptoms.

- Ask the patient to break daytime parafunctional and muscle-tensing habits, which may require a referral to a psychologist to assist the patient.
- Ask the patient to continually keep the masticatory muscles relaxed throughout the day, which may require a referral to a psychologist to train the patient. The psychologist may escalate therapy and use biofeedback to help the patient understand how to relax the masticatory muscles.
- Refer the patient to a psychologist to learn stress management and coping skills for life's irritations and frustrations.
- Provide the patient with a stabilization appliance to wear during the day (as a temporary reminder about daytime habits and keeping the masticatory muscles relaxed throughout day, and to increase the occlusal stability for when the patient clenches).
- Prescribe a tricyclic antidepressant that does not cause drowsiness (e.g. desipramine – 25 mg, 1 tab in the morning and 1 tab in the afternoon).

Some treatment effects generally carry over to the other portion of the day, so patients who awake with mild daytime pain may find these therapies provide them with satisfactory improvement.

Source: Wright (2014).

Table 8.6 Therapies beneficial for both TMD symptoms that occur upon awaking and during the daytime

- Prescribe medications (e.g. topical [e.g. Voltaren Gel] or oral NSAIDs, muscle relaxants, tricyclic antidepressants, etc.)
- Ask the patient to perform physiotherapy at home or receive them from a physical therapist (e.g. heat, ice, ultrasound, iontophoresis).
- Ask the patient to perform jaw exercises.
- Ask the patient to perform head and neck posture improvement exercises.
- Refer the patient for cervical therapies provided by a physical therapist to relieve neck pain.

Source: Adapted from Wright (2014).

When treating a patient with both TMD and cervical pain, depending on the severity of pain in each domain, the practitioner must decide whether to treat one or both components. Although, the diagnosis and treatment of cervical pain is within the scope of dental practice, it is recommended that patients with cervical pain be referred to a physical therapist with extensive experience with treating pain in this region of the body.

Finally, if the patient's pain is determined to most likely be neuropathic, the patient should be referred for evaluation by a neurologist or a practitioner experienced in the management of craniofacial pain.

8.4 Summary

Patients with orofacial pain rightfully expect that their dentist will be able promptly diagnose and manage their pain. The correct diagnosis, and subsequent therapeutic intervention, requires that the practitioner correctly interprets and correlates the historical and clinical findings to establish a coherent, defendable, relevant, and timely diagnosis. While in most cases, this expectation will be easily met, some patients will present with pain for which the etiology will be a challenge to determine. Furthermore, some patients will present with multiple, overlapping pain conditions further challenging the diagnostic acumen of the practitioner.

Suggested Reading

Bell, G.W., Joshi, B.B., and Macleod, R.I. (2011). Maxillary sinus disease: diagnosis and treatment. *Br. Dent. J.* 210 (3): 113–118.

Bendixen, K.H., Terkelsen, A.J., Baad-Hansen, L. et al. (2012). Experimental stressors alter hypertonic saline-evoked masseter muscle pain and autonomic response. *J. Orofac. Pain* 26 (3): 191–205.

Benjamin, P. (2011). Pain after routine endodontic therapy may not have originated from the treated tooth. *J. Natl. Dent. Assoc.* 142 (12): 1383–1384.

Clark, G.T. (2012). Nocebo-responsive patients and topical pain control agents used for orofacial and mucosal pain. In: *Orofacial Pain: A Guide to Medications and Management*, 2e

(eds. G.T. Clark and R.A. Dionne), 84–94. Ames, IA: Wiley Blackwell.

Cooper, B.C. and Kleinberg, I. (2007). Examination of a large patient population for the presence of symptoms and signs of temporomandibular disorders. *Cranio. J Craniomandib Sleep Pract* 25 (2): 114–126.

Dental Practice Act Committee (1997). The scope of TMD/orofacial pain (head and neck pain management) in contemporary dental practice. Dental Practice Act Committee of the American Academy of Orofacial pain. *J. Orofac. Pain* 11 (1): 78–83.

Haribabu, P.K., Eliav, E., and Heir, G.M. (2013). Topical medications for the effective management of neuropathic orofacial pain. *J. Natl. Dent. Assoc.* 144 (6): 612–614.

Khan, J., Heir, G.M., and Quek, S.Y. (2010). Cerebellopontine angle (CPA) tumor mimicking dental pain following facial trauma. *Cranio* 28 (3): 205–208.

de Leeuw, R. and Klasser, G.D. (2013). *Orofacial Pain: Guidelines for Assessment, Diagnosis and Management*, 5e. Chicago: Quintessence Publishing Co.

Murrary, G.M. and Peck, C.C. (2010). Etiopathogenesis of muscle disorders. In: *Current Concepts on Temporomandibular Disorders* (ed. D. Manfredini), 61–80. Chicago: Quintessence.

Nasri-Heir, C., Khan, J., and Heir, G.M. (2013). Topical medications as treatment of neuropathic orofacial pain. *Dent. Clin. N. Am.* 57 (3): 541–553.

Okeson, J.P. (2013). *Management of Temporomandibular Disorders and Occlusion*, 7e. St. Louis: CV Mosby Co.

van Selms, M.K., Lobbezoo, F., and Naeije, M. (2009). Time courses of myofascial temporomandibular disorder complaints during a 12-month follow-up period. *J. Orofac. Pain* 23 (4): 345–352.

Vickers, E.R. and Zakrzewska, J.M. (2009). Dental causes of Orofacial pain. In: *Orofacial Pain* (ed. J.M. Zakrzewska), 69–81. London: Oxford University Press.

Walton, R.E. (1986). Distribution of solutions with the periodontal ligament injection: clinical, anatomical, and histological evidence. *J. Endod.* 12 (10): 492–500.

Wright, E.F. (2000). Referred craniofacial pain patterns in patients with temporomandibular disorders. *J. Natl. Dent. Assoc.* 131 (9): 1307–1315.

Wright, E.F. (2008). Pulpalgia contributing to temporomandibular disorder-like pain: a literature review and case report. *J. Natl. Dent. Assoc.* 139 (4): 436–440.

Wright, E.F. (2014). *Manual of Temporomandibular Disorders*, 3e. Ames, IA: Wiley Blackwell.

Wright, E.F. and Gullickson, D.C. (1996). Identifying acute pulpalgia as a factor in TMD pain. *J. Natl. Dent. Assoc.* 127 (6): 773–780.

9

Evidence-Based Treatment Planning in Restorative Dentistry

9.1   Historical Perspective

Efforts to restore teeth have occurred since ancient times, but the modern history of restorative dentistry began when Dr. G.V. Black outlined principles of cavity preparation more than 100 years ago. During the 1890s, Dr. Black and Dr. W.D. Miller observed the positive relationship between plaque and dental caries. Due to limitations of the available science at the time, it was assumed that all plaque was odontopathic. This theory, which has become known as the "nonspecific plaque theory," was accepted well into the twentieth century.

The "surgical model" of dental caries management was a natural outgrowth of the nonspecific plaque theory. The surgical model focused on corrective and reparative interventions for teeth that were damaged by acid-producing oral bacteria. Caries were considered to be the result of ineffective oral hygiene, thus placing the burden of prevention on the patient.

By the 1970s Dr. Walter Loesche determined that only specific bacteria within the dental plaque were odontopathic, resulting in the proposal of the "specific plaque hypothesis." The "medical model of caries" which grew

Physical Evaluation and Treatment Planning in Dental Practice, Second Edition.
Géza T. Terézhalmy, Michaell A. Huber, Lily T. García and Ronald L. Occhionero.
© 2021 John Wiley & Sons, Inc. Published 2021 by John Wiley & Sons, Inc.
Companion Website: www.wiley.com/go/terezhalmy/physical

from the "specific plaque hypothesis" focuses on modifying the oral ecosystem to reduce the level of odontopathogens. The emphasis in the medical model is placed on diagnosis, early intervention, and prevention. Understanding the difference between the surgical and the medical model of caries management is essential to understanding the modern approach to treatment planning.

The contemporary dentist systematically assesses caries risk as an integral component in developing the restorative treatment plan. It is important to discriminate between carious lesions that are likely to advance from lesions that may be successfully remineralized. This strategy is consistent with the concept of minimally invasive dentistry (MID), a concept that emphasizes the conservation of healthy tooth structure wherever possible.

Efforts to reduce caries risk continue to focus on addressing those factors considered to be essential for the development of caries. The Venn diagram in Figure 9.1 illustrates the well-known factors that contribute to the development of caries: odontopathogenic bacteria, a susceptible tooth, time, and a fermentable substrate.

Conventional preservative treatments have focused on altering the factors shown in Figure 9.1. The teeth can be made less

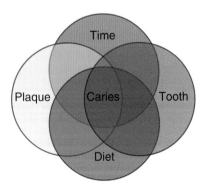

Figure 9.1 The Venn diagram shows that cavities are the result of the interaction between a susceptible tooth, a dietary substrate (fermentable carbohydrate), a chronic bacterial infection in plaque, and time.

susceptible to demineralization through the use of fluorides, fissure sealants, and other non-fluoride agents that promote remineralization. Proper hygiene measures to remove plaque by brushing and flossing have been the focus of anti-caries strategies since the days of G.V. Black. Dietary measures to limit the intake of refined carbohydrates and limiting the duration of carbohydrate exposure reduces the extent of acid challenge to the teeth.

Advances, particularly those of Dr. P.D. Marsh who developed the Ecological Plaque Hypothesis, have improved our understanding of the complex ecosystem of dental plaque biofilms. This has pointed the way for the development of novel therapeutic measures to prevent the attachment of cariogenic bacteria to the teeth, manipulate cell signaling mechanisms, genetically alter acid producing bacteria, deliver effective antimicrobials, and enhance host defenses. In addition, the search for protective probiotic solutions and a caries vaccine continues.

9.2 Etiology of Dental Caries

In a healthy caries-free mouth a homeostatic balance between protective and pathologic factors is maintained. The development of dental caries represents a failure of homeostasis in which the scale is tipped toward disease (Figures 9.2 and 9.3).

Dental caries occur when, in the presence of other factors, normal healthy bacteria are replaced by acid-producing bacteria. Acid-producing bacteria such as *Streptococcus mutans* and *Lactobacillus* have been implicated as a mixed infection and thrive in acidic pH environments, whereas favorable "healthy" bacteria thrive in neutral to slightly alkaline pH environments. Thus, a diet rich in fermentable carbohydrates that lowers the pH of the oral cavity for repeated or prolonged periods of time promotes the growth of cariogenic bacteria.

Homeostasis

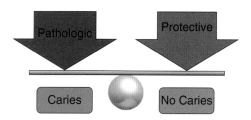

Figure 9.2 Dental homoeostasis is a balance between protective and pathologic factors and there is an equilibrium between the minerals that are lost from the tooth and those that are replaced. (Source: Reproduced with permission from Featherstone 1999 Community Dent Oral Epidemiol Copyright © 1999, John Wiley and Sons All rights reserved.)

Dental Caries

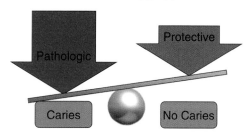

Figure 9.3 Dental caries represents an imbalance between protective and pathologic factors when more minerals are lost from the tooth than are replaced. (Source: Reproduced with permission from Featherstone 1999 Community Dent Oral Epidemiol Copyright © 1999, John Wiley and Sons All rights reserved.)

Early colonization by mutans streptococci in infants is considered to be a major risk factor for future caries development. Genotype analysis has confirmed that mutans streptococci infection is transmitted from the mother to the infant, although other sources of infection are possible. Once introduced, cariogenic bacteria including mutans streptococci and lactobacillus species compete with the normal healthy microorganisms already established in the mouth. These acid-producing microorganisms populate the biofilm that forms on and tenaciously clings to the teeth. The thicker and more mature a biofilm is, the more difficult it is for saliva to buffer the acid generated by the cariogenic bacteria within it.

With a biofilm that contains high numbers of cariogenic bacteria, the eating and drinking of carbohydrates will initiate a rapid drop in the oral cavity pH. The return to normal pH is largely dependent on the buffering efficacy of the saliva and the time necessary to clear the carbohydrates from the oral cavity. During the periods of time that the pH drops below 5.5, calcium and phosphate ions are removed beneath the surface of the enamel of the teeth. When the pH rises back to normal, calcium, and phosphate ions are reabsorbed from the saliva back into to the subsurface of the tooth (remineralization). The more the teeth are exposed to a low pH, such as may occur with frequent snacking, the more likely mineral loss will outpace remineralization. The same imbalance and net loss of minerals can occur if the saliva is of poor quality or quantity and thus unable to adequately buffer an acid challenge.

As more minerals are lost from beneath the surface, the carious lesion eventually presents as an incipient or "white spot" lesion, which is characterized as a smooth intact surface that becomes chalky white when air dried. The white spot lesion will progress as more and more minerals are lost to the tooth. Lost minerals under the tooth surface can be replaced as long as the surface is not cavitated. Cavitation occurs when the weakened subsurface can no longer support the overlying enamel.

Cavitation creates a protective environment for the biofilm in which bacteria may grow undisturbed, accelerating the caries process. Kidd and colleagues have stated that caries can be arrested in advanced lesions where the exposed tooth structure is cleansable and the biofilm can be disturbed. However, cavitated enamel cannot be replaced by remineralization and restorative intervention is usually required to restore function and/or esthetics.

9.3 Caries Lesion Detection, Assessment and Diagnosis

Caries lesion detection involves identifying whether or not a lesion is present by objectively observing a change in the mineral content in the tooth. Assessment of the lesion involves evaluation of physical criteria such as size, depth, and presence or absence of cavitation, and whether or not the damage to the tooth is reversible or irreversible. It takes into account the activity of the lesion and the likelihood of lesion progression. If the lesion is active, preventive or possibly operative, treatment is indicated to arrest lesion progression and to remove and restore diseased tooth structure. In summary, caries diagnosis entails a comprehensive summation of all available data to include an evaluation of the environmental and patient-related risk factors that have contributed to the carious lesion in the first place.

Primary Caries Lesion Detection

G.V. Black classified carious lesions into groups based on their location on the teeth. Class I lesions occur in pits and fissures on the facial, lingual or occlusal surfaces of teeth. Class II lesions occur within the proximal surfaces of posterior teeth. Proximal lesions in anterior teeth, which do not involve the incisal edge, are classified as Class III. Class IV lesions involve the proximal surfaces of anterior teeth which include the incisal edge. Class V caries lesions occur on smooth facial and lingual surfaces. Class VI lesions are in pit or wear defects on the incisal edges of anterior teeth or the cusp tips of posterior teeth. The Black classification system identifies where a lesion occurs, but does not address the extent of damage to the tooth. Modern caries detection systems attempt to assess both the size and activity of the lesion.

Generations of dentists were taught that a detailed examination of teeth included vigorous probing of the pits and fissures with a sharp explorer. Caries were considered to be detected when the explorer that had been forced into a pit or fissure experienced resistance on removal. Ekstrand and others determined that the heretofore classical aggressive or forceful use of sharp explorers may produce irreversible traumatic defects in demineralized areas in occlusal fissures favoring conditions for lesion progression. In keeping with the concept of MID, the use of explorers should be confined to removing plaque and lightly assessing surface hardness.

An ideal caries detection system would provide high sensitivity (the ability to detect the disease when present) as well as high specificity (the ability to eliminate false positives). Dentists have long relied on visual examination aided by radiography to identify caries. Adjuncts to caries lesion detection include fiber optic transillumination (FOTI), electronic caries monitors (ECM), and fluorescence-based devices. When additional tools or devices are used, the clinician must be cognizant to remember that a diagnosis should not be made based solely on a single parameter, but instead, on the totality of the evidence obtained.

Visual Evaluation

For visual evaluation the teeth must be clean and dry, to allow for adequate lesion detection. Drying the tooth with the air water syringe not only removes the superficial saliva from the tooth, but also removes water from the porous subsurface demineralized tissue in a white spot lesion, rendering it more opaque due to increased light scattering. Typically, non-cavitated lesions that are visible even before air-drying have penetrated more deeply into teeth than those that are only visible after five seconds of air-drying. The use of magnification has also been shown to significantly improve upon the accuracy of caries lesion detection as compared to unaided visual examination.

Visual examination is considered the only effective method available to assess caries lesion activity in a single visit. Its use, of course, is best for tooth surfaces that can be visualized directly. Clinical studies using visual examination to detect caries lesions on the proximal surfaces of permanent teeth reveal a sensitivity of only 30%. Therefore 70% of proximal lesions could be missed using visual inspection alone. Another limiting factor of a visual examination is that it is a subjective assessment. Unless the practitioner uses a detailed visual index that describes the characteristics of clinically relevant stages in the caries process, it is difficult to reliably monitor lesion progression over time. In an effort to facilitate monitoring lesions over time, several visual indices have been proposed.

Among the visual indices that have been proposed over the years only a few have been validated in the literature. In an effort to create a standardized, internationally accepted visual caries detection index, a group of cariologists, researchers, educators, and epidemiologists proposed the International Caries Detection Assessment System (ICDAS) in 2002. ICDAS is a two-digit identification system (see Table 9.1 and Figure 9.4). The first digit records the status of the surface as unrestored, sealed, restored, or crowned. The second digit measures the range of involvement from the first

visual changes in the enamel to extensive cavitation. A plus or minus sign is used to record the suspected activity of the lesion based on the visual appearance of the lesion, its surface roughness and the level of plaque stagnation.

ICDAS examinations are conducted on clean dry teeth with adequate light, compressed air and a ball-ended probe that is not used for probing lesions but for gentle detection of surface texture or for removing debris. ICDAS was devised as a detection matrix for primary caries and has been validated for its accuracy in correlating and predicting the histologic progression of the caries lesion into the tooth (Table 9.2).

Ekstrand and others have also related the severity of carious lesions and their histological depth. White spot lesions which require air-drying to be observed are most likely to be limited to the outer 1/2 depth of the enamel. When a white or brown spot lesion is visible without air-drying, its depth is somewhere between the inner 1/2 of the enamel and the outer 1/3 of the dentin. Localized enamel breakdown due to caries, with no visible dentin, indicates that the lesion extends to the middle 1/3 of the dentin. A grayish, brownish or bluish shadow of the dentin shining up through seemingly intact enamel also indicates

Table 9.1 The first digit of the ICDAS scoring system records the restoration status of the tooth; the second digit records the severity of the caries lesion. A plus or minus sign is used to record the suspected activity of the lesion.

Restoration status	Caries severity
0 = Sound: i.e. surface not restored or sealed	0 = sound tooth surface
1 = Sealant, partial	1 = First visual change in enamel (when dry)
2 = Sealant, full	2 = Distinct visual change in enamel (when wet)
3 = Tooth colored restoration	3 = Localized enamel breakdown
4 = Amalgam restoration	4 = Underlying dentin shadow
5 = Stainless steel crown	5 = Distinct cavity with visible dentin
6 = Porcelain or gold or PFM crown or veneer	6 = Extensive cavity with visible dentin
7 = Lost or broken restoration	
8 = Temporary restoration	
Activity	ICDAS Activity +/−

Source: Modified from Ismail et al. (2007).

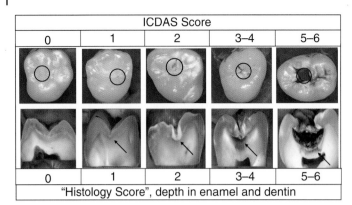

ICDAS Score				
0	1	2	3–4	5–6
0	1	2	3–4	5–6
"Histology Score", depth in enamel and dentin				

Figure 9.4 The ICDAS score as it relates to the clinical depth of the lesion. (Source: Images provided courtesy of Dr. Andrea Ferreira Zandona.)

a lesion extending to the middle 1/3 of dentin. Frank cavities with visible dentin indicate that a lesion extends to inner 1/3 of dentin.

In older adults, arrested non-cavitated lesions may represent a sclerotic response or scars from disease activity occurring years or even decades earlier; however, these scars do not provide useful information about the current disease status of an individual unless they reflect a recent documented change from an active lesion status. Adjunct criteria were subsequently devised for assessing caries lesion activity. Training exercises for using the ICDAS matrix can be found at the ICDAS web homepage.

Radiographic Evaluation

Bitewing radiography is more sensitive than clinical visualization in revealing proximal caries lesions in dentin and is also a reliable way of monitoring caries lesion progression over time. However, radiographs are not without their own set of disadvantages. In addition to the potential hazards of exposure to ionizing radiation, bitewing radiographs underestimate the actual lesion depth (measured histologically) and are unable to accurately show the very early stages of enamel caries lesions. They are also not able to reveal the presence of cavitations or lesion activity, which are both important considerations in planning treatment.

In 1992, Pitts and others correlated bitewing radiography with cavitation. They demonstrated that when the radiolucency was confined to the outer half of enamel, cavitation was not present. If the radiolucency appeared in the inner half of enamel, the presence of cavitation was about 10%. In both situations, preventive non-surgical measures are appropriate.

When the radiolucency had reached the internal half of dentin in the radiograph, the probability of cavitation was 100% and surgical intervention is the treatment of choice. A therapeutic gray zone exists in situations where the radiolucency is just entering into outer half of dentin where the probability of cavitation is about 41%. For such scenarios, knowledge of the patient's caries risk and compliance will help the clinician judge whether to implement preventive measures and monitor the situation or to intervene surgically.

Fiber Optic Transillumination

FOTI is an enhanced visual technique that uses a high-intensity white light to detect caries lesions. The method is more appropriately used for proximal surfaces than occlusal surfaces and for anterior rather than posterior teeth. Demineralized enamel and dentin appear as shadows when transilluminated, but the appearance is not quantitative and interpretation is subjective.

Digital fiber optic transillumination (DIFOTI) is a technique that builds on FOTI but which allows the recording of images of carious lesions during illumination. It also employs a

Table 9.2 The ICDAS severity of lesion score relates the visual appearance of the lesion to the lesion's actual depth.

ICDAS lay terms	Sound	Early stage decay		Established decay		Severe decay	
ICDAS dental terms	Sound	First visual change in enamel	Distinct visual change in enamel	Localized enamel breakdown	Underlying dentin shadow	Distinct cavity with visible dentin	Extensive cavity within visible dentin
ICDAS Detection	0	1	2	3	4	5	6
Depth of lesion	No enamel demineralization or a narrow surface zone of opacity	Demineralization limited to outer 50% of the enamel layer	Demineralization involving between 50% of the enamel and 1/3 of the dentin	Demineralization involving middle 1/3 of the dentin, clinically microcavitated	Demineralization involving middle 1/3 of the dentin, clinically shadowed	Demineralization involving inner 1/3 of the dentin, ± into the pulp, clinically cavitated. Cavitation <1/2 the surface	Demineralization involving inner 1/3 of the dentin, ± into the pulp, clinically cavitated. Cavitation >1/2 the surface
ICDAS activity	ICDAS Activity +/−						

Source: Modified from Ekstrand et al. (1995).

high intensity light and a gray scale camera. Images recorded on a computer allow the clinician to monitor progression of the lesion over time. The advantage of FOTI and DIFOTI over radiographs is the fact that the patient is not subjected to ionizing radiation, and it readily indicates the presence of very early carious lesions, cracks, or imperfections in the tooth surface. However, it may reveal demineralization that does not correlate with cavitation and results should not be interpreted in the same manner as bitewing radiographs.

Electronic Caries Monitors

ECM detect a decrease in electrical resistance or impedance of porous tooth structure relative to sound tooth structure through the use of an alternating current. The ECM uses a probe applied to a specific site on the occlusal surface to register the electrical resistance of the site as a number. Unfortunately, only fair reliability has been reported using this novel device.

Fluorescence-Based Methods

Fluorescence is a phenomenon by which an object is excited by a particular wavelength of light and the fluorescent (reflected) light is of a larger wavelength. When the excitation light is in the visible spectrum, the fluorescence will be of a different color. Caries lesions create a change in the fluorescence properties of dental hard tissues. As a result, several fluorescence-based methods for detecting and quantifying caries lesions have been developed and marketed to assist the clinician in caries assessment. It should be noted that the value and acceptance of these novel products in clinical practice remains a topic of ongoing debate.

The DIAGNOdent laser device (KaVo Dental GmbH, Biberach, Germany) uses laser fluorescence to detect incipient caries. It emits a wavelength of 655 nm through one of two intra-oral tips; one designed for pits and fissures and the other for smooth surfaces. The tip both emits the excitation light and registers the resultant fluorescence. Factors that may influence the outcome of the measurements include the degree of dehydration of tooth, the presence of plaque, calculus, and/or staining on the tooth surface.

Since the system detects fluorescent organic molecules that can be present in any surface deposits, there is an elevated chance of obtaining false positive results. When assessing occlusal surfaces, it is important that the tip be tilted over a range of several different angles in order to access all relevant subsurface regions.

The quantitative light-induced fluorescence (QLF) device emits a blue light (wavelength 370 nm) to excite the tooth surface causing the dental tissues to emit fluorescence in the green spectrum, which is recorded in a computer. Mineral loss in the tooth causes a decrease in the fluorescence and a proprietary computer program is used to quantify the mineral loss. Live images are displayed on a computer screen and individual images of the teeth of interest may be captured and stored. QLF can image all tooth surfaces except proximal surfaces.

9.4 Primary Caries Lesion Diagnosis and Risk Assessment

Once carious lesions have been detected and assessed (Figures 9.5–9.9), the dentist must assimilate all of the data collected in the context of the environment in which the carious lesions developed. All forms of carious lesions (cavitated and pre-cavitated) should be thought of as "symptoms" of the caries disease process itself, with the real cause of the tooth damage being bacterial infection, poor dietary habits, and possibly xerostomia. Thus, treatment should focus on addressing the root causes of caries, not just repairing the symptoms by restoring teeth.

Caries Risk Assessment (CRA) protocols measure the caries status of a patient at a point in time and the information that is gathered

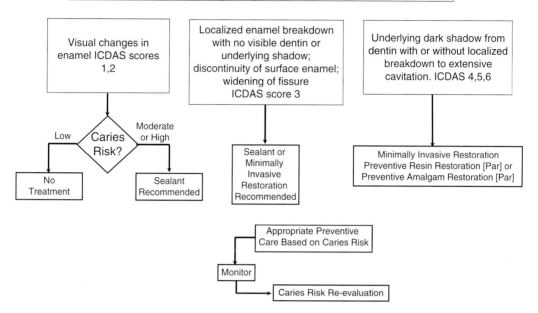

Figure 9.5 Protocol for assessment and management of initial caries lesions in fissured surfaces of permanent teeth. (Source: Courtesy of the Department of Comprehensive Dentistry, University of Texas Health Science Center at San Antonio.)

drives the decision-making process regarding clinical treatment. An example of a CRA form is seen in Table 9.3, which is one of two downloadable CRA forms found on the ADA website. One form is for patients 0–6 years of age and the other is for patients over 6 years of age. The CRA results can be used to help classify patients into categories of low, moderate, or high caries risk based upon the number of risk factors with which they present.

The ADA CRA forms were developed through the efforts of the Councils on Dental Practice (CDP) and Councils on Scientific Affairs (CSA), along with cariology subject matter experts, and with input from the Council on Access, Prevention and Interprofessional Relations (CAPIR). Other CRA forms are available at the California Dental Association's website. Once the caries risk of the patient has been assessed, a meaningful treatment plan can be created. Treatment strategies should

be evidence-based and tailored to address the needs of each individual patient.

9.5 Developing a Minimally Invasive Evidence-Based Treatment Plan Predicated on Caries Risk

The caries risk category of the patient is used to develop a preservative treatment plan. Caries Management by Risk Assessment (CAMBRA) provides a method of selecting preservative interventions and management strategies that are based on the patient's needs. CAMBRA was initially started in 2003 among a coalition of California Dental Schools, but has since grown into a national effort under the auspices of the American Dental Education Association. CAMBRA identifies the cause of disease through the assessment of risk factors

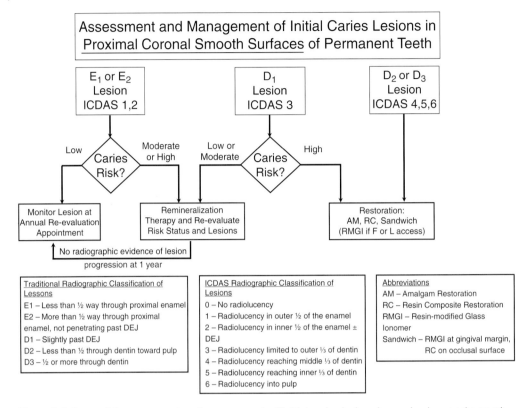

Figure 9.6 Protocol for assessment and management of initial caries lesions in proximal coronal smooth surfaces of permanent teeth. (Source: Courtesy of the Department of Comprehensive Dentistry, University of Texas Health Science Center at San Antonio.)

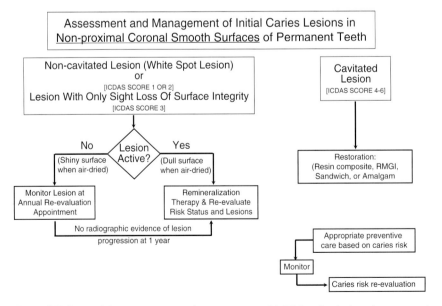

Figure 9.7 Protocol for assessment and management of initial caries lesions in non-proximal coronal smooth surfaces of permanent teeth. (Source: Courtesy of the Department of Comprehensive Dentistry, University of Texas Health Science Center at San Antonio.)

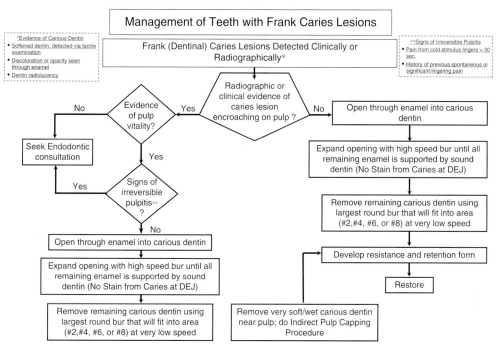

Figure 9.8 Protocol for assessment and management of teeth with frank caries lesions. (Source: Courtesy of the Department of Comprehensive Dentistry, University of Texas Health Science Center at San Antonio.)

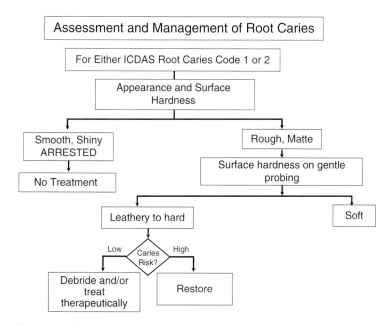

Figure 9.9 Protocol for assessment and management root caries lesions. (Source: Courtesy of the Department of Comprehensive Dentistry, University of Texas Health Science Center at San Antonio.)

Table 9.3 Caries risk assessment forms can be downloaded from the ADA website to help dentists evaluate a patient's risk of developing caries.

ADA American Dental Association®

America's leading advocate for oral health

Caries Risk Assessment Form (Age >6)

Patient name:		

Birth date:	**Date:**

Age:	**Initials:**

		Low risk	**Moderate risk**	**High risk**
Contributing conditions		**Check or circle the conditions that apply**		
I.	Fluoride exposure (through drinking water, supplements, professional applications, toothpaste)	☐Yes	☐No	
II.	Sugary foods or drinks (including juice, carbonated or non-carbonated soft drinks, energy drinks, medicinal syrups)	Primarily at meal times ☐		Frequent or prolonged between meal exposures/day ☐
III.	Caries experience of mother, caregiver and/or other siblings (for patients ages 6–14)	No carious lesions in last 24 months ☐	Carious lesions in last 7–23 months ☐	Carious lesions in last 6 months ☐
IV.	Dental home: established patient of record, receiving regular dental care in a dental office	☐Yes	☐No	
General health conditions		**Check or circle the conditions that apply**		
I.	Special health care needs (developmental, physical, medical or mental disabilities that prevent or limit performance of adequate oral healthcare by themselves or caregivers)	☐No	Yes (over age 14) ☐	Yes (ages 6–14) ☐
II.	Chemo/radiation therapy	☐No		☐Yes
III.	Eating disorders	☐No	☐Yes	
IV.	Medications that reduce salivary flow	☐No	☐Yes	
V.	Drug/alcohol abuse	☐No	☐Yes	

Table 9.3 (Continued)

Clinical conditions		Check or circle the conditions that apply		
I.	Cavitated or non-cavitated (incipient) Carious lesions or restorations (visually or radiographically evident)	No new carious lesions or restorations in last 36 months □	1 or 2 new carious lesions or restorations in last 36 months □	3 or more carious lesions or restorations in last 36 months □
II.	Teeth missing due to caries in past 36 months	□No		□Yes
III.	Visible plaque	□No	□Yes	
IV.	Unusual tooth morphology that compromises oral hygiene	□No	□Yes	
V.	Interproximal restorations – 1 or more	□No	□Yes	
VI.	Exposed root surfaces present	□No	□Yes	
VII.	Restorations with overhangs and/or open margins; open contacts with food impaction	□No	□Yes	
VIII.	Dental/orthodontic appliances (fixed or removable)	□No	□Yes	
IX.	Severe dry mouth (xerostomia)	□No		□Yes
Overall assessment of dental caries risk:		**□Low**	**□Moderate**	**□High**
Patient instructions:				

for each individual patient and then seeks to manage those risk factors through behavioral, chemical, and minimally invasive procedures. CAMBRA emphasizes the application of minimally invasive, evidence-based care.

Another available resource for the clinician is the ADA Center for Evidence Based Dentistry website. This site lists current best evidence summaries of available evidence addressing the use of topical and systemic fluoride, non-fluoride caries preventive agents, sealants, and other topics.

Caries management strategies include therapies documented to be very effective such as sealants and fluoride as well as adjunctive therapies to enhance remineralization of lesions that are not cavitated. Potential adjunctive therapies might include xylitol-containing products; buffering rinses for xerostomic patients to replace the cleansing and buffering functions of normal saliva; and calcium and phosphate pastes to replace the normal salivary components for remineralization of tooth structure following the acid production of food ingestion.

The management strategy for the low-risk patient is geared to maintain the balance of protective factors they currently have and to make them aware that their risk for caries can change over time. For this reason, dentists should educate the patient and perform a CRA periodically.

A moderate-risk patient is one who has some risk factors identified and whose caries balance could easily shift to high risk. The goal here is to prevent or arrest any new caries lesion formation. In addition to daily fluoride toothpaste use, the daily use of an over-the-counter (OTC) fluoride rinse such as 0.05% sodium fluoride rinse may be prescribed. Other potential risk factor interventions to consider include dietary counseling, oral hygiene instruction and more frequent recall. Finally, the use of sealants as a preventive measure may be justifiable in this risk category.

Patients in the high risk group must be more aggressively managed and recalled more frequently than those in the moderate risk group. Consideration should be given to prescribing high concentration 1.1% sodium fluoride (NaF) toothpaste to be used twice daily in lieu of OTC fluoride toothpaste. In addition, the application of fluoride varnish should be accomplished at all dental appointments.

The decision to manage an existing carious lesion by remineralization or by surgical means (excision and restoration) is influenced by the location, extent, and activity status of the lesion (active or arrested). If surgical treatment is indicated for a cavitated lesion, the principles of MID should apply.

The MID strategy chosen to treat a carious lesion is based on where the lesion occurs (occlusal fissured surfaces, proximal smooth surfaces, or non-proximal smooth surfaces); its extent (cavitated or not); and its caries activity. Although the pathogenesis of the caries process is the same at all sites, the differences in site morphology, mineral content, and detection accessibility generate different management strategies.

Occlusal Fissured Surfaces of Teeth

Using the ICDAS scoring system, pits, and fissures identified as codes 0–2 do not require sealants. Sealants are considered optional. Pits and fissures classified as two to three should have a minimally invasive "caries biopsy" (conservative fissure widening) to determine whether a sealant or restoration should be placed. Aggressive prevention and early minimal intervention is indicated for those at higher risk.

Proximal Coronal Smooth Surface Lesions

If the surface of a smooth surface lesion is not cavitated, then remineralization is the recommended treatment. Based on the probability of cavitation associated with the radiographic appearance, enamel-only lesions should be remineralized and carious lesions that extend to the inner half of the dentin should be restored. Lesions that extend to the outer half of dentin have a 41% chance of being cavitated and so other factors such as the patient's caries risk and the site's susceptibility to biofilm stagnation should be factored into the decision to remineralize or to restore.

Non-Proximal Coronal Smooth Surfaces of Permanent Teeth

Unlike proximal smooth surface carious lesions, non-proximal coronal smooth surfaces of permanent teeth can be visualized and an assessment of activity can be made. If the lesion is arrested, and appears smooth and shiny when air dried, no treatment is indicated. However, if the lesion is dull when air dried, remineralization should be initiated. Cavitated lesions usually require surgical intervention and restoration to prevent the biofilm from stagnating in the irregular surface of the cavitation.

Frank Cavitation

Depending upon their depth, caries lesions with frank cavitation should be assessed for vitality, and depending upon the findings, restored appropriately.

9.6 Diagnosis and Treatment of Root Caries Lesions

The incidence of root caries lesions has significantly increased with the aging of the population and the increased retention of teeth. It has been estimated that 60–90% of adults are affected. The challenge to develop evidence based protocols to both diagnose and effectively manage this ubiquitous disease persists.

There are a number of risk factors that contribute to root caries lesion formation: high coronal caries rates, exposed root surfaces, subgingival restoration margins, inadequate oral hygiene, cariogenic diets, lack of fluoride in water system, clasp location with removable partial dentures, advanced age, smoking, alcoholism, and illicit drug use. Hyposalivation caused by such conditions as Sjögren's syndrome, head and neck radiation treatment, or xerogenic medications also contribute to increased root caries risk.

The etiopathogenesis of root caries is similar to coronal caries lesion formation. However, the acid concentration that causes demineralization in dentin is weaker than the acid that causes demineralization in enamel. Dentin and cementum have a critical pH of 6.2 and enamel has a critical pH of 5.5. Root surfaces are six times more soluble because of the increased organic matrix. The demineralization cycle is found to be more intensive and lasts longer with root caries. This demineralization process is additionally exacerbated by reduced salivary buffering capacity and flow.

To more adequately detect root caries lesions, a thorough dental prophylaxis to remove debris and tooth accumulated material is recommended before the clinical examination. Root caries often occur supragingivally, and close to the cement-enamel junction. These lesions are most commonly found on proximal surfaces, followed by facial surfaces. Clinicians detect root caries lesions by evaluating color changes that range from yellow to brown to black, textural surface changes ranging from regular to irregular and from hard to soft. The International Caries Detection and Assessment System (ICDAS), using visual criteria, can also been applied to root caries lesions. Though a description of coding criteria based on clinical appearance has been shown to provide a predictable combination of specificity and sensitivity for root caries detection, there is no consensus on the correlation between color and underlying caries activity.

In combination with risk assessment, judicious probing of root caries allows the operator to determine if no treatment is needed, if the lesion can be arrested, or if a restoration is indicated. The tactile feel of softness noted on gentle exploration correlates well with the microbiologic activity of the root caries lesion. However, the clinician should be aware that probing root surfaces may create defects that may not respond to remineralization efforts. Active lesions that are soft, highly infected, and found close to the gingival margin are normally scheduled for restoration. Leathery to hard lesions should be considered for restoration or therapeutic remineralization depending on the patient's level of caries risk.

Bitewing radiographs, preferably vertical, can aid in the detection of early caries lesions in interproximal areas. Proper radiographic technique minimizes the occurrence of cervical burnout, which can compromise diagnostic accuracy.

The management protocol for patients at risk for root caries is depicted in Figure 9.9. This includes eliminating the sources of active infection (cavitations), implementing preventive measures, and re-examining the patient at appropriate intervals. The clinical presentation of the lesion and the patient's caries risk status are both considered when determining the treatment options. Dietary counseling is appropriate for all caries risk categories, as is the use of a daily fluoride.

For moderate or high-risk patients, OTC fluoride rinses are recommended. Fluoride applications including fluoride varnishes and APF or 2% sodium fluoride gels in trays are encouraged. Prescription home fluoride dentifrices in the 5000 ppm range have been found to be more effective than OTC 1100 ppm dentrifices. There is also limited evidence to support the use of Xylitol containing sugarless gums or mints; triclosan; and calcium/phosphate containing toothpastes to further protect the teeth.

Cavitated lesions require caries excavation and restoration and the extent of the preparation is dictated by the extent of the lesion. There is an obvious challenge for the clinician is to establish proper isolation and access to the lesions. Root caries may be restored satisfactorily with amalgam, resin modified glass ionomer, conventional glass ionomer or resin composite. Fluoride-releasing materials are the preferred restorative choice due to their ability to re-charge after exposure to topical fluorides, and proven adhesive bonding properties. These may be particularly beneficial when managing xerostomic patients or patients whose compliance with daily fluoride use is in doubt.

The recall interval for a patient with root caries lesions should be carefully determined based on the patient's caries risk and response to treatment. The low caries risk patient may be re-examined once a year, the moderate risk patient at six months, and the high risk patient every three months. At recall appointments, oral hygiene should be reinforced along with diet considerations and preventive measures.

9.7 Clinical Detection and Diagnosis of Secondary or Recurrent Caries Lesions

The terms secondary or recurrent caries denotes the presence of dental caries at the margins of an existing restoration. Numerous studies have investigated restoration longevity and causes for replacement. One systematic review on restoration longevity reported a mean survival time (MST) of 6–10 years for both amalgam and resin composite restorations. The most frequent reason for failure of either an amalgam or resin composite restoration was secondary caries followed by restoration fracture. Predictably, Class I restorations survived longer than multi-surface restorations. Negative survival factors for resin composites, included young patient age at time of placement and a high caries risk status.

Whether due to secondary caries or mechanical failure, the need for replacement dentistry is high. Various investigators have reported that from 50 to 80% of restorative procedures in general practice involve replacement dentistry. Resin composites fail more frequently than amalgam, multi-surface restorations fail more frequently than single surface restorations, and high caries risk patients experience more restoration failure than low caries risk patients. Historically, amalgam has performed significantly better than resin composite in large posterior restorations. In one study assessing recurrent caries and overhanging margins radiographically with bitewings, the resin composite failure rate was 3.5 times greater than the failure rate of amalgam.

The tools to clinically assess restoration status include many of the same standard tools used for detecting primary caries lesions. Visualization with magnification, use of the air syringe to thoroughly dry the tooth, careful use of the explorer, bitewing radiographs with archival series to assess lesion progression, and FOTI, have all been proven to be effective.

Visualization requires teeth to be clean and dry with an excellent light source and magnification. Subtle color changes such as opacity around the restoration margin can help detect demineralization of dentin while the overlying enamel is still intact. The general use of the explorer when dealing with primary caries lesions has been extensively debated and found to not improve diagnostic accuracy when compared to a visual exam with a carefully dried tooth and appropriate bitewing radiographs to determine presence of mineral loss. However, when evaluating recurrent caries lesions, the explorer can help remove debris, check margin integrity and determine dentin hardness.

With amalgam margins, it has been shown that there is no clear correlation between marginal ditching and staining as a predictor for the presence of recurrent caries. It has been proven that margin gap size and the probability of caries associated with a restoration occurs only when the defect is very large (250–400 μ). Gaps of less than 35–50 μ are inconsequential. The periodontal probe tip diameter (0.4 mm) is an easy way to assess margin gap size and potential need for intervention.

A clinical carious defect with radiographic evidence of demineralization indicates the presence of soft dentin, not a narrowly ditched margin. Overall, the caries incidence for occlusal ditching of a restoration is low, while the caries incidence for cervical ditching is high. Clinically assessing resin composite margins is more challenging than assessing amalgam margins. One clinical study found soft dentin beneath tooth-colored restorations was heavily infected with mutans streptococci and lactobacilli. However, intervention is recommended only for frank carious lesions that are marginally located.

There are number of considerations and challenges when using radiographs to aid in the detection of recurrent caries lesions. Examples include the "Mach Band" effect (an optical illusion of radiolucency between the abutting edges of the differing shades of gray produced by enamel and dentin), improper angulation techniques that can create distortion, and the possible misinterpretation of the phenomenon of cervical burnout versus actual root caries. Thick radiolucent adhesives under composite restorations, also referred to as "pseudo" lesions, may be misinterpreted as recurrent caries. If it appears there is a uniform radiolucent border around the restoration, one should consider that it represents the dentin bonding agent film thickness, and not an actual recurrent caries lesion. For such cases,

it may be prudent, in light of the patient's caries risk status, to radiographically monitor for lesion progression over time before considering replacement.

9.8 Repair Versus Replacement of Direct Restorations

The restoration survival rate for a direct posterior restoration is estimated to be 6–10 years. As a consequence, a posterior restoration placed in a teenage dental patient may have to be replaced as many as 10 times during that patient's lifetime. When a restoration is removed and replaced, a number of negative results can occur. Significant non-carious tooth structure may be inadvertently removed, thus weakening the remaining tooth structure, and potential pulpal insult can occur if the cavity preparation is deepened.

This phenomenon has been appropriately referred to as the "cycle of re-restoration" in which, as an example, the replacement cycling of an occlusal restoration may result in the eventual need for a full coverage crown. Multiple operative insults to the tooth may stress pulp, resulting in the need for endodontic intervention. Additionally, current patient demands to replace amalgam restorations for esthetic reasons and continued unsubstantiated concerns about mercury safety are contributing to a faster re-restoration cycle. It cannot be clinically justified to remove an entire restoration if only a small portion of it is defective. In an effort to dampen the cycle of re-restoration, protocols to repair or refurbish a restoration have been developed. Prior to attempting repair or refurbishment, a careful assessment of the surrounding restoration and tooth surfaces is necessary (Figure 9.10).

Three choices besides restoration replacement should be considered when considering less than total replacement. The first is *repair*, where there is removal of portion of the restoration to include the localized defect and then the prepared access is restored. Amalgam and resin composites can be used and the use of

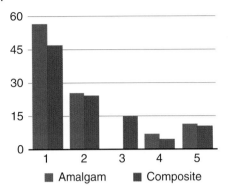

1. Secondary caries
2. Restorative fracture
3. Discoloration
4. Tooth fracture
5. Other reasons
   (missed proximal contact, overhang, poor anatomic form)

■ Amalgam ■ Composite

Figure 9.10 Reasons for replacement of amalgam and composite resin restorations. (Source: Modified from Mjor, I.A. (2005) Reasons for Replacement of Restorations, Recommendations for Clinical Practice. Operative Dentistry, 30 (4), 409-416.)

dental bonding agents and surface roughening can increase retention and marginal seal. A second alternative is the application of a pit and fissure *sealant,* such as a flowable resin composite, to close a non-carious marginal gap on the occlusal surface. Third, *refurbishment* is an alternative way to re-contour and reshape the existing restoration to proper anatomic form and/or remove surface margin stain that may have been caused by flash. Polishing of the existing amalgam restoration margins may be sufficient to smooth the margin gap and ultimately avoid replacement considerations.

A number of studies have investigated the use of minimal intervention techniques to repair, seal or refurbish amalgam or resin composite restorations, and several have compared the clinical results against replacement for up to seven years. The current consensus is that these conservative techniques increase the longevity of restorations that presented with marginal discrepancy, anatomic form problems, surface roughness, and marginal staining. More recently, the use of repair versus replacement therapies was investigated in the Dental Practice-Based Research Network (DPBRN) of 197 dental practices. Of the 9484 defective restorations occurring in 7502 patients, 75% were replaced, while 25% were repaired. As in previous studies, recurrent caries was the main need for intervention. It was also noted that the decision to repair rather than replace a defective restoration occurred more frequently in large group practices and among recent dental school graduates.

9.9 Summary

The principles of preservative dentistry can be equally applied to coronal and root caries lesions and to the management of existing defective restorations. MID represents a holistic approach to caries disease management that identifies and manages the etiological factors that cause dental caries, applies conservative principles in preparation design, and addresses where possible the multitude of factors that influence restoration longevity.

Suggested Reading

Amaechi, B.T., van Amerongen, J.P., van Loveren, C. et al. (2013). Caries management: diagnosis and treatment strategies. In: *Summitt's Fundamentals of Operative Dentistry: A Contemporary Approach*, 4e (eds. T.J. Hilton, J.L. Ferracane and J.C. Broome), 93–130. Chicago: Quintessence Publishing Co, Inc.

Anderson, M.H., Bales, D.J., and Omnell, K.A. (1993). Modern management of dental caries, the cutting edge is not the dental bur. *J. Am. Dent. Assoc.* 124: 37–44.

Bader, J.D. and Brown, J.P. (1993). Dilemmas in caries diagnosis. *J. Am. Dent. Assoc.* 124 (6): 48–50.

Banting, D.W. (2001). The diagnosis of root caries. *J. Dent. Educ.* 65 (10): 991–995.

Baysan, A., Ellwood, R., Davies, R. et al. (2001). Reversal of primary root caries using dentifrices containing 5000 and 1100 PPM fluoride. *Caries Res.* 35: 41–46.

Berkowitz, R.J. (2003). Acquisition and transmission of mutans streptococci. *J. Calif. Dent. Assoc.* 31 (2): 135–138.

Black, G.V. (1908). *A Work on Operative Dentistry in Two Volumes. Volume One. The Pathology of Hard Tissues of the Teeth. Volume Two. The Technical Procedures in Filling Teeth.* Medico-Dental Publishing Co.

Braga, M.M., Mendex, F.M., and Ekstrand, K.R. (2010). Detection activity assessment and diagnosis of dental caries lesions. *Dent. Clin. N. Am.* 54 (3): 479–493.

Brantley, C.F., Bader, J.D., Shugars, D.A. et al. (1995). Does the cycle of re-restoration Lead to larger restorations? *J. Am. Dent. Assoc.* 126 (10): 1407–1413.

Burgess, J.O. (1995). Dental materials for the restoration of root surfaces caries. *Am. J. Dent.* 8 (6): 342–351.

Burgess, J.O. and Gallo, J.R. (2002). Treating root surface caries. *Dent. Clin. N. Am.* 46: 385–404.

Cochran, M.A. and Matis, B.A. (2004). Root caries: recommendations for clinical practice. *Oper. Dent.* 29 (6): 601–607.

Coppa, A., Bondioli, L., Cucina, A. et al. (2006). Paleontology: early neolithic tradition of dentistry. *Nature* 440 (7085): 755–756.

Downer, M.C., Azil, N.A., Bedi, R. et al. (1999). How long do routine dental restorations last? A systematic review. *Br. Dent. J.* 187 (8): 432–439.

Duane, B. (2015). Xylitol and caries prevention. *Evid. Based Dent.* 16 (2): 37–38.

Ekstrand, K., Qvist, V., and Thylstrup, A. (1987). Light microscope study of the effect of probing in occlusal surfaces. *Caries Res.* 21 (4): 368–374.

Ekstrand, K.R., Kuzmina, I., Bjørndal, L. et al. (1995). Relationship between external and histologic features of progressive stages of caries in the occlusal fossa. *Caries Res.* 29 (4): 243–250.

Ericson, D. (2004). What is minimally invasive dentistry? *Oral Health Prev. Dent.* 2 (Suppl 1): 287–292.

Featherstone, J.D. (1999). Prevention and reversal of dental caries: role of low level fluoride. *Community Dent. Oral Epidemiol.* 27 (1): 31–40.

Featherstone, J.D. (2004). The continuum of dental caries – evidence for a dynamic disease process. *J. Dent. Res.* 83 (Spec Iss C): C39–C42.

Fogie, A.H., Pine, C.M., and Pitts, N.B. (2002). The use of magnification in a preventive approach to caries detection. *Quintessence Int.* 33 (1): 13–16.

Gordan, V.V., Garvan, C.W., Blaser, P.K. et al. (2009). Long-term evaluation of alternative treatments to replacement of RC restorations: 7 year study. *J. Am. Dent. Assoc.* 140: 1476–1484.

Gordan, V.V., Riley, J.L., Geraldeli, S. et al. (2012). Repair or replacement of defective restorations by dentists in the dental practice-based research network (DPBRN). *J. Am. Dent. Assoc.* 143 (6): 593–601.

Hamilton, J.C. and Stookey, G. (2005). Should a dental explorer be used to probe suspected carious lesions? *J. Am. Dent. Assoc.* 136: 1526–1532.

Haveman, C.W., Summitt, J.B., Burgess, J.O. et al. (2003). Three restorative materials and topical fluoride gel used in Xerostomic patients. *J. Am. Dent. Assoc.* 134: 177–183.

Hillman, J.D., McDonell, E., Cvtikovitch, D., and Hillman, C.H. (2007). Modification of an effector strain for replacement therapy of dental caries to enable safety trials. *J. Appl. Microbiol.* 102 (5): 1209–1219.

Ismail, A.I., Sohn, W., Tellez, M. et al. (2007). The international caries detection and assessment system (ICDAS): an integrated system for measuring dental caries. *Community Dent. Oral Epidemiol.* 35: 170–178.

Karlsson, L. and Tranæus, S. (2008). Supplementary methods for detection and quantification of dental caries. *Int. J. Laser Dent.* 16 (1): 6–14.

Keyes, P.H. and Jordan, H.V. (1963). Factors influencing the initiation, transmission and inhibition of dental caries. In: *Mechanisms of Hard Tissue Destruction* (ed. R.J. Harris), 261–283. New York: Academic Press.

Kidd, E.A.M. and Beighton, D. (1996). Prediction of secondary caries around tooth-colored restorations: a clinical and microbiological study. *J. Dent. Res.* 75 (5): 1206–1211.

Kidd, E.A.M. and O'Hara, J.W. (1990). The caries status of Occlusal amalgam restorations with marginal defects. *J. Dent. Res.* 69: 1275–1277.

Kidd, E.A.M., Joyston-Bechal, S., and Beighton, D. (1995). Marginal ditching and staining as a predictor of secondary caries around amalgam restorations: a clinical and microbiological study. *J. Dent. Res.* 74 (5): 1206–1211.

Leake, J.L. (2001). Clinical decision-making for caries management in root surfaces. *J. Dent. Educ.* 65 (10): 1147–1153.

Levin, L., Coval, M., and Geiger, S.B. (2007). Cross-sectional radiographic survey of amalgam and resin-based composite posterior restorations. *Quintessence Int.* 38 (6): 511–514.

Li, Y. and Caufield, P.W. (1995). The fidelity of initial acquisition of mutans streptococci by infants from their mothers. *J. Dent. Res.* 74 (2): 681–685.

Loesche, W.J. (1976). Chemotherapy of dental plaque infections. *Oral Sci. Rev.* 9: 65–107.

Loesche, W.J. (1979). Clinical and microbiological aspects of chemotherapeutic agents used according to the specific plaque hypothesis. *J. Dent. Res.* 58 (12): 2404–2412.

Manhart, J., Chen, H.Y., Hamm, G. et al. (2004). Review of the clinical survival of direct and indirect restorations in posterior teeth of the permanent dentition. *Oper. Dent.* 29 (5): 481–508.

Marsh, P.D. (2003). Are dental diseases examples of ecological catastrophes. *Microbiology* 149 (2): 279–294.

Marsh, P.D. (2006). Dental plaque as a biofilm and microbial community – implications for health and disease. *BMC Oral Health* 6 (Suppl 1): S14.

Marsh, P.D. (2009). Dental plaque as a biofilm: the significance of pH in health and caries. *Compendium* 30 (2): 76–87.

Matis, B.A., Gonzalez-Cabezas, C., and Cochran, M.A. (2013). Diagnosis and treatment of root caries. In: *Summittt's Fundamentals of Operative Dentistry: A Contemporary Approach*, 4e (eds. T.J. Hilton, J.L. Ferracane and J.C. Broome), 369–371. Chicago: Quintessence Publishing Co, Inc.

Millar, B.J., Robinson, P.B., and Davies, B.R. (1992). Effects of removal of composite resin restorations on class II cavities. *Br. Dent. J.* 173 (6): 210–212.

Miller, W.D. (1890). *Micro-Organisms of the Human Mouth*. Philadelphia, PA: S.S. White Dental Manufacturing.

Mjor, I.A. (2005). Clinical diagnosis of recurrent caries. *J. Am. Dent. Assoc.* 136: 1426–1433.

Mjor, I.A. (2005). Reasons for replacement of restorations, recommendations for clinical practice. *Oper. Dent.* 30 (4): 409–416.

Mjor, I.A., Jokstad, A., and Qvist, V. (1990). Longevity of posterior restorations. *Int. Dent. J.* 40: 11–17.

Moncada, G., Martin, J., Fernandez, E. et al. (2009). Sealing, repair and refurbishment of class I and class II defective restorations: a three year clinical trial. *J. Am. Dent. Assoc.* 140 (4): 425–432.

Peters, M.C. (2010). Strategies for noninvasive demineralized tissue repair. *Dent. Clin. N. Am.* 54 (3): 507–525.

Pitts, N. (2004). "ICDAS" – an international system for caries detection and assessment being developed to facilitate caries epidemiology, research and appropriate clinical management. *Community Dent. Health* 21 (3): 193–198.

Pitts, N.B. and Rimmer, P.A. (1992). An in vivo comparison of radiographic and directly assessed clinical caries status of posterior approximal surfaces in primary and permanent teeth. *Caries Res.* 6 (2): 146–152.

Rodrigues, J.A., Lussi, A., Seemann, R. et al. (2000). Prevention of crown and root caries in adults. *Periodotology* 55: 231–249.

Saha, S., Tomaro-Duchesneau, C., Tabrizian, M. et al. (2012). Probiotics and oral health biotherapeutics. *Expert Opin. Biol. Ther.* 12 (9): 1207–1220.

Semecek, J.W., Diefenderfer, K.E., and Cohen, M.E. (2009). An evaluation of replacement rates for posterior RC and AM restorations: US navy and marine corps recruits. *J. Am. Dent. Assoc.* 140 (2): 200–2009.

Shivakumar, K.M., Prasad, S., and Chandu, G.N. (2009). International caries detection and assessment system: a new paradigm in detection of dental caries. *J. Conservative Dent.* 12 (1): 10–16.

Smith, D.J. (2012). Prospects in caries vaccine development. *J. Dent. Res.* 91 (3): 225–226.

Tyler, D.W. and Thurmeier, J. (2001). Amalgam bonding: visualization and clinical implications of adhesive displacement during amalgam condensation. *Oper. Dent.* 26 (1): 81–86.

Warren, J.J., Levy, S.M., and Wefel, J.S. (2003). Explorer probing of root caries lesions: an in vitro study. *Spec. Care Dentist.* 23 (1): 18–21.

Wenzel, A. (2004). Bitewing and digital bitewing radiography for detection of caries lesions. *J. Dent. Res.* 83(Spec Issue, No C): C72–C75.

White, S.N., MacEntree, M.I., and Cho, G. (1994). Restoration treatment for geriatric root Carie. *J. Calif. Dent. Assoc.* 22 (3): 55–61.

Young, D.A. and Featherstone, J.D. (2005). Digital imaging fiber-optic trans-illumination, F-speed radiographic film and depth of approximal lesions. *J. Am. Dent. Assoc.* 136 (12): 1682–1687.

Zambon, J.J. and Kaspazak, S.A. (1995). The microbiology and histopathology of human root caries. *Am. J. Dent.* 8 (6): 342–351.

Zandona, A.F. (2011). Evolution of caries diagnosis. *Dimens. Dent. Hyg.* 9 (9): 84–87.

Zeckel, I., Zandona, A.F., Eckert, G. (2008) Comparing ICDAS on Root Surfaces with Unconventional Caries Detention Tools. IADR/AADR/CADR 87th General Session and Exhibition, Abstract #3362.

10

Periodontal and Peri-Implant Examination

As a result of improvement in understanding and treatment of periodontal diseases over the years, recent epidemiological studies suggest that their respective prevalence have slightly decreased (Borrell et al. 2005; Hugoson and Norderyd 2008). Despite these encouraging results, some studies also suggest that this trend is limited to cases of gingivitis and mild to moderate chronic periodontitis, while prevalence of more advanced and severe cases remain unchanged (Borrell et al. 2005; Hugoson et al. 2008). In fact, the percentage of advanced disease cases referred to specialists has increased over the years (Cobb et al. 2003; Dockter et al. 2006).

Collectively, these studies stress the importance for general practitioners to be adequately trained to examine, diagnose, and either initiate periodontal disease treatment or refer the patient to a specialist in a timely manner. The goals of periodontal therapy as defined by the American Academy of Periodontology (AAP) (Greenwell 2001) are to "preserve, improve and maintain the natural dentition, dental implants, periodontium and peri-implant tissues in order to achieve health, comfort esthetic and function."

Periodontal treatment is part of a comprehensive approach to dental care. The present chapter will focus on the periodontal

Physical Evaluation and Treatment Planning in Dental Practice, Second Edition.
Géza T. Terézhalmy, Michaell A. Huber, Lily T. García and Ronald L. Occhionero.
© 2021 John Wiley & Sons, Inc. Published 2021 by John Wiley & Sons, Inc.
Companion Website: www.wiley.com/go/terezhalmy/physical

examination and diagnosis, while it is assumed that the reader will perform the other examinations necessary to a comprehensive dental treatment planning including recording of the medical history, extra- and intraoral examinations to detect abnormalities, and dental examinations to detect caries and other hard and soft tissue problems.

10.1 Periodontal Evaluation

Comprehensive periodontal evaluation includes: (i) full mouth periodontal charting; (ii) occlusal examination, (iii) comprehensive radiographic evaluation; and (iv) endodontic assessment of teeth, when indicated.

Full-Mouth Periodontal Charting

Only full mouth periodontal charting accurately reflects the extent of periodontal diseases and conditions, and provides the basis for appropriate treatment planning. It is of note that the AAP recommends full-mouth periodontal charting as part of standard of care on an annual basis (Greenwell 2001).

Probing Depth, Clinical Attachment Level and Gingival Recession

In order to measure probing depths (PD), clinical attachment levels (CALs) and recession, a calibrated periodontal probe (such as a UNC-15) is utilized. The probe runs along the gingival sulcus of each tooth and measurements (rounded off to the nearest millimeter) are recorded at six sites per tooth. The PD represents the measurement from the free gingival margin to the base of the probable gingival crevice or the periodontal pocket (in case of an infected site) while applying a force of approximately 0.25N (Newton) to the probe. This amount of force allows for optimal detection of PD changes (Mombelli et al. 1992) and represents a light force which is most often well tolerated by the patients without the use of local anesthesia.

The CAL represents the measurement from a fixed point, i.e. the cementoenamel junction (CEJ) to the base of the probable gingival crevice. In a periodontally healthy individual with no attachment loss, CAL is at the level of the CEJ. If the CEJ is not readily detectable or is missing because of the presence of a restoration, then another fixed reference point (e.g. restoration margin) can substituted in order to measure the relative attachment level. While CAL is essential to establish a diagnosis and evaluate the efficacy of periodontal therapy, it is unlikely to be measured directly by the examiner. Rather, the PDs and recession are commonly recorded.

The CAL is then calculated by summing up the PD and the gingival recession measurements. The latter represents the distance from the CEJ to the gingival margin. In situations where the gingival margin has moved apically to the CEJ, a readily measurable recession is observable and a positive value is given to the recession measurement. However, in pristine periodontal situations, the measurement might be more challenging as the CEJ is located apically to the gingival margin and the examiner must feel for it by running the tip of the probe below the gingival margin. In this case the recession value is negative. Consequently, in cases where the gingival margin and the CEJ are at the same level (recession is 0 mm) PD and CAL have the same value (Figure 10.1).

The reference point from which PDs are measured is the gingival margin. Since this reference point can vary over time (e.g. when the gingiva is inflamed and swollen its location will be more coronal and conversely if a gingival recession occurs its position will be more apical than in a non-inflamed situation) the PD does not represent the ideal measurement to monitor patients' periodontal status over time. Conversely, since CAL is measured repeatedly from a fixed and stable reference point, i.e. the CEJ, attachment levels allow the clinician to assess the extent and severity of the periodontal destruction and are

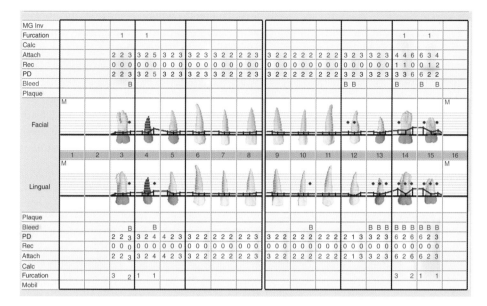

Figure 10.1 Example of comprehensive periodontal charting in the maxilla.

key for establishing a proper diagnosis and to evaluate the patients' periodontal status over time.

Bleeding on Probing

Bleeding on probing (BoP), using light force of 0.25N, is indicative of gingival inflammation. The use of excessive force will result in bleeding, which reflects mechanical trauma instead of gingival inflammation. BoP is usually recorded immediately after PD measurement. A few seconds following probing might be necessary to observe the actual bleeding. Therefore, the clinician usually measures the PD on all the teeth in a quadrant, e.g. facial surface of teeth #1–8, then return to #1 to assess for bleeding from 1 to 8. BoP may be measured at four or six sites per tooth. If BoP recording is done at four sites, three sites are recorded for the facial aspect of the tooth and one site on the palatal aspect, although recording BoP at six sites per tooth provides a more accurate representation of the gingival inflammatory status.

BoP is important to record since it has been shown that the absence of bleeding is a good indicator of clinical stability. In other words,

sites that do not bleed on probing are unlikely to experience future attachment loss (Lang et al. 1986, 1990). Gingivitis is a reversible gingival inflammation. Classic studies have demonstrated that in the absence of good oral hygiene measures, plaque will accumulate around teeth and marginal gingivitis with BOP develops within two to three weeks. Following the resumption of good oral hygiene measures, gingivitis resolves to baseline in approximately one week (Loe et al. 1965).

It is of note that the amount of plaque a patient presents with at a given appointment is only a snapshot on how well the patient has been brushing just before coming to the appointment and not a reflection of how well the patient has been brushing over the last few weeks. This is likely to happen since the patient knows that the dentist may be looking at the quality of the plaque control. In this instance BoP may be a better indicator of the patient's oral hygiene performance since one to two weeks are necessary to eliminate plaque-induced gingivitis at a given site. If a site is BoP then plaque has not been consistently eliminated during the last couple of weeks (Loe et al. 1965; Saxe et al. 1967).

Suppuration

Suppuration is usually an incidental finding during full-mouth periodontal charting; although it may represent an acute symptomatic event reported by the patient. A purulent exudate signifies the presence of an acute bacterial infection originating in the deepened periodontal pocket. If drainage occurs through the periodontal sulcus, the patient may be asymptomatic, but may report a bad or foul taste in their mouth. If there is marginal closure of the periodontal pocket, lack of drainage will lead to swelling and pain. In both scenarios, immediate treatment is required to alleviate pain and/or avoid further periodontal tissues destruction (refer to the periodontal abscesses section under "Acute Conditions").

Furcation Involvement

When periodontitis progresses the furcation area of a multi-rooted tooth can become involved. Bone loss around the area becomes clinically probable not only vertically but also horizontally. Furcation involvement is typically determined using a furcation probe (e.g. Nabers Probe), a curved probe used to determine the degree of horizontal penetration. The degree of furcation involvement may be classified as follows (Hamp et al. 1975):

- Class I: tissue destruction extends up to 3 mm measured horizontally from the most coronal aspect of the furcation.
- Class II: tissue destruction extends deeper than 3 mm, measured horizontally from the most coronal aspect of the furcation, but does not totally pass through the furcation.
- Class III: Also called a "through-and-through involvement" in which tissue destruction extends through the entire furcation. A blunt instrument passed between the roots can emerge on the other side of the tooth.

Furcation areas are not readily accessible for plaque control and studies have shown that the outcomes of non-surgical treatment of furcation involved molars are less favorable when compared to molars with no furcation involvement and are more likely to be lost during the periodontal maintenance phase (Hirschfeld and Wasserman 1978; Nordland et al. 1987; Loos et al. 1989; Claffey and Egelberg 1994). The poorer prognosis of furcation involved teeth emphasizes the importance of detecting these periodontal lesions for proper treatment planning.

Mobility

One major cause of tooth mobility is loss of alveolar bone support due to periodontal diseases. Increase in tooth mobility over time may reflect the progression of periodontal disease, which has to be confirmed by attachment level measurement. Mobility of a tooth may also increase following surgical periodontal therapy because of surgical trauma and the intentional removal of attachment support (ostectomy). Tooth mobility may be classified as follows (Miller 1950):

- Class I: Total facial-lingual or mesio-distal tooth movement of less than 1 mm.
- Class II: Total facial-lingual or mesio-distal tooth movement of more than 1 mm, without movement in a vertical direction.
- Class III: Total facial-lingual or mesio-distal tooth movement of more than 1 mm and movement in a vertical direction (i.e. the tooth is depressible).

Tooth mobility may also be observed in association with traumatic occlusal forces (see section on "Occlusal Examination"), orthodontic treatment, or when extensive peri-apical endodontic lesions are present. Clinically, the assessment of tooth mobility is performed by using the ends of two instrument handles placed against the facial and lingual (palatal) crown surfaces of the tooth to be assessed. The tooth is then observed for movement when applying horizontal (in a bucco-lingual/palatal direction) forces back and forth between the two instruments.

Dental Biofilm (Bacterial Plaque)

The primary etiology for periodontal disease is the presence and maturation of a bacterial biofilm, which, in turn, triggers host responses (Haffajee and Socransky 1994; Socransky and Haffajee 1992). Periodontal disease treatment and prevention is largely based on the adequate removal of plaque (Axelsson et al. 2004). The general consensus indicates that brushing twice daily should be recommended in order to maintain gingival health and prevent dental caries (Davies et al. 2003).

Based on the importance of plaque control in disease prevention and treatment, plaque control recording is an integral part of the comprehensive periodontal examination and should be assessed regularly to document patient status at the beginning of treatment (baseline), during active periodontal therapy including the non-surgical and surgical phases of treatment and the maintenance phase. Application of a disclosing agent will reveal the level of plaque control and may serve as a visual method to educate and motivate the patient toward optimal self-performed oral hygiene.

Calculus

Calculus represents a hardened form of plaque due to the accumulation of minerals, mainly calcium, and phosphate. Topographically, calculus can be described as supragingival or subgingival, depending on whether it is located coronally or apically to the gingival margin. It is considered a secondary etiologic factor of periodontal disease, since its rough surface serves as a reservoir for bacteria and a scaffold for biofilm development (Schroeder 1960; Zander et al. 1960). While common clinical practice does not require recording the presence of calculus it is imperative that its presence be identified for proper removal.

Occlusal Examination

Traumatic occlusal forces may overwhelm the capacity of the periodontium to redistribute the occlusal forces in such a way that the tooth cannot be maintained in its original position. The "injury to the attachment or tooth as a result of excessive occlusal forces" is termed *Occlusal Trauma* (Hallmon 1999). Occlusal trauma is characterized by widening of the periodontal ligament (PDL) space, bone resorption of the walls of the socket subjected to pressure, and increased mobility. Occlusal trauma is further divided in:

a) Primary occlusal trauma: a result of excessive occlusal forces in a normal periodontium;

b) Secondary occlusal trauma: a result of excessive or normal occlusal forces in a reduced periodontium; and

c) Occlusal trauma due to orthodontic forces (Jepsen et al. 2018).

Histologically, vasculitis, collagen destruction, and osteoclastic activity can be observed (Svanberg and Lindhe 1974; Wentz et al. 1958). These physiologic responses in response to traumatic occlusal forces allow the tooth to move away from the mechanical assault. When this occurs, the vasculitis resolves and the osteoclastic activity returns to normal, but the PDL space remains widened and the tooth still displays increased mobility. However, these changes remain stable and a status quo is reached (Svanberg and Lindhe 1974).

If occlusal trauma occurs in the absence of plaque induced periodontal inflammation, despite the widened periodontal space and the visible radiographic bone resorption, no loss in attachment level or deepened PD (pocket formation) can be measured (Lindhe and Ericsson 1976). Conversely, in the presence of plaque induced periodontal inflammation, occlusal trauma will lead to the adaptive changes mentioned previously but, instead of reaching a plateau, mobility will progress and it will be combined with an accelerated rate of periodontal destruction (Lindhe and Svanberg 1974; Nyman et al. 1978).

Occlusal examination is important to detect signs of parafunctional habits (e.g. bruxism, clenching, nail biting, chewing on a pen, biting on a pipe) resulting in excessive occlusal/incisal wear and occlusal discrepancies including premature contact and interferences in lateral or protrusive movements. The presence of fremitus should also be identified. Fremitus is defined as any perceptible tooth movement when the teeth occlude into maximum intercuspation (MI) or submitted to lateral or protrusive movements.

In order to detect fremitus, the clinician's finger is placed against the facial surfaces of maxillary teeth and the patient is asked to slowly close his/her jaws and gently tap teeth in MI. The same technique is used to assess fremitus when the patient is performing lateral or protrusive movements. Fremitus is classified as follows (Ingervall 1972):

- Class I fremitus: Mild vibration detected.
- Class II fremitus: Easily palpable vibration but no visible movement.
- Class III fremitus: Movement visible with the naked eye.

If parafunctional habits and/or occlusal discrepancies are discovered in conjunction with increased mobility then it can be assumed that the involved teeth are subjected to occlusal trauma. Similarly the same assumption can be made if teeth have increased mobility and are in fremitus. Radiographic examinations of teeth revealing a vertical bony defect and/or widened PDL around a tooth in conjunction with increased mobility may be indicative of occlusal trauma (Glickman and Smulow 1962; Waerhaug 1979). Therefore, when such radiographic defects are present, a careful examination of the occlusion should be performed.

Among the changes due to occlusal trauma, tooth mobility is the most likely to impact the patient's ability to function. Mobile teeth due to occlusal trauma which are associated with a healthy, inflammation-free periodontium (intact or reduced) may not have to be treated unless there is a functional impairment expressed by the patient. In the latter case, the cause of occlusal trauma has to be addressed. If related to parafunctional habits, the patient has to be made aware of the detrimental effect of these parafunctional habits, advised to cease them and also be informed of the possible alternatives to manage them.

If the parafunctional habits are unconscious (e.g. nocturnal bruxism or clenching) then an occlusal guard is recommended to relax the jaw muscles and redistribute the forces on the guard and avoid continuous excessive wear of tooth substance. If occlusal discrepancies are present then occlusal adjustment by selective grinding can be performed in order to eliminate premature contact and/or occlusal interferences. These measures should help decrease tooth mobility. Splinting of teeth can further decrease tooth mobility and improve patient's comfort while functioning.

In cases which present occlusal trauma and plaque-induced periodontal inflammation the primary goal must be aimed at the control of periodontal diseases. Consequently, periodontal therapy must come first, which in turn may reduce some of the mobility. Although this latter point is controversial (Burgett et al. 1992; Polson and Zander 1983; Polson et al. 1983; Rosling et al. 1976), the potential benefit obtained from a simple and fairly conservative occlusal adjustment seems to justify the elimination of occlusal trauma in conjunction with anti-infective therapy.

Radiographic Examination

Radiographic evaluation is an integral part of a comprehensive periodontal examination. Clinical examination can disclose PD, attachment level, tooth mobility which radiographic examination cannot. Conversely, root anatomy, crown to root ratio, percentage of bone loss in relation to the total root length (sometimes called relative bone loss), periapical status are features that can only be assessed with a radiograph.

Bitewing radiographs facilitate the evaluation of the quality of restorations (if present) and their marginal integrity. This is of paramount importance since overhanging restoration margins promote plaque accumulation and a shift toward a more pathogenic flora, which in turn can favor the development of periodontal diseases (Lang et al. 1983). Ill-fitting restoration margins must be considered as contributing factors to periodontal diseases and should be eliminated as part of the initial therapy.

Bitewing radiographs also enable practitioners to assess the bone height level in relation to the tooth. In cases when patients have already lost a substantial amount of bone support due to ongoing or past history of periodontal disease, bitewings may have to be taken in a vertical fashion to enable the visualization of the alveolar crest (Figure 10.2). Periapical radiographs allow the clinician to record information along the whole length of the root(s) including crown to root ratio, anatomy of the roots, anatomy of the furcation, periodontal spaces, and periapical status.

The full mouth radiographs allow the clinician to observe and estimate the amount of remaining supporting alveolar bone around the teeth. The morphology of the bone loss can also be evaluated. Typically, "horizontal" bone loss is distinguished from "vertical" bone loss. Radiographically, horizontal bone loss is present when the amount of bone loss is similar on the mesial and distal surface of two adjacent teeth, giving a flat appearance to the crest between these two teeth.

If a tooth is tilted, an actual horizontal bone loss may have the appearance of a vertical defect. To avoid any confusion and misleading interpretation of the bone defect morphology, a mental reference line should be drawn between the CEJs of two adjacent teeth. If the radiographic appearance of the interproximal alveolar crest is parallel to that reference line then the pattern of bone loss is horizontal and there is no vertical defect (Ritchey and Orban 1953) (Figure 10.3).

Radiographic images tend to underestimate the amount of bone loss as compared to measurements made at the time of surgery, which allows for direct bone measurements (Grimard et al. 2009; Yun et al. 2005). Because

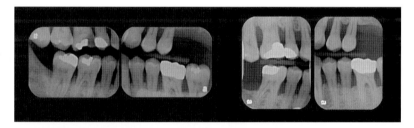

Figure 10.2 Vertical bitewings allow better visualization of alveolar bone loss.

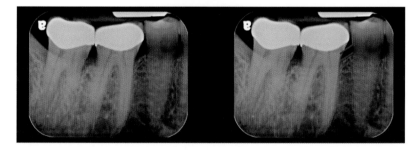

Figure 10.3 On left radiograph, the first impression could be given that there is a vertical bony defect on the mesial site of #30 (46 in the World Dental Federation [FDI] notation). However, since the reference line drawn between the CEJs of teeth #30 and 29 (46 AND 45 in the World Dental Federation [FDI] notation) runs parallel to the alveolar crest no vertical bony defect is actually present.

radiographs are a representation in two dimensions of a three dimensional reality, specific bony defects may not be seen on a radiograph or, if visible, the exact anatomy may be challenging to determine. For example, crater-like defects are often found between two adjacent posterior teeth.

Craters are two-wall bony defects, with the two remaining walls being the buccal/facial and the palatal/lingual bone walls. Craters are not readily visible because both buccal/facial and palatal/lingual cortical bone plates are still present. Furthermore, when a vertical defect is present, the exact anatomy of the defect, i.e. the number of bony walls encompassing the defect, may not be determined accurately based on radiographs.

Endodontic Status of Teeth

While endodontic and periodontal lesions are commonly two separate entities, there are instances where the two pathological conditions converge into one entity, i.e. a periodontal–endodontic lesion. Refer to periodontal-endodontic lesions in "Establishing a Periodontal Diagnosis" below. The reader is also referred to Chapter 12, Endodontic Evaluation.

10.2 Establishing a Periodontal Diagnosis

Based on the patient medical and dental history and a comprehensive periodontal evaluation, the clinician will establish a periodontal diagnosis. Not only does an accurate diagnosis allow the clinician to classify the condition but it also sets the stage for adequate treatment planning and implementation of care in order to successfully treat the patient's periodontal condition.

Establishing a periodontal diagnosis is currently based on the 2018 Classification of Periodontal and Peri-implant Diseases and Conditions. This classification was the outcome of a joint effort between the AAP and the European Federation of Periodontology (EFP) (Caton et al. 2018). Table 10.1 outlines

Table 10.1 Overview of the 2018 Classification of Periodontal and Peri-Implant Diseases and Conditions.

Periodontal diseases and conditions			Peri-implant diseases and conditions
Periodontal health, gingival diseases and conditions	Periodontitis	Other conditions affecting the periodontium	
I. Periodontal and gingival health	I. Necrotizing periodontal diseases	I. Systemic diseases or conditions affecting the periodontium	I. Peri-implant health
II. Gingivitis – dental biofilm induced	II. Periodontitis as manifestation of systemic diseases	II. Other periodontal diseases and conditions A. Periodontal abscesses B. Endodontal–periodontal lesions	II. Peri-implant mucositis
III. Gingival diseases non-dental biofilm induced	III. Periodontitis	III. Mucogingival deformities and conditions around teeth IV. Traumatic occlusal forces V. Prostheses and tooth related factors that modify or predispose to plaque-induced gingival diseases/periodontitis	III. Peri-implantitis IV. Peri-implant soft and hard tissue deficiencies

the main categories and subcategories of this classification system.

Dental biofilm-induced gingivitis and periodontitis are the most frequent clinical entities encountered among periodontal diseases. As such, the present section of this chapter will mainly focus on establishing diagnosis for plaque induced periodontal diseases as well as the acute periodontal conditions (in addition to the occlusal trauma that has already been described earlier in this chapter).

Classically, periodontal status can be been categorized as (i) healthy periodontium; (ii) gingivitis; and (iii) periodontitis.

Healthy Periodontium

Clinical periodontal health is defined as the absence of plaque induced periodontal disease. Clinically, the gingival tissues do not display signs of inflammation (absence of redness and/or swelling). More specifically, PDs are in the range of 1–3 mm and there is absence or very low levels (<10%) of sites with BOP. Periodontal health can be observed on an intact periodontium as well as on a reduced periodontium (as a result of history of periodontitis or due to non-periodontitis reasons, such as gingival recession).

Gingivitis (Dental Biofilm-Induced)

Gingivitis is defined as the presence of inflammation in the gingival tissue with no connective tissue attachment loss. Clinically, signs of inflammation are present (redness, swelling, BOP > 10%) but no true periodontal pocket can be measured. Similarly to periodontal health, dental biofilm-induced gingivitis, can also be diagnosed on intact or reduced periodontium. It can be further classified as localized or generalized (depending on if it involves less or more than 30% of the teeth respectively) and as mild, moderate or severe based on the severity of the clinical signs of inflammation (Chapple et al. 2018).

Periodontitis, Acute Conditions, and Combined Periodontal–Endodontic Lesions

Periodontitis is defined as the presence of inflammation at sites where the epithelium has migrated apically on the root surface in conjunction with loss of connective tissue attachment and alveolar bone. Signs of inflammation are observed and a true periodontal pocket can be measured. While the distinction between a healthy periodontium, gingivitis, and periodontitis is relatively straight forward, there is a number of periodontal diseases and conditions that may present with similar clinical and radiographic characteristics and these include: (i) periodontitis; (ii) acute conditions (such as necrotizing periodontal diseases or abscesses of the periodontium); and (iii) combined periodontal-endodontic lesions.

Periodontitis

Periodontitis (with periodic episodes of rapid progression) is the most frequent form of destructive periodontal disease. It is observed not only in adults, but also, in adolescents and children, although not as frequently. The combination of specific bacterial population with host susceptibility is necessary for the onset and progression of the disease. Patients present with plaque and calculus (subgingival calculus is often present), but the clinical characteristics may vary based on a number of local and systemic factors. Local predisposing factors include crowding of teeth and overhanging restoration margins, while smoking and uncontrolled diabetes are considered to be major systemic risk factors for periodontitis.

Following a comprehensive periodontal exam, the following criteria need to be met in order for the diagnosis of periodontitis to be made:

a) Clinical attachment loss in the interproximal surfaces of two or more non-adjacent teeth; or

b) Buccal/facial or lingual/palatal clinical attachment loss with PDs of 4 mm or more at two or more teeth.

The attachment loss, should only be attributed to periodontitis, and other reasons that can lead to attachment loss such as vertical root fracture, subgingival carious lesions or presence of an adjacent impacted tooth should be excluded. Once the diagnosis of periodontitis is established, it should be further classified as localized (affecting 30% of the teeth or less), generalized (affecting 30% of the teeth or more) or periodontitis with molar/incisor pattern.

The next steps are for the Stage and the Grade of the disease to be assigned. Staging of periodontitis ranges from I to IV and is suggestive of the severity of the disease as well as the complexity of management. Stages I and II represent slight to moderate cases that can be managed relatively easily from the general practitioner, whereas Stages III and IV are more complex cases that require advanced surgical treatment and interdisciplinary collaboration (Tonetti et al. 2018) (Table 10.2).

Finally, a case of periodontitis can be classified as Grade A, B or C. Grading is indicative of the rate of disease progression and the potential impact on systemic health. Initially, all cases may be classified as Grade B and as more information is collected, the grading can be changed to one of the other two categories (Tonetti et al. 2018) (Table 10.3).

Each case presents with *only one* Stage and Grade, as the goal of this classification system is to identify disease patterns on an individual, rather than focusing only on the clinical and radiographic characteristics of each case. Furthermore, the Stage for a given patient does not typically change over the years, whereas the Grade can be modified as the systemic factors implicated change (i.e. an uncontrolled diabetic that manages to lower and control the HbA1c levels may shift from Grade C to Grade B).

It should be highlighted that the distinction between chronic and aggressive periodontitis no longer exists. The three main characteristics of aggressive periodontitis were:

- A rapid rate at which the periodontal destruction, including attachment and bone loss, occurs (Figure 10.4).
- Familial aggregation.
- Typically, and other than the presence of periodontitis, patients were systemically healthy.

Despite the phenotypic differences between chronic and aggressive periodontitis, the 2017 World Workshop concluded that there is not enough evidence to support that the two diseases are in fact, two different entities (Fine et al. 2018). When a periodontitis case with molar-incisor pattern is noted, one should be suspicious of the possibility of accelerated rate of periodontal destruction and manage such cases appropriately (Albandar et al. 2002; Hoover et al. 1981; Kronauer et al. 1986; Saxen 1980; Van der Velden et al. 1989).

Acute Conditions

Acute conditions share the common feature of pain and include necrotizing periodontal diseases and periodontal abscesses. Necrotizing periodontal diseases are further classified as necrotizing gingivitis (NG) and necrotizing periodontitis (NP) and necrotizing stomatitis (NS). Patients presenting with NG and NP are typically 20–30 years of age (Horning and Cohen 1995). Risk factors including poor oral hygiene (Horning and Cohen 1995), smoking (Pindborg 1951, Stevens et al. 1984), stress (Cohen-Cole et al. 1983), malnutrition (Enwonwu 1994) and impaired immune system function associated with systemic disease, e.g. HIV (Glick et al. 1994; Melnick et al. 1988).

Necrotizing periodontal diseases are inflammatory diseases characterized by ulcerative and necrotizing lesions of the gingival margins and papillae. A yellowish, grayish layer of sloughing tissue (also called a pseudomembrane) covers the ulcerated papillae. In

Table 10.2 Staging of periodontitis.

Periodontitis		Stage I	Stage II	Stage III	Stage IV
Severity	**Clinical attachment loss**	1–2 mm	3–4 mm	≥5 mm	≥5 mm
	Radiographic bone loss	Coronal third of the root	Coronal third of the root	Middle or apical third of the root	Middle or apical third of the root
	Tooth loss due to periodontitis	No tooth loss		≤4 teeth	≥5 teeth
Complexity		PD ≤4 mm	PD ≤5 mm	In addition to Stage II:	In addition to Stage II:
		Mostly horizontal bone loss	Mostly horizontal bone loss	PD ≥6 mm	Need for complex rehabilitation due to: masticatory dysfunction, tooth mobility, bite collapse, pathologic migration, <20 remaining teeth
				Vertical bone loss ≥3 mm	
				Class II or III furcation involvement	
				Moderate ridge defects	
Extent and distribution		Localized (<30% of the teeth involved) Generalized (≥30% of the teeth involved) Molar-incisor pattern			

Source: Adapted with permission from Tonetti et al. (2018).

Table 10.3 Grading of periodontitis.

	Progression		Grade A: Slow Rate	Grade B:: Moderate Rate	Grade C:: Rapid Rate
Primary criteria (Direct evidence should be used when available)	Direct evidence of progression	Radiographic bone loss or CAL	No loss over 5 years	<2 mm over 5 years	≥2 mm over 5 years
	Indirect evidence of progression	% bone loss/age	<0.25	0.25–1	>1
		Case phenotype	Heavy biofilms with low levels of destructions	Destruction commensurate with biofilm deposits	Destruction inconsistent with biofilm deposits; clinical patterns suggestive of periods of rapid progression and/or early onset
Grade modifiers	Risk factors	Smoking	Non-smoker	<10 cigarettes/day	≥10 cigarettes/day
		Diabetes	Non-diabetic	Diabetic with HbA1c < 7%	Diabetic with HbA1c ≥ 7%

Source: Adapted with permission from Tonetti et al. (2018).

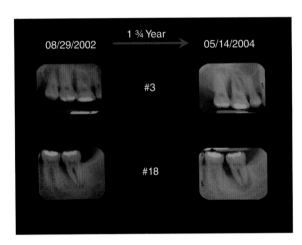

Figure 10.4 Radiographic examinations taken 1¾ years apart illustrating the rapid periodontal destruction in a patient diagnosed with generalized aggressive periodontitis (according to the previous classification system – Armitage (1999)).

addition to the typical clinical appearance, patients will also present with a fetid odor (fetor ex ore) and complain of pain in the gingiva. While the clinical features of NG and NP are similar, the hallmark of necrotizing ulcerative periodontitis is rapid bone destruction. NS is characterized by tissue necrosis extending beyond the mucogingival junction (in the alveolar mucosa) (Papapanou et al. 2018).

NG is not uncommon in healthy, younger individuals that undergo through a transient period of stress and/or malnutrition (such military personnel, college students during the exam periods). On the other hand, NP and NS are frequently associated with severely immunocompromised patients (e.g. HIV positive subjects).

A periodontal abscess is an acute bacterial infection (Gray et al. 1994). When a periodontal abscess is associated with a pre-existing deep periodontal pocket, clinical presentation may include swelling, pain, purulent exudate, and/or a sinus tract (McLeod et al. 1997). Teeth involved may be mobile, sensitive to percussion and slightly in supra-occlusion. When the marginal part of the pocket reattaches to the tooth surface, bacteria are trapped in the apical part of the pocket, and an abscess develops (Dello Russo 1985). This can frequently occur following inadequate non-surgical periodontal treatment, when calculus is not removed from the entire root surface of a periodontal pocket.

A periodontal abscess may also develop in sites without a pre-existing periodontal pockets. This is the case when foreign bodies (e.g. food particles, impression material, toothbrush bristles) are impacted into the gingival sulcus (Gillette and Van House 1980). Signs that will guide the clinician toward a periodontal etiology are: history of periodontal disease, localized deep PD, purulence through the gingival sulcus, vitality of the affected tooth is often positive, radiographic bone loss with deep angular bony defect or furcation involvement and localized sharp pain.

A differential diagnosis between periodontal abscesses and abscesses of endodontic origin is often required. The latter are associated with deep caries, extensive restorations, negative vitality test, periapical radiolucency, and/or diffuse pain that is difficult to relate to one specific tooth. When a tooth fracture is present the patient will often report pain on biting, which can be elicited by applying selective pressure on a specific cusp of the involved tooth. If the tooth is vital, it will usually be sensitive to cold while rarely to heat stimuli.

Combined Endodontic–Periodontal Lesion

The combined involvement of the periodontium and the pulp can result from: (i) an extension of a primary endodontic lesion with periodontal repercussions; (ii) an extension of a primary periodontal lesion with endodontic repercussions; and (iii) a combination of two separate lesions, endodontic, and periodontal, which have united.

Whenever a primary endodontic lesion is not diagnosed in a timely manner and is left untreated, the infection which started in the pulp and resulted in pulp necrosis can propagate to the root surface of the tooth through the root canal system. Typically, it reaches the apex of the root through the main root canals or the side of the root through lateral canals (Vertucci 1984). From there the infection may extend through the alveolar bone plate and give rise to an endodontic abscess or a sinus tract if it perforates the gingival or alveolar mucosa.

Another path for an infection of endodontic origin, once it has reached the root surface is through the PDL to the gingival sulcus. Thus, a sinus tract is created along the root surface and deep PDs are measurable on the affected tooth. If diagnosed early, before plaque and calculus have propagated apically from the gingival sulcus along the root surface, a conventional endodontic treatment will eliminate the endodontic infection.

If a primary endodontic lesion with a sinus tract through the gingival sulcus is left untreated, plaque, and calculus can extend apically creating a secondary periodontal lesion. In this case, the conventional endodontic therapy may resolve the endodontic problem. In order to achieve optimal reattachment, scaling, and root planning to remove plaque and calculus must be performed to promote reattachment of fibers and increase the chance for periodontal healing.

If a primary periodontal lesion is left untreated, over time it can display clinical and radiographic features similar to a primary endodontic lesion. For instance, a periodontal pocket can progress over time and involve the apex of a tooth similarly to an advanced primary endodontic lesion that has reached the gingival sulcus. The differential diagnosis is based on all vitality tests including thermal and electrical stimuli being within normal limits.

When a primary periodontal lesion reaches a lateral canal (accessory canal) or the apex of the root (more frequently), the infection can take a retrograde path and infect the pulp with subsequent loss of pulp vitality.

Table 10.4 Classification of endo-periodontal lesions.

Endo-periodontal lesion with root damage	Root fracture or cracking	
	Root canal or pulp chamber perforation	
	External root resorption	
Endo-periodontal lesion without root damage		Grade 1 – narrow deep periodontal pocket in 1 tooth surface
	Endo-periodontal lesion in periodontitis patient	Grade 2 – wide deep periodontal pocket in 1 tooth surface
		Grade 3 –deep periodontal pockets in >1 tooth surface
		Grade 1 – narrow deep periodontal pocket in 1 tooth surface
	Endo-periodontal lesion in non-periodontitis patient	Grade 2 – wide deep periodontal pocket in 1 tooth surface
		Grade 3 –deep periodontal pockets in >1 tooth surface

In this instance vitality test results may be inconclusive depending on whether the pulp is completely or partially necrotic, e.g. in a multi-rooted tooth, the pulp can be vital in one root canal and necrotic in the others. If the pulp is necrotic, clinical, and radiographic findings are similar to that of a primary endodontic lesion with a secondary periodontal lesion.

A combined periodontal–endodontic lesion represents the union of two distinct disease processes that have converged into one single entity. Unless previous radiographs showing two distinct lesions are available, recognizing combined lesions may be difficult. Treatment planning should include conventional endodontic therapy followed by appropriate non-surgical and surgical periodontal intervention. Prognosis is predicated on the nature of the periodontal defect.

In addition, vertical root fractures can also mimic the appearance of a combined lesion. Therefore, if a vertical root fracture is suspected, exploration of the root surface with a probe to detect the fracture or even an exploratory surgery may be necessary to exclude a possible root fracture before investing in costly attempts to save the tooth.

From the above information, one can conclude that oftentimes, it is a challenge for the clinician to determine the origin of the primary lesion, as all the information may not be available. A new classification of the combined endodontal–periodontal lesions has been proposed to address this issue, on the basis of the presence or absence of root damage (Table 10.4).

10.3 Basic Principles of Periodontal Treatment Planning

A basic understanding of periodontal treatment planning is helpful in order to determine when to refer a patient for specialized care. Classically, periodontal treatment is divided into six phases: (i) systemic phase; (ii) phase 1 or cause-related therapy; (iii) reevaluation after cause-related therapy; (iv) surgical phase; (v) reevaluation after surgical phase; and (vi) maintenance phase.

Systemic Phase

The main goal of the systemic phase is to ensure that the patient can undergo regular periodontal therapy without substantial risks related to his/her overall medical conditions.

Also, consultation with physicians may be necessary to limit the impact of systemic conditions on the treatment per se and/or its outcomes, e.g. diabetes.

Phase 1 or Cause-Related Therapy (Non-Surgical Treatment)

The aim of cause-related therapy, which has two sequential components, is to decrease the pathogenic microflora. Step one includes patient education, motivation, and instruction on how to perform good oral hygiene, i.e. remove plaque. Step two includes the elimination of possible contributing factors to the problem such as the removal of calculus and overhanging restorations (Socransky and Haffajee 1992). This is typically achieved by a non-surgical debridement of the teeth and root surfaces using a combination of hand and ultrasonic instruments.

Reevaluation after Cause-Related Therapy

Once cause-related therapy is completed, a comprehensive periodontal reevaluation is indicated to determine the need of further treatment. Stage I and Stage II periodontitis may resolve following cause-related therapy and the patient may be placed into the maintenance phase. More severe periodontitis cases (Stages III and IV) may require surgical intervention, interdisciplinary treatment, complex diagnostic, and therapeutic intervention. Early diagnosis and timely referral to a periodontist are key to the proper management of the case and improve the prognosis.

Surgical Phase

If the disease was more severe, reevaluation after cause-related therapy will indicate the presence of unresolved problems. Surgical therapy may be indicated to further decrease and eliminate PDs to improve CALs.

In addition, regeneration procedures may have to be implemented to potentially reverse the sequela of previous disease and reconstitute the integrity of the lost periodontal support.

Reevaluation after Surgical Phase

If the patient's cooperation is adequate, disease resolution might be expected and should be documented by a periodontal reevaluation, which will serve as the baseline data for the maintenance phase. If cooperation is inadequate, i.e. the patient still presents with a plaque infected dentition, periodontal destruction will occur following surgery (Nyman et al. 1977), which is therefore contraindicated. Consequently, periodontal disease resolution may not be achieved.

Maintenance Phase

The aim of this phase is to maintain reestablished periodontal health and prevent disease recurrence. Oral hygiene instructions and motivation are reinforced. The maintenance intervals vary but most commonly patients return periodically every three, four or six months. PDs and signs of inflammation around teeth and implants are repeatedly monitored at each recall appointment. If indicated, maintenance care includes instrumentation of deepened sites with BoP and caries prevention by means of topical fluorides. It should be noted, that patients must be placed in a periodontal maintenance program immediately after the non-surgical phase, even if the treatment plan includes some sort of corrective/surgical treatment. It is not uncommon for patients to schedule their surgical appointments several months later due to a number of reasons (finances, non-compliance, scheduling conflicts). That can lead to patients being overdue for a maintenance appointment with a negative effect on their periodontal status and the course of their treatment.

Table 10.5 Case definitions of peri-implant health and peri-implant diseases.

	Peri-implant health	Peri-implant mucositis	Peri-implantitis Presence of previous examination	Peri-implantitis Absence of previous examination
Clinical signs of inflammation	−	+/−	+/−	+/−
BOP/suppuration	−	+	+	+
Increase in PD comparing to previous visits	−	+/−	+	PD $\geq$ 6 m
Bone loss beyond the initial remodeling (normal range up to 2 mm)	−	−	+	$\geq$3 mm from the most coronal part of the intraosseous portion of the implant

Source: Based on Berglundh et al. (2018).

10.4 Peri-Implant Examination and Diagnosis

The peri-implant examination includes similar components to the periodontal examination (radiographic and clinical examination, occlusal analysis, etc.). However the following items need to be taken into consideration due to the differences between the periodontal and peri-implant tissues.

Probing around implants requires reduced force (approximately 0.15 N). Although it can be performed with either a metal or a plastic probe, the plastic probe has the advantage of being more flexible and therefore easier to adapt to the contour of the implant abutment/restorations. PDs in peri-implant health are slightly deeper (up to 5 mm) in comparison to those found in periodontal health.

While natural teeth can present with various degrees of mobility, no mobility should be noted on implants, irrespective of the amount of bone loss that may be present. Once implant mobility is noted, the implant is failed and should be removed.

Following implant placement, a degree of crestal bone remodeling can be anticipated. This remodeling will reach its maximum within the first year following the delivery of the implant prosthesis and typically should not exceed 2 mm.

Peri-implant mucositis and peri-implantitis are the equivalent diseases to gingivitis and periodontitis respectively. As discussed earlier in this chapter, the CEJ is most commonly the landmark used to calculate CAL around teeth. Around implants, different landmarks are used in order to longitudinally monitor the clinical stability of the peri-implant tissues (Table 10.5) (Berglundh et al. 2018).

10.5 Summary

Generally, most patients presenting in a general practice will have signs of gingivitis or Stage I–II periodontitis. Severe cases including Stage III, IV or periodontitis with molar-incisor pattern are more infrequent. Nonetheless, the general practitioner should be able to diagnose these entities and make a referral in a timely manner if needed.

Provided that the knowledge and the skills of the clinician are appropriate, no specific periodontal or peri-implant disease solely belongs in a specialist practice. However, it is the responsibility of the general practitioner to acknowledge their limitations and make a referral to a specialist keeping in mind the best interest of the patient.

References

Albandar, J.M., Muranga, M.B., and Rams, T.E. (2002). Prevalence of aggressive periodontitis in school attendees in Uganda. *J. Clin. Periodontol.* 29: 823–831.

Armitage, G.C. (1999). Development of a classification system for periodontal diseases and conditions. *Ann. Periodontol.* 4: 1–6.

Axelsson, P., Nystrom, B., and Lindhe, J. (2004). The long-term effect of a plaque control program on tooth mortality, caries and periodontal disease in adults. Results after 30 years of maintenance. *J. Clin. Periodontol.* 31: 749–757.

Berglundh, T., Armitage, G., Avila-Ortiz, G. et al. (2018). Peri-implant diseases and conditions: consensus report of workgroup 4 of the 2017 World Workshop on the Classification of Periodontal and Peri-Implant Diseases and Conditions. *J. Periodontol.* 89 (Suppl 1): S313–S318.

Borrell, L.N., Burt, B.A., and Taylor, G.W. (2005). Prevalence and trends in periodontitis in the USA: the [corrected] nhanes, 1988 to 2000. *J. Dent. Res.* 84: 924–930.

Burgett, F.G., Ramfjord, S.P., Nissle, R.R. et al. (1992). A randomized trial of occlusal adjustment in the treatment of periodontitis patients. *J. Clin. Periodontol.* 19: 381–387.

Caton, J., Armitage, G., Berglundh, T. et al. (2018). A new classification scheme for periodontal and Peri-Implant Diseases and Conditions – introduction and key changes from the 1999 classification. *J. Periodontol.* 89 (Suppl 1): S1–S8.

Chapple, I.L.C., Mealey, B.L. et al. (2018). Periodontal health and gingival diseases and conditions on an intact and a reduced periodontium: consensus report of workgroup 1 of the 2017 World Workshop on the Classification of Periodontal and Peri-Implant Diseases and Conditions. *J. Periodontol.* 89 (Suppl 1): S74–S84.

Claffey, N. and Egelberg, J. (1994). Clinical characteristics of periodontal sites with probing attachment loss following initial periodontal treatment. *J. Clin. Periodontol.* 21: 670–679.

Cobb, C.M., Carrara, A., El-Annan, E. et al. (2003). Periodontal referral patterns, 1980 versus 2000: a preliminary study. *J. Periodontol.* 74: 1470–1474.

Cohen-Cole, S.A., Cogen, R.B., Stevens, A.W. Jr., et al. (1983). Psychiatric, psychosocial, and endocrine correlates of acute necrotizing ulcerative gingivitis (trench mouth): a preliminary report. *Psychiatr. Med.* 1: 215–225.

Davies, R.M., Davies, G.M., and Ellwood, R.P. (2003). Prevention. Part 4: toothbrushing: what advice should be given to patients? *Br. Dent. J.* 195: 135–141.

Dello Russo, N.M. (1985). The post-prophylaxis periodontal abscess: etiology and treatment. *Int J Periodontics Restorative Dent* 5: 28–37.

Dockter, K.M., Williams, K.B., Bray, K.S. et al. (2006). Relationship between prereferral periodontal care and periodontal status at time of referral. *J. Periodontol.* 77: 1708–1716.

Enwonwu, C.O. (1994). Cellular and molecular effects of malnutrition and their relevance to periodontal diseases. *J. Clin. Periodontol.* 21: 643–657.

Fine, D.H., Patil, A.G., and Loos, B.G. (2018). Classification and diagnosis of aggressive periodontitis. *J. Periodontol.* 89 (Suppl 1): S103–S119.

Gillette, W.B. and Van House, R.L. (1980). Ill effects of improper oral hygiene procedure. *J. Am. Dent. Assoc.* 101: 476–480.

Glick, M., Muzyka, B.C., Salkin, L.M. et al. (1994). Necrotizing ulcerative periodontitis: a marker for immune deterioration and a predictor for the diagnosis of aids. *J. Periodontol.* 65: 393–397.

Glickman, I. and Smulow, J.B. (1962). Alterations in the pathway of gingival inflammation to the underlying tissues induced by excessive occlusal forces. *J. Periodontol.* 33: 7–13.

Gray, J.L., Flanary, D.B., and Newell, D.H. (1994). The prevalence of periodontal abscess.

J. Indian Dent. Assoc. 73 (18–20): 22–13. quiz 24.

Greenwell, H. (2001). Position paper: guidelines for periodontal therapy. *J. Periodontol.* 72: 1624–1628.

Grimard, B.A., Hoidal, M.J., Mills, M.P. et al. (2009). Comparison of clinical, periapical radiograph, and cone-beam volume tomography measurement techniques for assessing bone level changes following regenerative periodontal therapy. *J. Periodontol.* 80: 48–55.

Haffajee, A.D. and Socransky, S.S. (1994). Microbial etiological agents of destructive periodontal diseases. *Periodontology* 2000 (5): 78–111.

Hallmon, W.W. (1999). Occlusal trauma: effect and impact on the periodontium. *Ann. Periodontol.* 4: 102–108.

Hamp, S.E., Nyman, S., and Lindhe, J. (1975). Periodontal treatment of multirooted teeth. Results after 5 years. *J. Clin. Periodontol.* 2: 126–135.

Hirschfeld, L. and Wasserman, B. (1978). A long-term survey of tooth loss in 600 treated periodontal patients. *J. Periodontol.* 49: 225–237.

Hoover, J.N., Ellegaard, B., and Attstrom, R. (1981). Radiographic and clinical examination of periodontal status of first molars in 15–16-year-old danish schoolchildren. *Scand. J. Dent. Res.* 89: 260–263.

Horning, G.M. and Cohen, M.E. (1995). Necrotizing ulcerative gingivitis, periodontitis, and stomatitis: clinical staging and predisposing factors. *J. Periodontol.* 66: 990–998.

Hugoson, A. and Norderyd, O. (2008). Has the prevalence of periodontitis changed during the last 30 years? *J. Clin. Periodontol.* 35: 338–345.

Hugoson, A., Sjodin, B., and Norderyd, O. (2008). Trends over 30 years, 1973–2003, in the prevalence and severity of periodontal disease. *J. Clin. Periodontol.* 35: 405–414.

Ingervall, B. (1972). Tooth contacts on the functional and nonfunctional side in children and young adults. *Arch. Oral Biol.* 17: 191–200.

Jepsen, S., Caton, J.G. et al. (2018). Periodontal manifestations of systemic diseases and developmental and acquired conditions: Consensus report of workgroup 3 of the 2017 World Workshop on the Classification of Periodontal and Peri-Implant Diseases and Conditions. *J. Periodontol.* 89 (Suppl 1): S237–S248.

Kronauer, E., Borsa, G., and Lang, N.P. (1986). Prevalence of incipient juvenile periodontitis at age 16 years in Switzerland. *J. Clin. Periodontol.* 13: 103–108.

Lang, N.P., Kiel, R.A., and Anderhalden, K. (1983). Clinical and microbiological effects of subgingival restorations with overhanging or clinically perfect margins. *J. Clin. Periodontol.* 10: 563–578.

Lang, N.P., Joss, A., Orsanic, T. et al. (1986). Bleeding on probing. A predictor for the progression of periodontal disease? *J. Clin. Periodontol.* 13: 590–596.

Lang, N.P., Adler, R., Joss, A. et al. (1990). Absence of bleeding on probing. An indicator of periodontal stability. *J. Clin. Periodontol.* 17: 714–721.

Lindhe, J. and Ericsson, I. (1976). The influence of trauma from occlusion on reduced but healthy periodontal tissues in dogs. *J. Clin. Periodontol.* 3: 110–122.

Lindhe, J. and Svanberg, G. (1974). Influence of trauma from occlusion on progression of experimental periodontitis in the beagle dog. *J. Clin. Periodontol.* 1: 3–14.

Loe, H., Theilade, E., and Jensen, S.B. (1965). Experimental gingivitis in man. *J. Periodontol.* 36: 177–187.

Loos, B., Nylund, K., Claffey, N. et al. (1989). Clinical effects of root debridement in molar and non-molar teeth. A 2-year follow-up. *J. Clin. Periodontol.* 16: 498–504.

McLeod, D.E., Lainson, P.A., and Spivey, J.D. (1997). Tooth loss due to periodontal abscess:

a retrospective study. *J. Periodontol.* 68: 963–966.

Melnick, S.L., Roseman, J.M., Engel, D. et al. (1988). Epidemiology of acute necrotizing ulcerative gingivitis. *Epidemiol. Rev.* 10: 191–211.

Miller, S.C. (1950). *Textbook of Periodontia*, 3e. Philadelphia: The Blakeston Co.

Mombelli, A., Muhle, T., and Frigg, R. (1992). Depth-force patterns of periodontal probing. Attachment-gain in relation to probing force. *J. Clin. Periodontol.* 19: 295–300.

Nordland, P., Garrett, S., Kiger, R. et al. (1987). The effect of plaque control and root debridement in molar teeth. *J. Clin. Periodontol.* 14: 231–236.

Nyman, S., Lindhe, J., and Rosling, B. (1977). Periodontal surgery in plaque-infected dentitions. *J. Clin. Periodontol.* 4: 240–249.

Nyman, S., Lindhe, J., and Ericsson, I. (1978). The effect of progressive tooth mobility on destructive periodontitis in the dog. *J. Clin. Periodontol.* 5: 213–225.

Papapanou, P.N., Sanz, M. et al. (2018). Periodontitis: consensus report of Workgroup 2 of the 2017 World Workshop on the Classification of Periodontal and Peri-Implant Diseases and Conditions. *J. Periodontol.* 89 (Suppl 1): S173–S182.

Pindborg, J.J. (1951). Influence of service in armed forces on incidence of gingivitis. *J. Am. Dent. Assoc.* 42: 517–522.

Polson, A.M. and Zander, H.A. (1983). Effect of periodontal trauma upon intrabony pockets. *J. Periodontol.* 54: 586–591.

Polson, A.M., Adams, R.A., and Zander, H.A. (1983). Osseous repair in the presence of active tooth hypermobility. *J. Clin. Periodontol.* 10: 370–379.

Ritchey, B. and Orban, B. (1953). The crest of the interdental alveolar septa. *J. Periodontol.*: 75–87.

Rosling, B., Nyman, S., and Lindhe, J. (1976). The effect of systematic plaque control on bone regeneration in infrabony pockets. *J. Clin. Periodontol.* 3: 38–53.

Saxe, S.R., Greene, J.C., Bohannan, H.M. et al. (1967). Oral debris, calculus, and periodontal disease in the beagle dog. *Periodontics* 5: 217–225.

Saxen, L. (1980). Prevalence of juvenile periodontitis in Finland. *J. Clin. Periodontol.* 7: 177–186.

Schroeder, H.E. (1960). *Formation and Inhibition of Dental Calculus*. Berne: Hans Huber Publishers.

Socransky, S.S. and Haffajee, A.D. (1992). The bacterial etiology of destructive periodontal disease: current concepts. *J. Periodontol.* 63: 322–331.

Stevens, A.W. Jr., Cogen, R.B., Cohen-Cole, S. et al. (1984). Demographic and clinical data associated with acute necrotizing ulcerative gingivitis in a dental school population (anug-demographic and clinical data). *J. Clin. Periodontol.* 11: 487–493.

Svanberg, G. and Lindhe, J. (1974). Vascular reactions in the periodontal ligament incident to trauma from occlusion. *J. Clin. Periodontol.* 1: 58–69.

Tonetti, M.S., Greenwell, H., and Kornman, K.S. (2018). Staging and grading of periodontitis: framework and proposal of a new classification and case definition. *J. Periodontol.* 89 (Suppl 1): S159–S172.

Van der Velden, U., Abbas, F., Van Steenbergen, T.J. et al. (1989). Prevalence of periodontal breakdown in adolescents and presence of actinobacillus actinomycetemcomitans in subjects with attachment loss. *J. Periodontol.* 60: 604–610.

Vertucci, F.J. (1984). Root canal anatomy of the human permanent teeth. *Oral Surg. Oral Med. Oral Pathol.* 58: 589–599.

Waerhaug, J. (1979). The angular bone defect and its relationship to trauma from occlusion and downgrowth of subgingival plaque. *J. Clin. Periodontol.* 6: 61–82.

Wentz, F.M., Jarabak, J., and Orban, B. (1958). Experimental occlusal trauma imitating cuspal interferences. *J. Periodontol.* 29: 117–127.

Yun, J.H., Hwang, S.J., Kim, C.S. et al. (2005). The correlation between the bone probing, radiographic and histometric measurements of bone level after regenerative surgery. *J. Periodontal Res.* 40: 453–460.

Zander, H.A., Hazen, S.P., and Scott, D.B. (1960). Mineralization of dental calculus. *Proc. Soc. Exp. Biol. Med.* 103: 257–260.

11

Oral and Maxillofacial Surgery

11.1 Introduction

Office based oral surgery is an important aspect of dentistry. Nearly 50 % of adults between the ages of 20 and 64 have had at least one permanent tooth extracted (not included third molars) and approximately 20 % of people aged 65 and older are completely edentulous (Dye et al. 2015). Dentists must be able to evaluate patients and formulate appropriate treatment plans in order to treat patients with surgical needs. These treatment plans are often modified based on the overall health of each patient. A large portion the population has been diagnosed with at least one medical condition. 25 % of Americans suffer from multiple chronic medical conditions (US Department of Health and Human

Physical Evaluation and Treatment Planning in Dental Practice, Second Edition.
Géza T. Terézhalmy, Michaell A. Huber, Lily T. García and Ronald L. Occhionero.
© 2021 John Wiley & Sons, Inc. Published 2021 by John Wiley & Sons, Inc.
Companion Website: www.wiley.com/go/terezhalmy/physical

Services, 2010). Seventy five percentage of Americans who are 65 years or older have multiple chronic medical conditions (Gerteis et al. 2014). As an increasing number of Americans develop medical problems, more medications are being prescribed to treat these chronic medical conditions. Approximately 15 % of Americans take five or more prescription medications (Kantor et al. 2015). This number increases to 39 % for adults 65 and older (Kantor et al. 2015). It is the responsibility of the healthcare provider to be able to perform an adequate preoperative evaluation of the patient and request additional information from the patient's medical providers as needed. The dentist must obtain the needed medical information in order to appropriately treat the patient and to set appropriate expectations both from the dentist and from the patient. It is important to note that a patient may not have routine medical care and a dentist may be the first healthcare provider to notice that a patient requires further medical attention.

11.2 Medical History

Preparation for surgery begins with a complete medical history. The patient's medical history is obtained in order to establish the overall health of the patient. The dentist will also be able to assess risk factors associated with providing a specific treatment. This information can also be used to modify planned treatment. The medical history is usually obtained from the patient, but also may be obtained from the patient's parent, guardian, or previous medical providers. The dentist should consider consulting the patient's primary care physician if the patient's health history is complex.

An important portion of the patient evaluation is the pre-printed medical history questionnaire. This form is completed by the patient at the first clinical visit. The dentist may also elect to send the medical health questionnaire to the patient prior to the first visit, which will allow the patient the ability to fill out the form prior to the first visit. This allows the dentist to review the questionnaire prior to the dental appointment. Many of these forms are available through professional resources and the level of detail can vary from superficial to extremely detailed. It is better that the health history form err being overly detailed, rather than lacking detail. Many dentists develop their own health history forms once they are comfortable with the information they wish to gain from the patient. It is important to organize the information to make it easy to review. It is also best to format the questions so that either a positive or "yes" response will require follow up questions. This medical history is the basis for the dentist to interview the patient in order to complete an adequate assessment of the patient's health. The patient should be asked at each appointment if any changes have occurred in the health history. These changes, if any, should be documented in the patient's chart.

11.3 Chief Complaint (CC)

The chief complaint is a brief description of why the patient is seeking dental care. This is often written in the patient's own words. Examples may include: "I have a broken tooth," or "I have a filling that fell out."

11.4 History of Present Illness (HPI)

The HPI relates directly to the chief complaint. This is the story of what caused the complaint and often involves terms such as duration, location, intensity, worsening, improvement, and other descriptive terms. The patient should be asked to describe when the chief complaint started and if it has changed since the initial presentation. The HPI often begins when the last time the patient felt normal. The evolution of the HPI can often be obtained by asking the patients questions about the chief complaint. An example of an HPI: "I had a tooth that I lost a filling from and it broke off when I was eating some breadsticks three days ago and now it is really hurting."

11.5 Past Medical History

The past medical history should be investigated to determine the overall health of the patient presurgically. This should include questioning the patient specifically about any information that was marked on the medical history questionnaire. The patient should be asked when any disease process was first diagnosed and if the disease is being treated by a physician. It is important to know if the patient's medical comorbidities are optimized as much as possible. The dentist should also inquire about any previous hospitalizations as this may affect the planned treatment. If the patient is unable to answer, then a parent or caregiver may be needed to answer questions regarding the medical history. Contacting the patient's primary care physician may also be required for more detailed information that is unable to be obtained from the patient.

11.6 Past Surgical History

The past surgical history gives an indication of how the patient may respond to surgical insult. The patient should be asked about any complications with surgery or anesthesia. Local anesthetic is often used at some point during nearly every surgery even if it is just to start an IV. The surgeries the patient has undergone may also give an indication of the overall health of the patient. Although most previous surgeries will not alter the dental plan, some previous surgeries, such as a recent coronary artery bypass graft (CABG) or a prosthetic heart valve, may require a revision in the dental treatment plan.

11.7 Medications

Patients, particularly pre-surgical patients should be advised to bring all current medications to the consultation visit. Alternatively, the patient may bring a medication list, or the dentist can call the patient's pharmacy for an active list of medications. Reviewing the medications and dosage may fill in some of the missing parts of the medical history, particularly if the patient either can't or will not give a truthful answer to the medical history questions. Non-prescription supplements and over-the-counter (OTC) medications must also be considered as they may have adverse interactions with prescription medications or have side effects that affect the planned treatment. The dentist should inquire about herbal and "all natural" supplements as these can also have medication interactions and side effects that may alter treatment. It is also important to ask the patient if they routinely take the prescribed medications and if the patient took the medications the day of the procedure.

11.8 Allergies

Drug allergies and adverse effects should be investigated and considered pre-operatively as they may influence what medications are used during and after the surgery. Important drug allergies to consider in the dental office are allergies to local anesthetics, antibiotics, sedatives, or pain medications (NSAIDS, acetaminophen narcotics). Dentists must be aware of the difference between a sensitivity and allergy. A true allergy usually occurs immediately or within hours and may present with symptoms of hives, itching, difficulty breathing, or other severe symptoms. A sensitivity or intolerance often manifests gradually and can cause symptoms such as nausea, vomiting, stomach upset, or less severe symptoms. Obviously, drugs and related classes of drugs the patient is allergic to must be avoided. The prescriber must know all the components of the drugs prescribed so that none of the components cause allergic reactions.

11.9 Social History

The patient's social history pertains to information regarding occupation, living arrangements, diet, exercise habits, hobbies, tobacco use, alcohol use, and illicit drug use. The social history can introduce important modifiers into a treatment plan. The provider may encounter times where the patient lives in a nursing home or has another person who provides consent due to a mental incapacity. The provider may discover the patient abuses drugs or alcohol. A social history of drug use is important particularly if sedative drugs are to be used in treating the patient. Tobacco use can lead to pulmonary and cardiovascular disease as well as increase the patient's risk for oral cancer. Patients with chronic alcoholism may require significantly more sedative drugs to achieve the same level of sedation as a non-drinker (Chapman and Plaat 2009). Chronic alcohol use may also lead to liver dysfunction and possible excessive bleeding. Recreational drugs should be avoided pre-operatively to avoid any potential for drug interactions and so the patient can give informed consent.

11.10 Last Meal

It is always a good idea to ask if the patient has eaten prior to the surgical procedure. Patients are often in pain and do not eat or drink enough, which increases the risk of hypoglycemia or dehydration. A diabetic patient who has taken insulin but did not eat may become hypoglycemic and a medical emergency may arise. The term "NPO" (nil per os) means nothing by mouth. In general, a patient should only be NPO if an IV sedation or general anesthetic is planned.

11.11 Review of Systems (ROS)

The review of systems (ROS) allows the provider to ask the patient questions regarding symptoms the patient is experiencing, which allows the provider to check on the current status of the organ systems. This can be done quickly in most cases if a thorough medical history has already been taken or the patient is one of record and known history. Preoperative ROS may be as simple as asking if there has been any change in medical history since the last visit. Questioning the patient on the systems listed below will help avoid starting a surgery on an ill patient, which may lead to a medical emergency.

Constitutional – nausea, vomiting, chills, fever, sweats, weight loss, fatigue.

Neurological – headaches, dizziness, vision changes, hearing changes, weakness, depression.

Skin – itching, dryness, rash, pruritis, pigmentation, sores, hair loss.

Ear/Nose/Throat/Mouth – nasal discharge, dry mouth, dry eyes, oral pain, ear pain, hearing changes, neck tenderness.

Cardiovascular – angina, palpitations, peripheral edema, dyspnea, fainting.

Pulmonary – cough, sputum, dyspnea, wheezing.

Gastrointestinal – constipation, diarrhea, intolerance to foods, abdominal pain, blood in stools, difficulty swallowing, heartburn.

Genitourinary – frequent urination, incontinence, bladder problems.

Musculoskeletal – joint pain, muscle pain, swelling in joints, difficulty extending neck.

Endocrine – intolerance to hot/cold, hunger, thirst, frequent urination.

Psychiatric – depression, anxiety, memory loss.

11.12 Physical Examination

The physical examination of the dental patient focuses primarily on the oral cavity but may also include other areas of the face or body. It is important to document in detail any significant findings or pertinent negative findings. Physical examination of the patient involves visual inspection, percussion, palpation, and auscultation.

Table 11.1 Categories of BP in adults (Chobanian et al. 2003).

Blood pressure category	SBP (mm Hg)	DBP (mm Hg)
Normal	<120	<80
Pre-hypertension	120–139	80–89
Stage 1 Hypertension	140–159	90–99
Stage 2 Hypertension	≥160	≥100

Blood Pressure (BP)

The blood pressure should be taken at the initial visit, any visit a dental procedure is performed, or when local anesthesia is administered. The blood pressure should be taken if the patient experiences new symptoms of high or low pressure (lightheadedness or headache). Normal systolic blood pressure in an adult is <120 mmHg and normal diastolic blood pressure is <80 mmHg. Table 11.1 shows categories of BP in adults:

Consistently elevated blood pressure is an indication that the patient should be referred for evaluation by their physician. Elective dental treatment should be avoided in patients with blood pressures over 180/110. Treatment should also be avoided in patients who have symptoms of high blood pressure (headache, blurred vision, dizziness, confusion, chest pain) or a medical history that puts the patient at increased risk of adverse medical events. Consideration should be given to the difficulty and length of the procedure as well as the amount of local anesthesia with vasoconstrictor is to be given.

Pulse

The pulse should be taken every time the BP is taken. The pulse has two components, rate and rhythm.

Rate: The rate is the number of beats of the heart per minute. The normal rate is between 60 and 100. The dentist should take note if the rate falls outside this normal range. Higher than normal rate may be due to pain, anxiety, medications, physical activity, or related to a medical condition. A low heart rate can be normal and an athlete, but also could be secondary to a medical condition or medications.

Rhythm: Rhythm is also an important factor of evaluation. Taking the pulse may allow the provider to check the rhythm since electronic monitors do not always recognize an irregular rhythm. For the general dentist, if the rhythm is not regular treatment should be deferred until the rhythm is evaluated by a physician.

Respirations

Normal respiratory rate for the adult should be 12–18 breaths/minute. A dentist should be concerned and defer treatment if the respirations fall significantly outside this range.

Temperature

The normal temperature is 98.6°F or 37°C. A fever is present when the temperature is elevated to 100.4°F (38°C). The temperature should be taken when a patient has a suspected infection. If a patient has a significant swelling from a tooth and increased temperature, referral to an oral and maxillofacial surgery should be considered.

Height/Weight/BMI

Height and weight can be an important when they are at the extremes. Very tall or short adult patients may be a result of a genetic syndrome. Some syndromes can have physiologic problems that may need special management. Obesity can affect the patient's ability to lay flat in a dental chair due to difficulty breathing, but also because of the weight limit in dental chairs. Standard dental chair weight limits are generally around 350 pounds, although there are specialty chairs that can accommodate a larger weight.

Body mass index (BMI) is a relationship between the height and weight and is

Table 11.2 Categories of BMI in adults.

Category	BMI
Underweight	<18.5
Normal	18.5–24.9
Overweight	25–29.9
Obese	>30

calculated with the following equation where weight is measured in kilograms and height is measured in meters (Table 11.2).

$$BMI = weight/height^2$$

Clinical Examination

The clinical examination by a dentist is usually a focused evaluation of the oral cavity and surrounding structures. The examination may include the maxillofacial region or other organ systems such as the skin, heart, and lungs if indicated. The key methods in evaluating a patient consist of inspection, palpation, percussion, and auscultation. Clinical examination of the patient should include observing the overall appearance of the patient. The dentist would then inspect the face and neck looking for any abnormal changes. A detailed oral examination is then completed, which should include the lips, teeth, oral mucosa, tongue, floor of mouth, palate, and oropharynx.

ASA (American Society of Anesthesiologists) Classification

The ASA categories are related to the relative risk for anesthesia. The higher the ASA category, the greater the risk for the patient to have anesthesia.

ASA 1	Normal healthy patient
ASA 2	Patient with a mild systemic disease
ASA 3	Patient with a severe systemic disease, not incapacitating
ASA 4	Patient with a severe systemic disease that is a constant threat to life
ASA 5	A moribund patient not expected to survive without the operation
ASA 6	Organ donor

Laboratory Studies

General dentists generally do not rely on laboratory tests as often as they should. Being comfortable with a few laboratory tests can greatly increase the safety of practice and reduce the chance for a medical emergency happening in the dental office. Below are a few important labs that can be ordered if needed. Many other laboratory tests can be helpful in evaluating the preoperative patient and should be ordered as necessary depending on the patient's medical history.

Blood glucose: A blood glucose should be taken on all diabetic patients before treatment. This test can be done with a point-of-care glucometer in an office setting. A glucose of 250 dl/ml or more should be an indication for medical consult prior to elective general dentistry. The hemoglobin A1c (HbA1c) test measures the control of glucose over a period of two to three months. HbA1c values under 8 % show good levels of control while a value greater than 9 % shows poor control. The goal HbA1c for diabetic patients is less than 7.0 (Fauci 2008).

INR: The International Normalization ratio is a standardized reading for evaluating the anticoagulant therapy of Warfarin (Coumadin). The normal reading is 1 when the patient is not anticoagulated. A patient who is anticoagulated with Warfarin will have a therapeutic INR between 2.0 and 3.5. The appropriate INR will depend on the condition that is being treating. An INR of <3.5 is generally an accepted level for safe surgery. Strong consideration should be given to referral to a specialist for any surgical procedures on patients who are taking anticoagulants. Local hemostatic measures should be used and consultation with the patient's physician may be warranted if a larger procedure is being performed. Of note, there are new medications (factor Xa inhibitors) that are not able to be quantified using INR.

Platelet count: Platelets aggregate together to stop bleeding after surgery. Many diseases can affect the function and number of platelets. Normal platelet count is in the range of 150,000–450,000 platelets/μl of blood. Surgery should be avoided in patients with platelet counts less than 50,000 platelets/μl. Medications such as NSAIDS and clopidogrel (Plavix) can inhibit the effectiveness of platelets and must be considered preoperatively.

Radiographs

Radiographic examination is often needed prior to providing dental treatment. Periapical, bitewing, and panoramic radiographs are the most common radiographs that are utilized in dentistry. Other specialty radiographs may also be obtained such as occlusal and cephalometric radiographs. Cone beam computed tomography (CBCT) is also available and allows the dentist to study the three-dimensional relationships of the structures in the maxillofacial region. CBCT technology has helped to enhance the treatment of patients receiving oral surgery, orthodontic treatment, endodontic treatment, and other specialty treatment. The CBCT in Figure 11.1 shows a patient who sustained multiple mandible fractures.

11.13 Medical Status

Once all the appropriate medical information has been obtained, the dentist can make a determination as to how the patient can and should be managed. Healthy patients will not need any special precautions. Medically compromised patients may need to have additional precautions prior to treating the patient. This may include monitors (Blood pressure, pulse oximetry, electrocardiogram), modification of position such as treating the patient semi-upright, or the use of supplemental oxygen. Extremely ill patients or patients with significant medical comorbidities may need to be treated in a hospital setting.

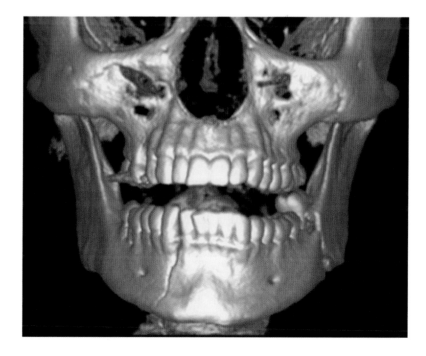

Figure 11.1 CBCT showing a patient who sustained multiple mandible fractures.

11.14 Anesthesia Requirements

The majority of dental patients can proceed safely with dental treatment using local anesthesia in an office setting. However, some patients may benefit from additional anesthesia methods such as the use of nitrous oxide, oral sedation, or IV sedation. There are also patients who will require general anesthesia to facilitate dental treatment due to either the inability to cooperate or due to significant medical comorbidities. The dental provider and patient can discuss the options. Referral to a specialist who can offer sedation or general anesthesia may be required in order to treat patients who are medically compromised, uncooperative, or who would otherwise not tolerate a procedure with local anesthesia.

Listed below are specific clinical and radiologic considerations that should be evaluated before starting a surgical case.

Clinical Analysis

Presence of Infection

No Infection Surgery in an area where there is no active infection is easier due to the ability obtain better local anesthesia and there is less bleeding (Figure 11.2). It is also easier to reflect a mucoperiosteal flap as the tissue is of normal consistency. Infected and inflamed tissue has the tendency to form mucosal tears.

Local Infection Localized infections will present according to where the infection erodes through the alveolar bone in relation to the facial and masticator muscles (Figure 11.3). Local anesthesia may be more difficult due to the change in the pH of the soft tissue and the increased pain that the patient is experiencing. Incision and drainage is often required to drain purulence that has accumulated.

Extensive Infection Extensive infections should be immediately referred to a specialist experienced in the management of head and neck

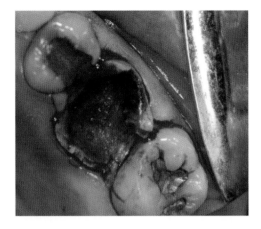

Figure 11.2 Surgical area with no infection.

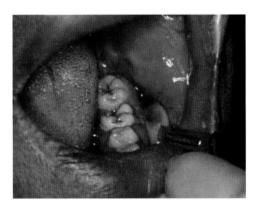

Figure 11.3 Surgical area with local infection.

infections. These patients are often extremely ill. These infections can spread quickly. If left untreated, the patient may develop airway compromise or the infection can spread the other parts of the body such as the neck, chest, eye, or brain. Although rare, death could result if an infection is not treated promptly. The patient in Figure 11.4 has a right submental and submandibular space infection secondary to a carious, infected mandibular molar.

Trismus

No Trismus A patient who can open wide will allow for access to preform nearly any intraoral procedure. Normal maximum incisal opening (MIO) is approximately 40 mm (Figure 11.5). Bite blocks are available in both pediatric and

Figure 11.4 Extensive infection secondary to a carious, infected mandibular molar.

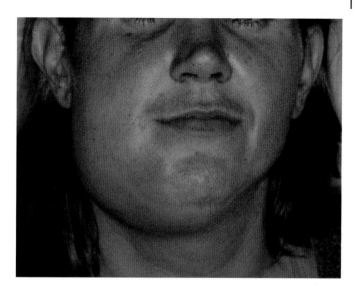

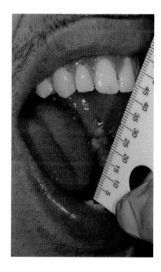

Figure 11.5 Normal maximum incisal opening (MIO).

adult sizes to help the patient's mouth stay open during procedures.

Trismus and Limited Opening Patients with significant trismus may best be referred to a specialist (Figure 11.6). Trismus can be due to temporomandibular disease, radiation therapy, tumors, or infections. Local anesthesia and access to the posterior areas of the oral cavity will be difficult in patients who have limited opening. Hospitalization and

intravenous antibiotics may be necessary if the trismus is due to infection. Advanced airway management techniques may be needed to treat the cause of the trismus and any other oral conditions.

Dental Caries

No Caries Teeth, such as premolars being removed for orthodontic reasons and do not have decay are generally easily removed with elevators and forceps (Figure 11.7).

Extensive Caries Teeth with extensive decay may be extremely difficult to remove particularly if the surrounding bone is dense and no clinical crown remains. Extensive decay will make tooth extraction more difficult due to the lack of tooth structure to engage with forceps. Mucoperiosteal flaps are often needed to gain access for elevation and removal of teeth with extensive caries. Bone removal may also be required. Some teeth that are grossly decayed, as depicted in the radiograph in Figure 11.8, may or may not be particularly difficult to extract due to the chronic periodontal and endodontic disease. These teeth likely have significant bone loss making elevation more effective.

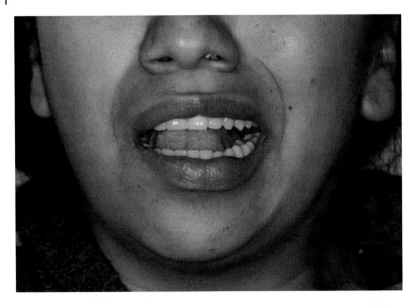

Figure 11.6 Patient with trismus showing limited opening.

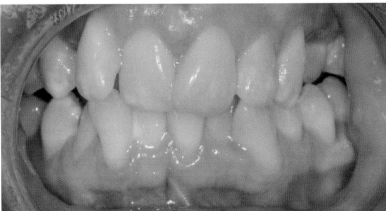

Figure 11.7 Patient showing teeth with no caries to be removed for orthodontic reasons.

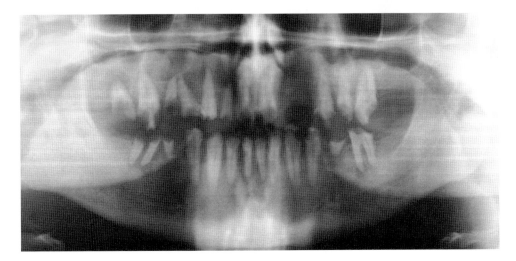

Figure 11.8 Radiograph showing gross decay of teeth.

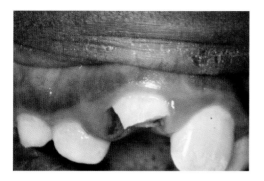

Figure 11.9 Patient with crown fracture secondary to trauma.

Tooth Fracture

Crown Fracture Teeth that are extracted due to a fracture secondary to trauma are usually difficult to remove (Figure 11.9). There are often secondary fractures and cracks, which complicates tooth removal. Often, there is not enough tooth structure to use forceps, so surgical removal is required. Any time a tooth is surgically removed consideration of the prosthodontic rehabilitation should be considered and socket preservation may be used.

Tooth Mobility

Minimal Extractions for patients with excessive one as shown in Figure 11.10 may be difficult. The surgical plan will likely include reflecting a tissue flap and bone removal.

Periodontally Involved Teeth Teeth with significant periodontal bone loss (Figure 11.11), either clinically or via radiographic review, are usually not overly difficult to extract if sound surgical principals are used. This includes soft tissue reflection, proper elevation technique, and proper forceps use.

Ankylosed Ankylosed teeth are rare. Teeth that have been reimplanted after being avulsed, transplanted teeth, or teeth that have been traumatized during development may become ankylosed. This is a pathologic diagnosis and not just a difficult extraction. If a tooth is truly ankylosed, a drill must be used to remove the ankylosed root.

Tooth Alignment

Good Alignment Tooth alignment should be considered as the majority of oral surgical

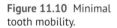

Figure 11.10 Minimal tooth mobility.

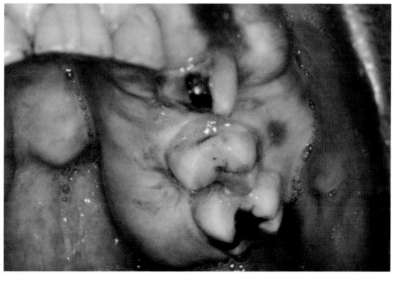

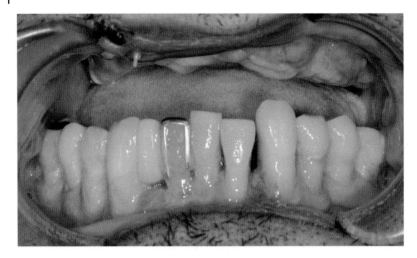

Figure 11.11 Teeth with significant periodontal bone loss.

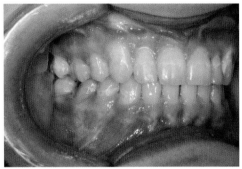

Figure 11.12 Normal alignment.

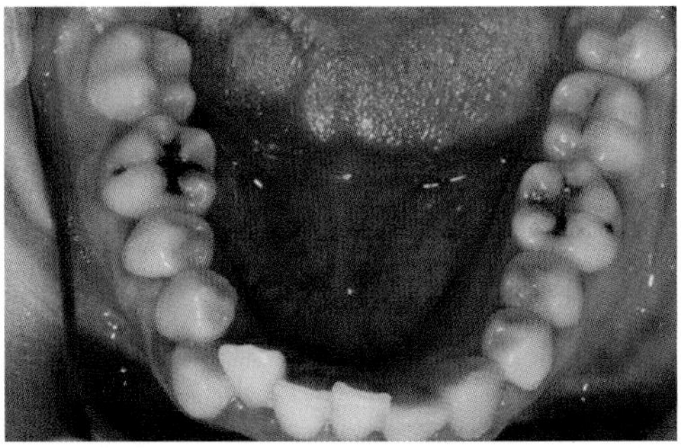

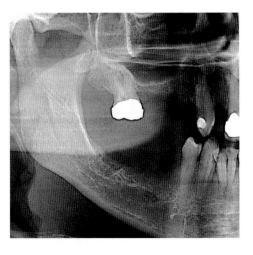

Figure 11.13 Misaligned mandibular anterior teeth.

instruments are designed to work best when the teeth are in normal alignment (Figure 11.12).

Misaligned Teeth Misaligned mandibular teeth can be challenging to extract (Figure 11.13). Normal dental forceps may not work well when significant crowding is present. Modification of the surgical plan to include bone removal or tooth sectioning may need to be considered. The right mandibular canine in Figure 11.13 would be difficult to remove due to the dental crowding that is present.

Isolated Teeth Thorough review and careful surgical technique must be used when there is an isolated posterior maxillary tooth (Figure 11.14). A tuberosity fracture or fracture

Figure 11.14 Radiograph showing isolated posterior maxillary tooth.

Figure 11.15 Tilted teeth.

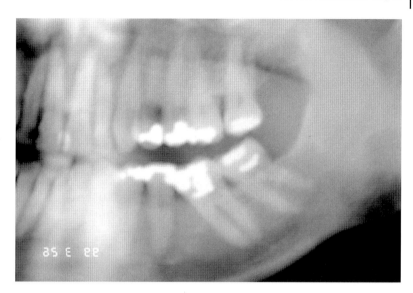

of the floor of the maxillary sinus may occur. Either of these complications can be accompanied by an oroantral communication. Tooth sectioning may be required even if a solid crown is present and a forceps could be used.

Tilted Teeth When a tooth is missing for a long period of time, the adjacent tooth may tilt into the space. Tilted teeth can be difficult to remove if the teeth are tilted to a significant extent. Care must be taken to be sure the correct tooth is removed. The incorrect number may be assigned clinically and appear to be different when the radiograph is reviewed. It is best to confirm which tooth is to be removed and contact the referring provider if needed. The panoramic radiograph in Figure 11.15 shows a patient who had tooth #19 (mandibular left first molar) removed many years ago, which has allowed teeth #17 and 18 to tilt into the space. Clinically this patient may appear to have a normal tooth relationship even though the first molar is missing.

Medication Related Osteonecrosis of the Jaw (MRONJ) and Osteoradionecrosis (ORN)

Medication Related Osteonecrosis of the Jaw (MRONJ) Certain antiresorptive medications such as bisphosphonates and the monoclonal antibody denosumab are used for the treatment of osteoporosis and treatment of certain cancers. Unfortunately, these medications can affect the ability of the maxillary and mandibular bones to heal (Figure 11.16). Patients on antiresorptive medications should be referred to an oral and maxillofacial surgeon if there are any concerns for non-healing ulcers, swelling, or exposed bone. Removal of teeth on patients on antiresorptive medications should be performed by and oral and maxillofacial surgeon. The surgeon may consider suspending use of or discontinuing these medications after discussion with the patient's primary care physician or oncologist.

Osteoradionecrosis (ORN) Head and neck radiation is often used as a primary or adjunctive treatment for the management of head and neck cancers. Radiation treatment involving the maxillofacial region and neck can affect the mandible and maxilla by decreasing the healing capacity of the bone and overlying soft tissue in these regions. Any patient who has had previous head and neck radiation and needs a surgical procedure or has exposed bone, increasing mobility of teeth, non-healing ulcers, or swelling should be referred to and oral and maxillofacial surgeon. The surgeon may consider hyperbaric oxygen to aid

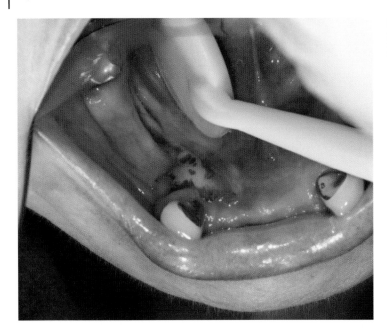

Figure 11.16 Medication related osteonecrosis of the jaw (MRONJ).

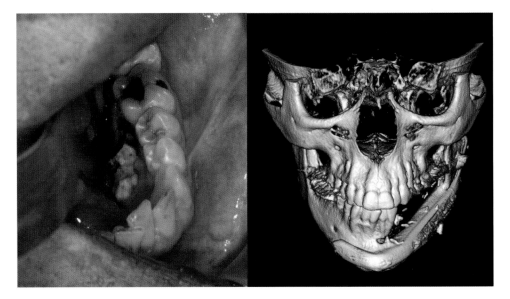

Figure 11.17 Patient with osteoradionecrosis (ORN).

in managing these patients. The patient in Figure 11.17 developed ORN following resection of a left tongue squamous cell carcinoma followed by radiation therapy. She was treated with several debridements with eventual resection and fibula free flap reconstruction.

Soft Tissue Lesions

Soft tissue lesions of the head and neck region should be identified on clinical examination and documented. Dentists should be cognizant of lesions of the eyes, face, neck, oral cavity, and throat. Patients with soft tissue lesions

Figure 11.18 Soft tissue lesion: ranula.

Ranula:

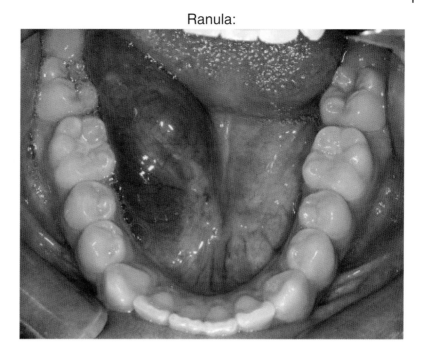

Figure 11.19 Soft tissue lesion: prominent maxillary frenum.

Prominent maxillary frenum:

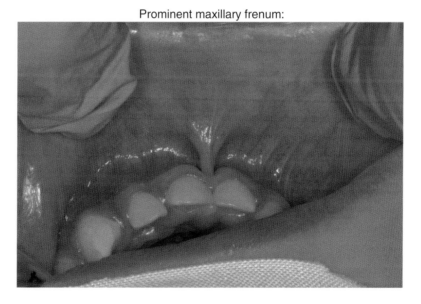

which do not resolve in the course of two to three weeks should be referred for a biopsy to an appropriate specialist (oral pathologist, oral and maxillofacial surgeon, otolaryngologist, dermatologist). Examples of soft tissue lesions are shown in Figures 11.18–11.22. The soft tissue lesions shown include ranula, prominent maxillary frenum, oroantral fistual, scalp cyst (trichilemmal cyst) and squamous cell carcinoma identified in the lower lip.

Oroantral Fistula

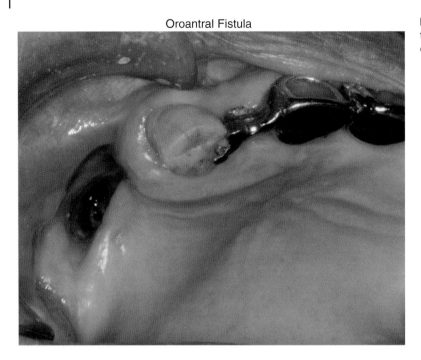

Figure 11.20 Soft tissue lesion: oroantral fistula.

Scalp Cyst (Trichilemmal Cyst)

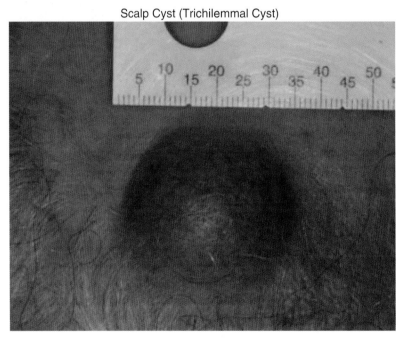

Figure 11.21 Soft tissue lesion: scalp cyst (trichilemmal cyst).

Radiographic Analysis

The standard of care for performing oral surgery is to have an adequate radiograph of the area of interest to review before beginning the surgery. Often, a periapical radiograph, which shows the entire roots, is all that is needed. A panoramic radiograph is often indicated for removal of posterior teeth, especially

Figure 11.22 Soft tissue lesion: squamous cell carcinoma (lower lip).

Squamous Cell Carcinoma (Lower Lip):

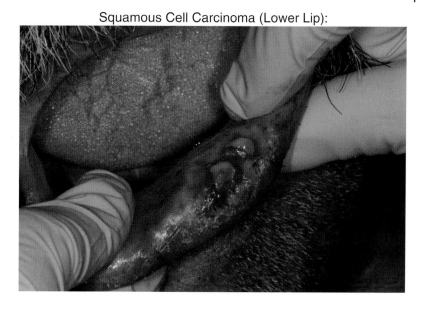

third molars. Panoramic radiographs allow for improved visualization of anatomic structures. CBCT can also be used to evaluate the proximity of vital structures, location of impacted teeth, and the extend of pathology. Radiographs are also useful in acquiring a complete and accurate informed consent by showing them to patients. Pathology on radiographs my warrant a referral to a specialist.

Adjacent Anatomy

Maxillary Sinus The maxillary premolars and molars are adjacent to or have roots extending into the maxillary sinus. Sinus perforations may occur in these areas. Roots of these teeth may also be displaced into the maxillary sinus, which may require direct access (Caldwell–Luc) into the sinus to retrieve to displaced root. The periapical radiograph in Figure 11.23 shows the close proximity of the maxillary left first molar to the maxillary sinus.

Nerves Close attention must be paid to the relationship of the inferior alveolar nerve and impacted and posterior teeth (Figure 11.24). Darkening of the roots, loss of the cortical border of the canal, or diversion of the canal

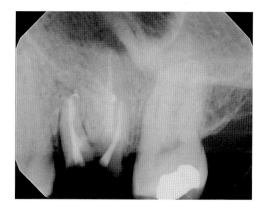

Figure 11.23 Radiograph showing close proximity of the maxillary left first molar to the maxillary sinus.

are risk factors for nerve injury. A CBCT can be used to evaluate the proximity of the inferior alveolar canal to adjacent teeth.

Caries, Large Restorations, Root Fracture, Previous Endodontic Therapy, Bone Structure

Extensive Caries Extensive caries can make tooth removal difficult as there is often little tooth structure to grasp with a forceps. Surgical removal of these teeth is often necessary (Figure 11.25).

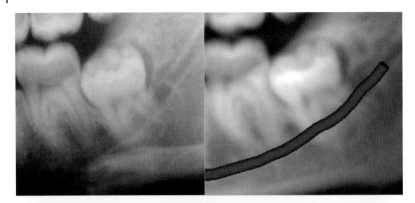

Figure 11.24 Cone beam computed tomography (CBCT) for evaluating proximity of the inferior alveolar canal to adjacent teeth.

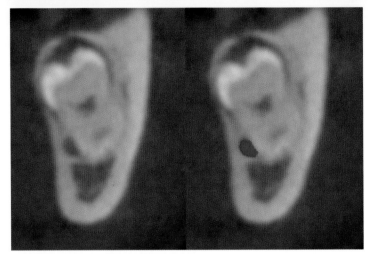

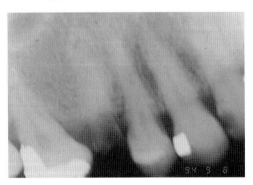

Figure 11.25 Surgical removal of tooth.

Large Restorations Teeth with crowns or large restorations often break or the crown or restoration can become dislodged when an elevator or forceps is used (Figure 11.26). A gauze throat screen should be used, and the surgeon and assistant should be prepared to retrieve any dislodged restoration.

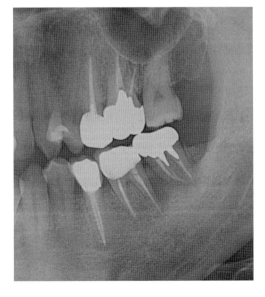

Figure 11.26 Large restoration.

Root Fracture Care should be taken during pre-operative review of the radiographs to identify root fractures (Figure 11.27). Root fractures can increase the difficulty of tooth extraction and will probably change the surgical plan. When a fracture of a tooth occurs, the surgeon should be mindful that the surrounding alveolar bone may also be fractured.

Previous Endodontic Therapy Previous endodontic therapy may make a tooth more likely to facture due to the decreased internal tooth structure. Endodontic material that has been extruded through the root apex may cause periapical pathology (Figure 11.28).

Periodontal Bone Loss Bone loss generally makes the extraction easier. Occasionally, the apical aspect of the root can fracture (Figure 11.29). A decision will need to be made if the root tip can or should be removed. A root fragment of 3 mm or less will generally not be a problem unless it is infected.

Figure 11.27 Root fracture.

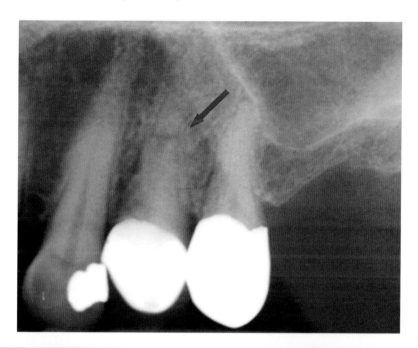

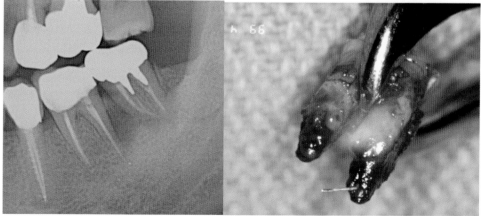

Figure 11.28 Effects of previous endodontic therapy.

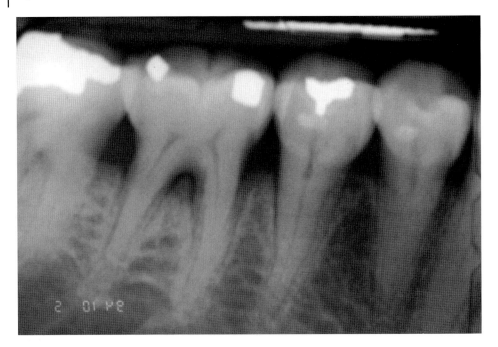

Figure 11.29 Periodontal bone loss and root fracture.

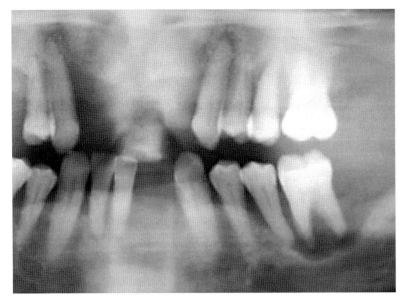

Figure 11.30 Severe bone loss.

Care must be taken when removing teeth with severe bone loss because the soft tissue may be easily torn (Figure 11.30).

Bone Density Increased bone density can make removal of teeth more difficult. Alveolar bone density often increases as the patient ages. Impacted third molars on patients over the age of 35 years should be removed after careful evaluation and if symptoms are present (Figure 11.31).

Figure 11.31
Impacted molars.

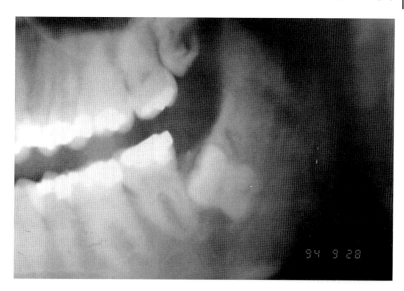

Figure 11.32
Radiograph to check number of roots.

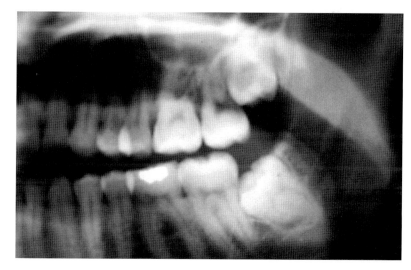

Root Morphology

Root Number Radiographs should be carefully reviewed to try to determine the number of roots that each tooth might have (Figure 11.32). Keep in mind that additional roots can be found on any tooth and that roots may be fused. In either case the surgery may be different then anticipate and may require a change in the surgical plan during the surgery.

Multi-Rooted Tooth Morphology Teeth with multiple roots which are divergent will be more difficult to remove than single rooted teeth or multi-rooted teeth with straight or fused roots. The retained deciduous mandibular left second molar in the radiograph in Figure 11.33 is an example of a tooth with divergent roots.

Dilacerated Roots Dilacerated or curved roots will be difficult. Most times with careful surgery the roots can be removed. The distal root of the mandibular left third molar in Figure 11.34 has a severe dilaceration, which is also in close proximity to the inferior alveolar canal.

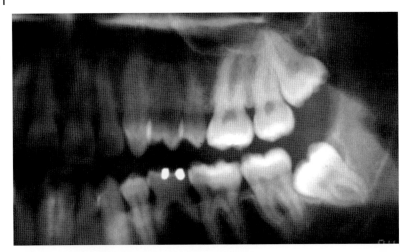

Figure 11.33 Tooth with divergent roots.

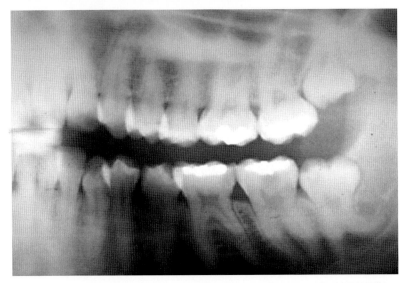

Figure 11.34 Severe dilaceration.

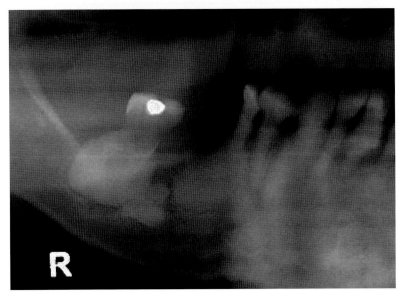

Figure 11.35 Enlarged roots: widespread hypercementosis of the mandibular teeth.

Enlarged Roots Bulbous roots or roots with hypercementosis may need to be sectioned several times or require have bone removal in order to extract the tooth. The radiograph in Figure 11.35 shows an example of a patient with widespread hypercementosis of the mandibular teeth.

Root Length Elongated roots can make tooth removal more difficult. Removal of bone around the tooth may be required in order luxate and remove the tooth. The radiograph in Figure 11.36 showed mandibular molars with elongated roots.

Root Resorption Root resorption can be secondary to many factors including impacted adjacent teeth, trauma, orthodontic treatment and pathology. Mandibular second molars can experience root resorption from impacted third molars as shown in Figure 11.37.

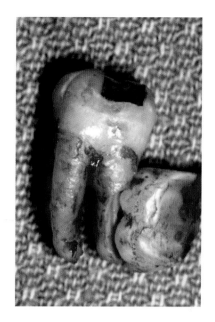

Figure 11.37 Root resorption.

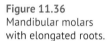

Figure 11.36 Mandibular molars with elongated roots.

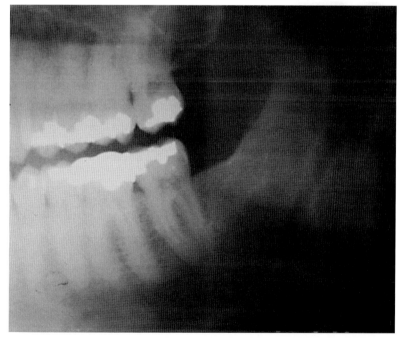

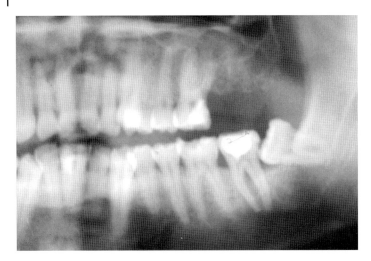

Figure 11.38
Impacted tooth next to tooth
to be removed.

Ameloblastoma:

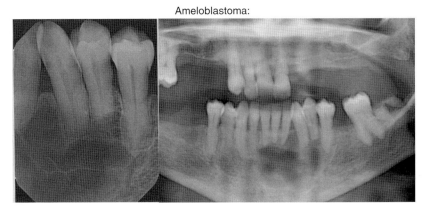

Figure 11.39
Ameloblastoma.

Keratyocystic odontogenic tumor:

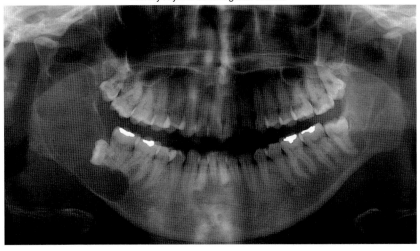

Figure 11.40 Keratocystic odontogenic tumor.

Nasopalatine duct cyst:

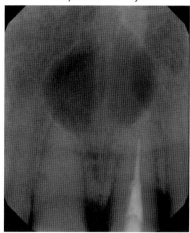

Figure 11.41 Nasopalatine duct cyst.

Impacted Tooth Next to the Tooth to Be Removed
The relationship of a tooth to an impacted

tooth must be considered as the impacted tooth may need to be removed at the same time (Figure 11.38). If the impacted tooth is uncovered or visualized in the extraction socket, it is usually advisable to remove the impacted tooth.

Pathology of Bone
Radiographs should be evaluated for bony pathology. Pathology of the jaw bones can range from simple periapical cysts associated with a necrotic tooth to large, deforming jaw tumors such as ameloblastomas. Consideration should be given to referral to an oral and maxillofacial surgeon if pathology is encountered on a radiograph. Often, a biopsy may be warranted for these cases. A few examples of radiographic findings are shown in Figures 11.39–11.42.

Figure 11.42 Osteradionecrosis.

Osteradionecrosis

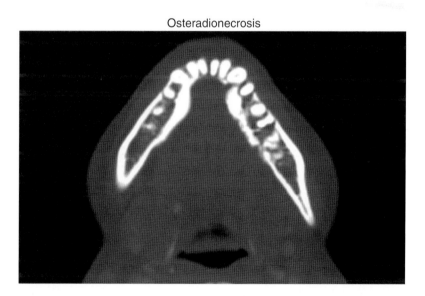

References

American Society of Anesthesiologists. (2020). ASA Physical Status Classification System. https://www.asahq.org/standards-and-guidelines/asa-physical-status-classification-system (accessed 13 December 2020).

Chapman, R. and Plaat, F. (2009). Alcohol and anesthesia. *Contin. Educ. Anaesth. Crit. Care Pain* 9 (1): 10–13.

Chobanian, A.V., Bakris, G.L., Black, H.R. et al. (2003). Seventh report of the joint National Committee on prevention, detection, evaluation and treatment of high blood pressure. *J. Am. Med. Assoc.* 289: 2560–2571.

Dye, B.A., Thornton-Evans, G., Li, X. et al. (2015). Dental Caries and Tooth Loss in Adults in the United States, 2011–2012. National Center for Health Statistics Data Brief. 197.

Fauci, A.S. (2008). *Harrison's Principles of Internal Medicine*, 2e, 2294. McGraw-Hill Professional Publishing.

Gerteis, J., Izrael, D., Deitz, D. et al. (2014). Multiple Chronic Conditions Chartbook. AHRQ Publications No, Q14-0038. Agency for Healthcare Research and Quality. Rockville, MD.

Kantor, E.D., Rehm, C.D., and Haas, J.S. (2015). Trends in prescription drug use among adults in the United States from 1999-2012. *J. Am. Med. Assoc.* 314 (17): 1818–1830.

US Department of Health and Human Services (2010). Multiple Chronic conditions – A Strategic Framework: Optimum Health and Quality of Life for Individuals with Multipole Chronic Conditions. Washington, DC.

12

Endodontic Evaluation

Diagnosis and Treatment Planning

12.1 Introduction

Successful treatment planning should be centered on an accurate and comprehensive diagnosis. An astute clinician must integrate the patient's chief complaint, history of present illness, medical history and a clinical evaluation in order to achieve an accurate diagnosis.

Previous clinical experiences are contributing factors that facilitate most diagnoses. However, diagnoses that rely solely on "experience" should be avoided at all costs. Instead, a thorough evaluation should be performed with the goal of reproducing the chief complaint, if existent, and formulating a diagnosis followed by the treatment plan. The focus of this chapter is to provide essential information to aid clinicians to achieve accurate endodontic diagnoses.

Determination of pulpal and periradicular status is not typically performed for every tooth in routine examination, but often is restricted to teeth believed to be "endodontically involved." This is a common mistake that may result in the delay of treatment and often disrupts the order of treatment planning. For example, a tooth with a necrotic pulp and normal periradicular tissues (no symptoms and normal radiographic presentation) may receive full cuspal coverage restoration such as a porcelain-fused metal crown (PFM) if

Physical Evaluation and Treatment Planning in Dental Practice, Second Edition.
Géza T. Terézhalmy, Michaell A. Huber, Lily T. García and Ronald L. Occhionero.
© 2021 John Wiley & Sons, Inc. Published 2021 by John Wiley & Sons, Inc.
Companion Website: www.wiley.com/go/terezhalmy/physical

not tested to determine its pulp and peri-radicular status prior to the formulation of treatment planning. This results in perpetuation of a disease state (infected pulp/tooth) and damage to the newly cemented crown when endodontic treatment is required due to signs or symptoms of disease. Unfortunately, this is often a finding in clinical practice (Figure 12.1). Thus, endodontic evaluation should be performed routinely for every tooth similarly to periodontal probing and caries detection.

Endodontic infections are polymicrobial in nature with complex microbial flora often present within biofilms (Sundqvist 1992; Jacinto et al. 2008; Montagner et al. 2010). The complexity of this microbial flora and its resistance to treatment is directly proportional to the duration of infection (Sundqvist 1992). Therefore, early detection and treatment increases successful outcome rates for endodontic treatments. Clinical success rates for endodontic therapies have been reported to be as high as 93–97% in large retrospective studies (Fonzar et al. 2009; Salehrabi and Rotstein 2010). Importantly, the survival of endodontically treated teeth also depends on the timely and adequate restoration of the tooth once the endodontic therapy is finished

(Ray and Trope 1995; Salehrabi and Rotstein 2010). This highlights the need for streamlined interdisciplinary treatment planning that aims to treat disease and increase the survival and functionality of a previously compromised tooth.

A primary reason a person seeks oral care is pain or discomfort involving a tooth. This is not surprising as teeth are one of the most nociceptive rich-tissues in the human body (Taylor and Byers 1990). It is estimated that approximately 22% of the population in the United States of America suffer from some kind of orofacial pain condition (Lipton et al. 1993). Noteworthy, not all these conditions are odontogenic and will not respond to endodontic therapy (Lipton et al. 1993; Nixdorf et al. 2010a, 2010b). Thus, attention must be given for the presentation of a patient's chief complaint.

The chief complaint must be expressed in the patient's own words. The oral care provider must refrain from interrupting the patient while he or she is explaining the chief complaint. Patients often use adjectives or descriptors of their symptoms that are particularly useful in deciding whether pain or another symptom is of odontogenic origin. Descriptors such as periodic, electric-like,

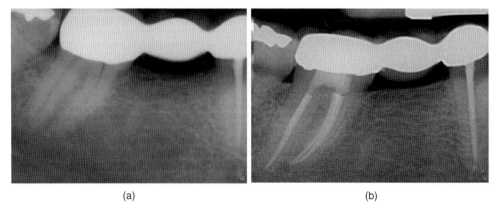

(a)   (b)

Figure 12.1 Tooth #30 received was used as an abutment for a fixed partial prosthesis (FPP; aka bridge) abutment without prior pulp and periradicular status testing. The tooth became increasingly tender to biting pressure and was referred to an endodontist who determined that the pulp was necrotic despite the normal radiographic appearance of the periradicular tissues (a). The root canal therapy was completed after access was made in the newly cemented crown and the chief complaint resolved (b).

lancinating, stabbing and "lightening bolt" provide qualitative information that does not match the seldom sharp (short duration) and mostly dull-aching odontogenic pain. Thus, allowing the patient to express himself may provide great information of the quality and intensity of the symptoms. It is important to note that while patients can precisely describe the quality and intensity of the pain, they often fail to associate the pain to a specific tooth. This is due to the common diffuse pain felt by most patients. In fact, only approximately 50% of the patients were able to accurately identify the tooth responsible for the pain. Thus, the oral care provider is charged with the task of identifying the tooth or teeth as the source(s) of the chief complaint. This tasks starts with the determination of the pulpal and periradicular status of the suspected tooth and/or adjacent teeth.

12.2 Pulp Status

The next step in an endodontic clinical examination after the evaluation of the chief complaint and history of present illness is the determination of the pulp status. This can be easily accomplished for most situations. However, in teeth with crowns or which are heavily restored, this can be a challenging task. The pulp diagnosis can be divided into four main categories: (i) vital or healthy; (ii) irreversible pulpities (symptomatic or asymptomatic); (iii) necrotic; (iv) previous initiated therapy; or (v) previously treated (see the definition of endodontic diagnostic terms below under "Diagnosis"). For teeth without history of treatment only the two first categories apply. Thus, most not previously treated teeth will have either a vital or necrotic pulp.

Vitality/sensitivity tests must be employed in order to determine the pulp status. The two main types of vitality tests are thermal and electrical tests. For thermal testing, cold is by far the most used stimulus to test the pulp status. This is largely due to cold being part of most chief complaints, and the easiness by which is performed. Also, cold tests are known to have diagnostic accuracy of approximately 90% versus 48% for heat testing (Petersson et al. 1999). Commercial available products containing compressed gas refrigerants such as Hygienic Endo-Ice® (Coltène/Whaledent Inc. Cuyahoga Falls, OH) and Frigident® (ELLMAN international MFG CO; Hewlett, NY) allow for easy access to very low temperatures (approx. −26°C) for cold testing in a consistent and predictable way.

The cold test must be performed on teeth that have been partially isolated with cotton rolls and air-dried. Next, a cotton pellet, larger than half the surface area of the tooth where the test will be applied, should be sprayed copiously with refrigerant immediately prior to testing each tooth (Figure 12.2).

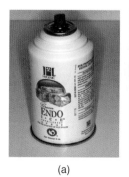
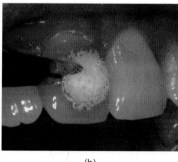
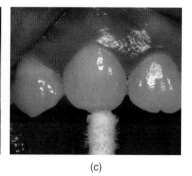

| (a) | (b) | (c) |

Figure 12.2 Commercially available Endo-Ice ® (a); Proper placement of a frozen cotton pellet placed on a dried tooth surface (b); Improper placement of frozen a cotton swab on a tooth (c).

A new cotton pellet may be required if it becomes wet with saliva. First, the stimulus (frozen cotton pellet) should be applied to a healthy contralateral tooth, as a comparative method, in order to demonstrate to the patient the type of response that is expected to be "normal." If an adjacent tooth is not present, another healthy tooth with similar anatomy could be tested. This approach allows the clinician to determine what is the basal response for the patient. This practice is particularly important since every patient will respond differently to the same stimulus due to multi-factorial factors such as anatomical features, neurobiological responses and psychological factors (e.g. fear and anxiety). Once the baseline is established, the clinician should proceed to testing the tooth suspected to originate the chief complaint. The application of the frozen cotton pellet to a surface of a tooth (e.g. buccal surface) may cool the surrounding tissues if kept on the tooth for a long period of time. Typically the cold stimulus should be applied onto a tooth no longer than five seconds. The clinician should pay close attention to the intensity and duration of the response in comparison to the baseline established previously (healthy teeth). Also, patients often provide verbal descriptors of their sensation such as very sharp followed by a dull-aching response seen in symptomatic irreversible pulpitis cases.

Another valuable vitality/sensitivity test is the use of an electric pulp tester (EPT). This device sends electric current through the tooth structure that activates voltage-gated sodium channels in the dental pulp eliciting a nociceptive response. This test does not provide quality (e.g. sharp vs. dull), or quantity (e.g. intensity) of the response. In fact, only a dichotomous response (i.e. "yes" or "no") should be considered from an EPT. The number displayed on the testing device when the patient feels the stimulus may be recorded but it does not relate to the intensity of pulpal inflammation or lack thereof. The EPT is reported to have an accuracy similar to the cold test (Petersson

et al. 1999; Weisleder et al. 2009). However, unlike the cold test, it does not reproduce the patient's chief complaint, nor provides additional information (e.g. intensity, quality of pain, etc.). Thus, the cold test is still the preferred test for most clinical presentations and EPT is only used when a negative response to cold is detected serving as secondary test. The exceptions are teeth with substantial deposition of secondary or tertiary dentin due to aging or trauma, respectively. In these teeth, EPT is considered the primary diagnostic tool to determine pulp vitality, since the cold test responds as negative in the majority of cases (Andreasen and Andreasen 1985; Andreasen et al. 1987; Biggs and Sabala 1990; Pileggi et al. 1996; Flores et al. 2001).

The electric pulp test should be performed on teeth that are isolated and air-dried. The probe of the EPT device should be placed on the occlusal 2/3 of either the buccal or lingual surfaces as this allows for more predictable responses and minimizes false positive responses arising from the periodontal ligament (PDL) if the probe was positioned at the cervical 1/3 of these surfaces (Jacobson 1984). Also, the speed by which the current rises should be set at approximately 50%, as too fast a voltage increase may lead to false-positive responses. Moreover, the placement of a small dab of toothpaste on the tip of the probe increases the surface contact between the probe and the tooth, and the conduction of electricity through the dental structure (Figure 12.3).

Similar to the cold test, the clinician should first test teeth that are believed healthy. This ensures that the device is functional prior to testing the tooth in question. A potential pitfall of this test is the possibility of electrical transfer between adjacent teeth resulting in false positive responses. Thus, the interproximal region must be free of saliva films that may serve as a conduit transferring electrical stimulus between adjacent teeth resulting in loss of diagnostic value (Figure 12.4).

Figure 12.3 Electric Pulp Tester (a); Partial isolation of the teeth that should be tested and placement of the EPT tip on the 2/3 of the buccal surface with toothpaste (b).

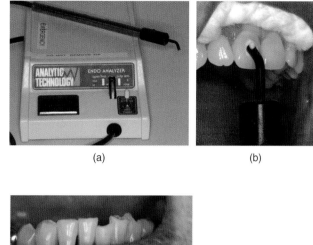

(a)   (b)

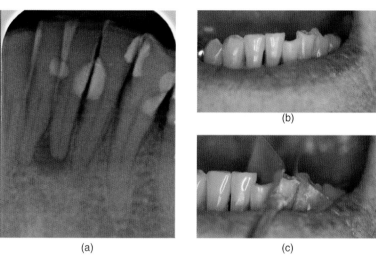

(a)   (c)

Figure 12.4 A patient with chief complaint of dull, aching pain on the anterior mandibular teeth. Teeth #25 and #26 did not respond to cold or EPT and were diagnosed with necrotic pulp. However, tooth #23 responded repeatedly to EPT despite having radiographic radiolucency (a). It was suspected that due to anterior crowding (b), leading to transference of electrical stimulus between adjacent teeth. The interproximal contacts were isolated with pieces of rubber dam (c), resulting in repeated negative responses to EPT, confirming the diagnosis of necrotic pulp and refuting the previous false positive responses.

12.3   Periradicular Status

The determination of the periodontal status is a key component of the correct endodontic diagnosis. It provides insight into the endodontic–periodontal relationship of the clinical presentation. Both clinical (pain or discomfort) and radiographic (e.g. radiolucency) may be either of primary endodontic with secondary periodontal source, or primary periodontal with or without endodontic involvement. In addition, clinical and radiographic evaluation of the periodontal status sheds light on the degree of inflammation of the tooth to be treated by the clinician. Based on these findings, the clinician must use his/her best clinical judgment and modify the treatment planning as appropriate (e.g. multiple visit endodontic therapy with intracanal medicament in teeth with extreme percussion sensitivity).

Approximately 67% of teeth diagnosed with irreversible pulpitis and 56% of teeth diagnosed with necrotic pulp will present with percussion sensitivity and/or tenderness to biting (Paheco et al. 2011). This is an interesting finding that suggests that pulpal inflammation is of enough intensity that leads to the accumulation of inflammatory mediators in the apical region of teeth far in advance of total pulpal necrosis and formation of periapical radiolucencies. Thus, percussion and palpation tests are a straightforward way to determine the degree of inflammation in the diseased tooth.

The clinician must first determine if the periodontal probing depths are within normal limits (approximately 3 mm, or greater if generalized in other teeth). It is important that this probing is performed along the whole sulcular circumference and in selected areas of the sulcus. This approach ensures that the whole PDL attachment is evaluated. Isolated probing defects are highly indicative or either a crown-to-root fracture, vertical fracture or sulcular sinus tract (Figure 12.5).

The definitive diagnosis of radicular fractures may be difficult to achieve, and these cases may require referral to an endodontist who may elect to create access to the tooth's pulp chamber and perform a microscopic evaluation of the remaining dental structure (Figures 12.6 and 12.7).

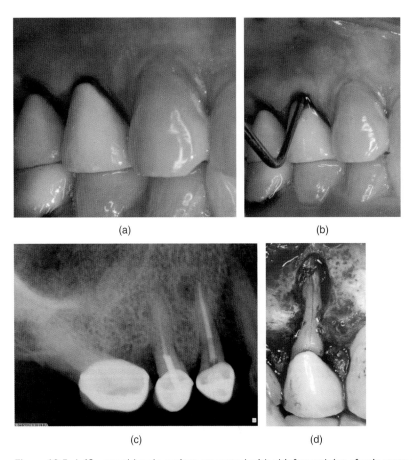

(a) (b)

(c) (d)

Figure 12.5 A 62-year-old male patient presented with chief complaint of pain upon mastication on the posterior maxillary right quadrant. Teeth #4 and #5 did not respond to cold or EPT but tooth #5 had moderate response to percussion (a) and (c). Also, tooth #5 had a localized, narrow defect of 12 mm on buccal surface (b). It was suspected that a vertical root fracture (VRF) was present and an exploratory surgery recommended. Upon surgical intervention, the root surface was stained with methylene blue and the VRF was confirmed with the operating microscope, as the etiology of the endo-perio lesion (d).

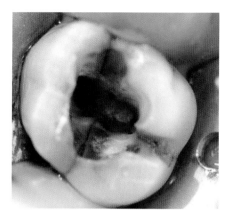

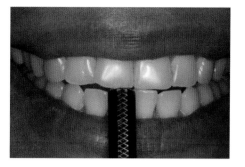

Figure 12.8 Percussion test being performed on tooth #8.

Figure 12.6 Patient had pulpal a diagnosis of irreversible pulpitis and periradicular diagnosis of symptomatic apical periodontitis. A longitudinal mesial-distal fracture was observed upon access. The extension of fracture must be assessed, after being stained, through the operating microscope. The prognosis of these teeth will change based on the extension of these fracture lines.

Next, the percussion test must be performed. The tooth should be gently tapped with the mirror handle parallel to the long axis of the tooth, and sensitivity level recorded as compared to healthy contralateral teeth (Figure 12.8). As mentioned previously, this simple test provides information as to whether the periapical region of a given tooth is inflamed.

The palpation test should be performed by applying digital pressure (a cotton swab may be used) on the buccal or lingual/palatal surfaces over the anatomical position of the roots and apical regions. This test is particularly useful to provide information as to whether there has been erosion of the cortical plates.

Tenderness to biting is the main chief complaint of patients with symptomatic apical periodontitis. This simple test can be easily performed by instructing the patient to bite over a cotton roll one tooth at time while recording the level of discomfort for each tooth. Alternatively, a tooth sleuth may be used. This simple diagnostic tool focuses the biting force on a single tooth and allows for testing individual cusps on posterior teeth, a crucial step in diagnosing fractured teeth. Thus, the use of the tooth sleuth allows for more predictable results and should be the preferred method to test teeth (Figure 12.9).

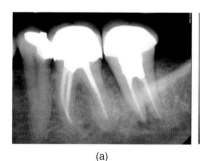
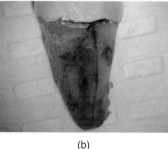

(a)   (b)

Figure 12.7 Patient presents one year after root canal therapy was performed on tooth #18 with pain upon biting and a sinus tract. A radiolucency is seen around the apices of tooth #18 (a). Photograph of the extracted tooth #18 shows evident vertical fracture after staining with a blue dye (b).

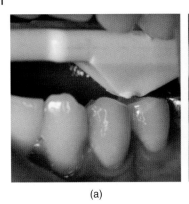 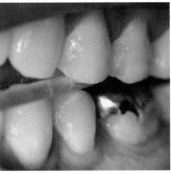

(a)   (b)

Figure 12.9 Tooth sleuth testing the lingual cusp of a mandibular bicuspid (a); cotton tip applicator is used if a tooth sleuth is not available (b).

12.4 Imaging Assessment

The use of radiographs to complement the clinical findings is extremely valuable. However, they do not always reflect the existence of normal or altered conditions of the tissues surrounding the tooth. The capability of existing radiographic systems to perceive periapical radiolucent lesions is essential for diagnosis and determination of a prognosis. Unfortunately, radiographs are a two-dimensional representation of a three-dimensional object.

In terms of diagnosis, radiographs will concentrate on modifications taking place on hard tissues or on the lack of mineralized substance. The use of the term "intact lamina dura" in dentistry to represent a normal radiographic appearance of healthy periradicular tissues is universal. According to some classic evidence, the best radiographic features for accuracy in diagnosis are lamina dura continuity and PDL width and shape (Kaffe and Gratt 1988). All the radiographic techniques recommend that the clinician should follow this structure all the way around examined teeth, at the specific area, confirming its normality. However, there is some evidence demonstrating that the inability to take parallel radiographs in certain conditions may result in an increase or decrease of perception of the "intact lamina dura," or even result in the inability to detect radiolucencies (Huumonen and Ørstavik 2002).

An additional term commonly used in dentistry to validate the presence of apical periodontitis at initial stages is called "widened"

PDL. The radiographic expansion of the PDL space near to the apex of a tooth is often considered abnormal. However, any factor that causes inflammation of the periodontal tissues such as bruxism or occlusal interferences can lead to a widened PDL that may not progress as long as the stimulus is removed (i.e. management of the parafunction or occlusal adjustment). Thus, a widened PDL alone without evidence of pulpal disease does not constitute reason for endodontic therapy.

The percentage of mineral bone loss that is required to produce a radiolucent area is between 30 and 50% in osteoporotic bone. Moreover, the amount of mineral bone loss in cancellous bone does not significantly affect the radiographic results (Bender 1982). According to the author, radiographic visualization of radiolucencies is influenced by the location of the lesions in different types of bone. A periapical lesion is radiographically visualized most promptly when it is near or in the cortex, less likely when it is located in the endosteal region, and least likely when it is in the region of the cancellous structure. Also, the cortical plate is one of the reasons why the radiographic size of the periapical lesion is under-estimated when compared with its actual size (Scarfe et al. 1999). Therefore, it has been demonstrated that two-dimension regular or digital radiographs both lack in accuracy.

Cone beam computed tomography (CBCT) has been implemented in dentistry to overpower the limitations of conventional radiography. Despite some disadvantages such as high radiation doses and the cost of the equipment, the ability to construct three-dimensional scans has changed the way we practice endodontics. There are basically two types of CBCT, the large volume allowing the entire maxilla and/or mandible to be scanned, and focus CBCT scanners, which have a smaller field of view. This is a foremost advantage over CT scanners, because the smaller the field of view, the lower the radiation.

The CBCT accuracy on the detection of periapical radiolucencies compared to periapical radiographs has been extensively reported. A study that compared CBCT and periapical radiographs found that the frequency of periapical lesions was 31% higher when CBCT was applied (Lofthag-Hansen et al. 2007). This result has been confirmed by other studies (Estrela et al. 2008; Patel et al. 2009), and some authors stated that CBCT should be used as a "gold standard" to detect the presence or absence of periradicular diseases (Low et al. 2008). However, it is important to emphasize that the "As Low As Reasonably Achievable" (ALARA) radiation exposure concept should still be applied to all patients.

The importance of CBCT in endodontics as an additional imaging technique for diagnosis is unquestionable but it should be properly used. The American Association of Endodontists (AAE) released a position statement addressing the discriminating use of CBCT scanners that needs to be taken in consideration. The statement says: "All radiographic examinations must be justified on an individual needs basis whereby the benefits to the patient of each exposure must outweigh the risks." In no case may the exposure of patients to x-rays be considered "routine," and certainly CBCT examinations should not be done without initially obtaining a thorough medical history and clinical examination. CBCT should be considered an adjunct to two-dimensional imaging in dentistry.

12.5 Additional Clinical Evaluations

Extraoral examination is an important step toward determining the severity of an endodontic infection. Facial swelling (cellulitis) is readily evident upon extraoral examination, and demonstrates the spreading of pus through the fascial planes. Also, local lymph nodes must be palpated to check for lymphadenopathies. Body temperature should be always assessed in emergency situations, or when there is suspected systemic involvement. The presence of facial swelling, lymphadenopathies and/or fever is (are) an indication that the endodontic infection presents with systemic involvement. Besides prophylactic antibiotic regimen (when indicated), this is the only endodontic clinical presentation that should require oral antibiotic (systemic) coverage.

Intraoral examination should include tissues surrounding the offending tooth. The clinician must carefully examine for the presence of erythema, swelling, or sinus tract(s) (Figures 12.10 and 12.11). In addition, the suspected tooth and adjacent teeth must be examined for the presence of occlusal interferences and fracture lines. Intraoral swelling, when associated with an endodontically involved tooth, is sign of an acute apical abscess. This clinical presentation benefits from an incision and drainage procedure to allow for alleviation of symptoms, reduction in the microorganisms load and increase in periradicular vascularity (important for healing and antibiotic efficacy). Although oral antibiotics may be required if there is further systemic involvement, the definitive treatment and outcome rely on the intracanal disinfection and obturation achieved in a complete root canal therapy.

Sinus tracts are defined as a pathway from an enclosed area of infection to an epithelial surface; opening or stroma may be intraoral or extraoral and represents an orifice through which pressure or pus is discharged. This clinical presentation has been often incorrectly

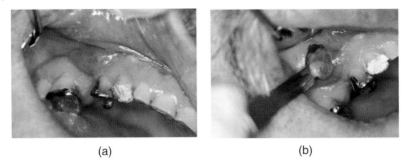

(a)   (b)

Figure 12.10 Presence of an intraoral swelling was seen upon examination. Despite its location distal to tooth#4, the abscess is associated with tooth #5 (a). Incision and drainage was performed after root canal instrumentation and placement of calcium hydroxide in tooth #5 (b).

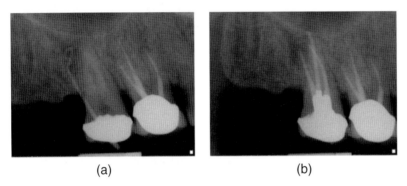

(a)   (b)

Figure 12.11 A 62-yo male patient presented with a chief compliant of pain upon mastication after crown was cemented on tooth #2 months prior. Upon intraoral examination, a sinus tract was detected and traced (a). The sinus tract closed and symptoms subsided after root canal therapy was performed through the newly cemented crown (b). Pulpal and periradicular diagnosis should have been performed for this tooth prior to restorative treatment.

called "fistulas." The presence of a sinus tract is the hallmark feature of a chronic apical abscess. The tracing of a sinus tract is an important diagnostic tool that a clinician must utilize to achieve the highest level of accuracy as possible. This is typically done, after local anesthesia, by carefully placing a gutta-percha master cone (sizes between 25 and 30) through the opening of the sinus tract until firm resistance is felt. A radiograph must be taken with care not to remove the GP master cone from its position. This approach allows for the visualization of the sinus tract path that always leads to the offending tooth. Noteworthy, sinus tracts appear in areas of least tissue resistance. It is typically around the apices of the teeth originating the abscess. However, they can be found anywhere in the adjacency of the offending tooth, including around the apices of healthy adjacent teeth. Thus, tracing the sinus tract points to the tooth with the chronic abscess and prevents misdiagnosis (Figure 12.12).

12.6   Diagnosis

In 2008 the AAE assembled a committee formed by world renowned endodontists to establish a consensus diagnostic terminology in endodontics. This initiative was propelled by the lack of standardization used in diagnostic terms impairing communication between clinicians. Also, most previously used diagnostic terms emphasized the radiographic presentation (e.g. chronic apical periodontitis

Figure 12.12
Pulpal diagnostic decision diagram. Determination of pulp status is directly related to responses achieved during diagnostic testing.

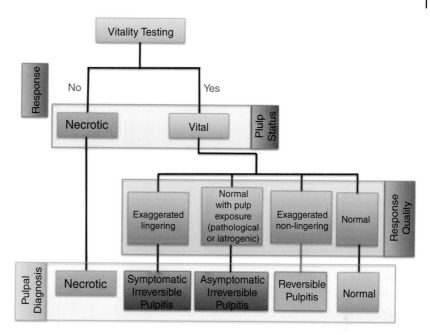

for teeth with *apical radiolucencies*). However, the focus should be on patients' symptoms and chief complaint. The consensus on the diagnostic term was reached and endorsed by the American Board of Endodontics (ABE). Listed below are the consensus diagnostic terms.

Pulpal

Normal pulp	A clinical diagnostic category in which the pulp is symptom-free and normally responsive to pulp testing.
Reversible pulpitis	A clinical diagnosis based on subjective and objective findings indicating that the inflammation should resolve and the pulp return to normal.
Symptomatic irreversible pulpitis	A clinical diagnosis based on subjective and objective findings indicating that the vital inflamed pulp is incapable of healing. Additional descriptors: lingering thermal pain, spontaneous pain, referred pain.
Asymptomatic irreversible pulpitis	A clinical diagnosis based on subjective and objective findings indicating that the vital inflamed pulp is incapable of healing. Additional descriptors: no clinical symptoms but inflammation produced by caries, caries excavation, trauma.
Pulp necrosis	A clinical diagnostic category indicating death of the dental pulp. The pulp is usually nonresponsive to pulp testing.
Previously treated	A clinical diagnostic category indicating that the tooth has been endodontically treated and the canals are obturated with various filling materials other than intracanal medicaments.
Previously initiated therapy	A clinical diagnostic category indicating that the tooth has been previously treated by partial endodontic therapy (e.g. pulpotomy, pulpectomy).

Periradicular

Normal apical tissues	Teeth with normal periradicular tissues that are not sensitive to percussion or palpation testing. The lamina dura surrounding the root is intact, and the periodontal ligament space is uniform.
Symptomatic apical periodontitis	Inflammation, usually of the apical periodontium, producing clinical symptoms including a painful response to biting and/or percussion or palpation. It might or might not be associated with an apical radiolucent area.
Asymptomatic apical periodontitis	Inflammation and destruction of apical periodontium that is of pulpal origin, appears as an apical radiolucent area, and does not produce clinical symptoms.
Acute apical abscess	An inflammatory reaction to pulpal infection and necrosis characterized by rapid onset, spontaneous pain, tenderness of the tooth to pressure, pus formation, and swelling of associated tissues.
Chronic apical abscess	An inflammatory reaction to pulpal infection and necrosis characterized by gradual onset, little or no discomfort, and the intermittent discharge of pus through an associated sinus tract.
Condensing osteitis	Diffuse radiopaque lesion representing a localized bony reaction to a low-grade inflammatory stimulus, usually seen at apex of tooth.

It is important to note that the new accepted diagnostic terms are symptom-centric and better describe the patient clinical presentation. These diagnoses can be easily achieved after careful clinical evaluation and diagnostic testing. The algorithms presented in this chapter can be used to help the clinician to reach both pulpal (Figure 12.13) and periradicular diagnosis (Figures 12.14 and 12.15).

12.7 Endodontic Treatment Planning

A thoughtful clinician must be ready to institute a treatment plan as soon as the diagnosis

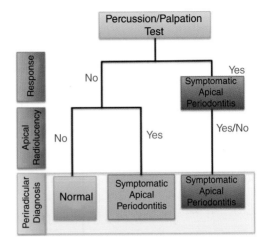

Figure 12.13 Periradicular diagnosis decision diagram. Determination of periradicular diagnosis depends mainly on symptoms. Radiographic presentation only dictates the diagnosis when a radiolucency is detected in an asymptomatic tooth.

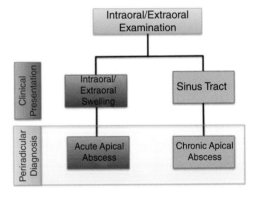

Figure 12.14 Periradicular diagnosis for abscesses decision diagram. Determination of abscess diagnosis depends directly on the clinical presentation and intraoral/extraoral examination (presence of swelling or sinus tracts).

is reached. This is particularly important in cases of emergencies. Patients in distress due to severe pain or systemic signs of infection (cellulitis, fever and/or edema) may require immediate treatment. This can be a stressful situation for patients, clinicians, and practice staff. Thus, a well-prepare dentist is ready to take action appropriately depending on the diagnosis and clinical preparation.

The endodontic treatment procedures may vary from simple pulpotomies, to pulpectomies, partial root canal debridement, full

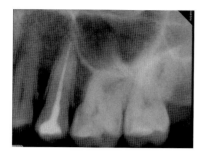 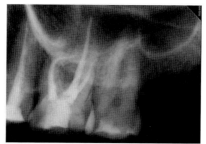

Figure 12.15 A 45-yo female patient was for irreversible pulpitis in tooth #14 due to an incomplete crown fracture (a). The severe curvature and complex anatomy of tooth #14 can be appreciated in the post-operative radiograph with "S" shaped mesial and distal canals.

debridement and obturation (1-visit endodontics), debridement followed by intracanal medicament and obturation in different visit (2-visit endodontics) or periapical surgeries (aka, apicoectomies).

Certainly for most cases the appropriate treatment course is the definitive treatment (full root canal therapy) in either a single visit or multiple visits. As stated previously, this treatment modality has high rates of clinical success resulting in resolution of patient's chief complaint (Salehrabi and Rotstein 2010). However, in certain situations, the clinician may elect not definitive treatment but emergency treatments such a pulpotomies, pulpectomies, or partial debridement procedures. These are aimed to provide immediate attenuation of the etiologic factor(s) behind the chief complaint. Typically, these are temporary solutions that should be followed through with completion of the root canal therapy procedure. The exceptions are immature teeth with vital pulps that could benefit from pulpotomies when appropriate to allow for complete root development.

Pulpotomies are procedures aimed to remove all the pulp tissue from the pulp chamber to the canal orifice level (full pulpotomy) or a portion of the pulp believed to be inflamed (partial pulpotomy or Cvek pulpotomy) (Cvek 1978). It should be stressed that pulpotomies, like pulpectomies, are vital pulp therapies that are capable of immediately reducing the pain level of symptomatic irreversible pulpitis. In fact, in a clinical trial, pulpotomies alone were capable of producing 96% pain relief with 85% of patients reporting at least a 50% (Hasselgren

and Reit 1989). This beneficial procedure for symptomatic irreversible pulpitis in conjunction with pharmacological pain management represents a relatively simple method by which clinicians are able to reduce pain sensitivity in the majority of patients diagnosed with irreversible pulpitis in a fast and effective method.

Similarly to pulpotomies, pulpectomy procedures are intended to be performed in emergency situations in teeth diagnosed with irreversible pulpitis (Figure 12.16). The term "pulpectomy" is often misused when describing incomplete debridement of root canals in teeth with in necrotic pulps. In most cases diagnosed with necrotic pulp the tissue has been dissolved due to liquefaction necrosis. Thus, the pulp cannot be removed as a whole or partially from the root canal system. Instead, these cases require either a partial debridement or full debridement.

Partial debridement procedures are intended to reduce the etiological factors (i.e. bacteria) of symptoms in teeth diagnosed with necrotic pulps. This procedure requires significant more dedication from the clinician since microorganisms in endodontic infections are hard to eradicate due to high virulence and anatomical challenges (root canal anatomical morphology and variations). Thus, it is safe to state that partial debridements are not accomplished by simply using small sized, not properly tapered hand files or barbed broaches. Although the use of these instruments could be appropriate in pulpectomies (vital pulp cases), it gives no benefit in cases with infected, necrotic

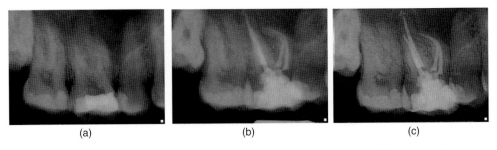

(a) (b) (c)

Figure 12.16 A 25-yo patient was referred by a general dentist who unsuccessfully attempted a pulpectomy procedure on tooth #3 (a). The severe curvature of the mesial root with 2 canals exiting separate foramina can be appreciated in the post-operative radiographs (b) and (c) of the same tooth imaged from two perspectives.

pulp with symptoms (clinical indication for debridement). It is well-established that these teeth have complex microflora that may be present in biofilms with strong antigenic components such as endotoxin (lipopolysaccharides, LPS) or lipoteic acid (LTA). To treat these cases as simple pulpectomies, represent a serious clinical mistake since hand files or barbed broaches do not remove the bulk of bacteria (coronal and middle 1/3 of the root canal space) and may push bacteria and their toxins out the apex into the periradicular tissue evoking robust immunological responses (aka flare-ups) (Siqueira 2003).

Partial debridement procedures must be only performed in teeth with necrotic pulps when symptoms are of intensity sufficient to justify an emergency procedure, as the best option for these teeth is always complete debridement and inter-appointment medication with a calcium hydroxide paste (2-visit endodontic therapy). Thus, when elected, partial debridement must always involve cleaning and shaping of the coronal and middle 1/3 of the root canal system to allow for the bulk of bacteria to be removed, appropriate access of irrigants and intracanal medicaments into the root canal system, both key components of intracanal disinfection.

The complete debridement of a canal system and obturation (complete root canal therapy) is always the main treatment course for teeth that are endodontically involved. The clinician must be up-to-date with evidence-based cleaning and shaping and disinfection techniques in order to achieve success in this treatment modality. There is no reason why endodontics should not be an integral part of a general dental practice. However, endodontic cases should only be treated if they fall within the level of training and comfort of the oral care provider. The decision to treat or refer is often difficult. It requires clinical experience to decide that a case may be too difficult requiring referral to an endodontist. For this reason, the AAE created a Case Difficulty Assessment Form that can be found at: www.aae.org/guidelines and is shown in Figure 12.17. This form was designed to help general practitioners to identify potential challenges in a systematic way avoiding delays in referral, costly multiple visits, patient dissatisfaction, and possible procedural accidents and liability.

Several factors are taken into account on the AAE's Case Difficulty Assessment Form. These are clustered under (i) Patient's considerations (e.g. complex medical histories, high level of anxiety or gag reflex and, etc.); (ii) Diagnostic and treatment considerations (e.g. diagnosis difficulty, moderate to severe canal curvatures or calcifications and, etc.); and (iii) Additional considerations (history of trauma, previous root canal therapy and complex endo-periodontal relationships). The AAE Case Difficulty Assessment Form represents a valuable tool for assessing the difficulty of a case.

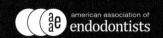

AAE Endodontic Case Difficulty Assessment Form and Guidelines

Patient Information

Full Name

Street Address   Suite/Apt

City   State/Country   Zip

Phone

Email

Disposition

Treat in Office: ○ Yes   ○ No

Refer Patient to:

Date

Guidelines for Using the AAE Endodontic Case Difficulty Assessment Form

The AAE designed the Endodontic Case Difficulty Assessment Form for use in endodontic curricula. The Assessment Form makes case selection more efficient, more consistent and easier to document. Dentists may also choose to use the Assessment Form to help with referral decision making and record keeping.

Conditions listed in this form should be considered potential risk factors that may complicate treatment and adversely affect the outcome. Levels of difficulty are sets of conditions that may not be controllable by the dentist. Risk factors can influence the ability to provide care at a consistently predictable level and impact the appropriate provision of care and quality assurance.

The Assessment Form enables a practitioner to assign a level of difficulty to a particular case.

Levels of Difficulty

MINIMAL DIFFICULTY
Preoperative condition indicates routine complexity (uncomplicated). These types of cases would exhibit only those factors listed in the MINIMAL DIFFICULTY category. Achieving a predictable treatment outcome should be attainable by a competent practitioner with limited experience.

MODERATE DIFFICULTY
Preoperative condition is complicated, exhibiting one or more patient or treatment factors listed in the MODERATE DIFFICULTY category. Achieving a predictable treatment outcome will be challenging for a competent, experienced practitioner.

HIGH DIFFICULTY
Preoperative condition is exceptionally complicated, exhibiting several factors listed in the MODERATE DIFFICULTY category or at least one in the HIGH DIFFICULTY category. Achieving a predictable treatment outcome will be challenging for even the most experienced practitioner with an extensive history of favorable outcomes.
Review your assessment of each case to determine the level of difficulty. If the level of difficulty exceeds your experience and comfort, you might consider referral to an endodontist.

Criteria and Subcriteria	MINIMAL DIFFICULTY	MODERATE DIFFICULTY	HIGH DIFFICULTY
A. PATIENT CONSIDERATIONS			
MEDICAL HISTORY	☐ No medical problem (ASA Class 1*)	☐ One or more medical problem (ASA Class 2*)	☐ Complex medical history/serious illness/disability (ASA Classes 3-5*)
ANESTHESIA	☐ No history of anesthesia problems	☐ Vasoconstrictor intolerance	☐ Difficulty achieving anesthesia
PATIENT DISPOSITION	☐ Cooperative and compliant	☐ Anxious but cooperative	☐ Uncooperative
ABILITY TO OPEN MOUTH	☐ No limitation	☐ Slight limitation in opening	☐ Significant limitation in opening
GAG REFLEX	☐ None	☐ Gags occasionally with radiographs/treatment	☐ Extreme gag reflex which has compromised past dental care
EMERGENCY CONDITION	☐ Minimum pain or swelling	☐ Moderate pain or swelling	☐ Severe pain or swelling

The contribution of the Canadian Academy of Endodontics and others to the development of this form is gratefully acknowledged. The AAE Endodontic Case Difficulty Assessment Form is designed to aid the practitioner in determining appropriate case disposition. The American Association of Endodontists neither expressly nor implicitly warrants any positive results associated with the use of this form. This form may be reproduced but may not be amended or altered in any way. © American Association of Endodontists, 180 N. Stetson Ave., Suite 1500, Chicago, IL 60601; Phone: 800-872-3636 or 312-266-7255; Fax: 866-451-9020 or 312-266-9867; E-mail: info@aae.org; Website: aae.org

Access additional resources at aae.org

Figure 12.17 The American Association of Endodontists (AAE) AAE Case Difficulty Assessment Form.

Criteria and Subcriteria	MINIMAL DIFFICULTY	MODERATE DIFFICULTY	HIGH DIFFICULTY
B. DIAGNOSTIC AND TREATMENT CONSIDERATIONS			
DIAGNOSIS	☐ Signs and symptoms consistent with recognized pulpal and periapical conditions	☐ Extensive differential diagnosis of usual signs and symptoms required	☐ Confusing and complex signs and symptoms: difficult diagnosis ☐ History of chronic oral/facial pain
RADIOGRAPHIC DIFFICULTIES	☐ Minimal difficulty obtaining/interpreting radiographs	☐ Moderate difficulty obtaining/interpreting radiographs (*e.g.*, high floor of mouth, narrow or low palatal vault, presence of tori)	☐ Extreme difficulty obtaining/interpreting radiographs (*e.g.*, superimposed anatomical structures)
POSITION IN THE ARCH	☐ Anterior/premolar ☐ Slight inclination (<10°) ☐ Slight rotation (<10°)	☐ 1st molar ☐ Moderate inclination (10-30°) ☐ Moderate rotation (10-30°)	☐ 2nd or 3rd molar ☐ Extreme inclination (>30°) ☐ Extreme rotation (>30°)
TOOTH ISOLATION	☐ Routine rubber dam placement	☐ Simple pretreatment modification required for rubber dam isolation	☐ Extensive pretreatment modification required for rubber dam isolation
CROWN MORPHOLOGY	☐ Normal original crown morphology	☐ Full coverage restoration ☐ Porcelain restoration ☐ Bridge abutment ☐ Moderate deviation from normal tooth/root form (*e.g.*, taurodontism microdens) ☐ Teeth with extensive coronal destruction	☐ Restoration does not reflect original anatomy/alignment ☐ Significant deviation from normal tooth/root form (*e.g.*, fusion dens in dente)
CANAL AND ROOT MORPHOLOGY	☐ Slight or no curvature (<10°) ☐ Closed apex (<1 mm in diameter)	☐ Moderate curvature (10-30°) ☐ Crown axis differs moderatel from root axis. Apical opening 1-1.5 mm in diameter	☐ Extreme curvature (>30°) or S-shaped curve ☐ Mandibular premolar or anterior with 2 roots ☐ Maxillary premolar with 3 roots ☐ Canal divides in the middle or apical third ☐ Very long tooth (>25 mm) ☐ Open apex (>1.5 mm in diameter)
RADIOGRAPHIC APPEARANCE OF CANAL(S)	☐ Canal(s) visible and not reduced in size	☐ Canal(s) and chamber visible but reduced in size ☐ Pulp stones	☐ Indistinct canal path ☐ Canal(s) not visible
RESORPTION	☐ No resorption evident	☐ Minimal apical resorption	☐ Extensive apical resorption ☐ Internal resorption ☐ External resorption
C. ADDITIONAL CONSIDERATIONS			
TRAUMA HISTORY	☐ Uncomplicated crown fracture of mature or immature teeth	☐ Complicated crown fracture of mature teeth ☐ Subluxation	☐ Complicated crown fracture of immature teeth ☐ Horizontal root fracture ☐ Alveolar fracture ☐ Intrusive, extrusive or lateral luxation ☐ Avulsion
ENDODONTIC TREATMENT HISTORY	☐ No previous treatment	☐ Previous access without complications	☐ Previous access with complications (*e.g.*, perforation, non-negotiated canal, ledge, separated instrument) ☐ Previous surgical or nonsurgical endodontic treatment completed
PERIODONTAL-ENDODONTIC CONDITION	☐ None or mild periodontal disease	☐ Concurrent moderate periodontal disease	☐ Concurrent severe periodontal disease ☐ Cracked teeth with periodontal complications ☐ Combined endodontic/periodontic lesion ☐ Root amputation prior to endodontic treatment

*American Society of Anesthesiologists (ASA) Classification System **Class 1:** No systemic illness. Patient healthy. **Class 2:** Patient with mild degree of systemic illness, but without functional restrictions, e.g., well-controlled hypertension. **Class 3:** Patient with severe degree of systemic illness which limits activities, but does not immobilize the patient. **Class 4:** Patient with severe systemic illness that immobilizes and is sometimes life threatening. **Class 5:** Patient will not survive more than 24 hours whether or not surgical intervention takes place. www.asahq.org/clinical/physicalstatus.htm

Access additional resources at aae.org

Figure 12.17 (*Continued*)

In summary, the form is an excellent tool for familiarizing the clinician with potential treatment challenges, and helps in the decision making of when to treat or refer. Examples of difficult cases that may require referral are presented below.

12.8 Concluding Remarks

- Pulp and periradicular status should be established for every tooth undergoing any kind of treatment (restorative, periodontal, orthodontic, etc.).

- Clinical testing when done in a systematic and adequate way leads to accurate diagnoses.
- "Proper diagnosis leads to appropriate treatment and a successful outcome."
- Not every chief complaint is odontogenic.
- The use of standardized consensus diagnostic terms is imperative to better describe the clinical presentation and improve communication among clinicians.
- A thoughtful clinician must perform difficulty assessment for every tooth undergoing endodontic therapy. Cases that fall outside the expertise levels of the general dentist must be referred to an endodontist.

References

Andreasen, F.M. and Andreasen, J.O. (1985). Diagnosis of luxation injuries: the importance of standardized clinical, radiographic and photographic techniques in clinical investigations. *Endod. Dent. Traumatol.* 1: 160–169.

Andreasen, F.M., Zhijie, Y., Thomsen, B.L., and Andersen, P.K. (1987). Occurrence of pulp canal obliteration after luxation injuries in the permanent dentition. *Endod. Dent. Traumatol.* 3: 103–115.

Bender, I.B. (1982). Factors influencing the radiographic appearance of bony lesions. *J. Endod.* 8: 161–170.

Biggs, J.T. and Sabala, C.L. (1990). Endodontic management of trauma to permanent teeth. *Compendium* 11 (538): 540–534.

Cvek, M. (1978). A clinical report on partial pulpotomy and capping with calcium hydroxide in permanent incisors with complicated crown fracture. *J. Endod.* 4: 232–237.

Estrela, C., Bueno, M.R., Azevedo, B.C. et al. (2008). A new periapical index based on cone beam computed tomography. *J. Endod.* 34: 1325–1331.

Flores, M.T., Andreasen, J.O., Bakland, L.K. et al. (2001). Guidelines for the evaluation and management of traumatic dental injuries. *Dent. Traumatol.* 17: 49–52.

Fonzar, F., Fonzar, A., Buttolo, P. et al. (2009). The prognosis of root canal therapy: a 10-year retrospective cohort study on 411 patients with 1175 endodontically treated teeth. *Eur. J. Oral Implantol.* 2: 201–208.

Hasselgren, G. and Reit, C. (1989). Emergency pulpotomy: pain relieving effect with and without the use of sedative dressings. *J. Endod.* 15: 254–256.

Huumonen, S. and Ørstavik, D. (2002). Radiological aspects of apical periodontitis. *Endod. Top.* 1: 3–25.

Jacinto, R.C., Montagner, F., Signoretti, F.G. et al. (2008). Frequency, microbial interactions, and antimicrobial susceptibility of Fusobacterium nucleatum and *Fusobacterium necrophorum* isolated from primary endodontic infections. *J. Endod.* 34: 1451–1456.

Jacobson, J.J. (1984). Probe placement during electric pulp-testing procedures. *Oral Surg. Oral Med. Oral Pathol.* 58: 242–247.

Kaffe, I. and Gratt, B.M. (1988). Variations in the radiographic interpretation of the periapical dental region. *J. Endod.* 14: 330–335.

Lipton, J.A., Ship, J.A., and Larach-Robinson, D. (1993). Estimated prevalence and distribution of reported orofacial pain in the United States. *J. Am. Dent. Assoc.* 124: 115–121.

Lofthag-Hansen, S., Huumonen, S., Grondahl, K., and Grondahl, H.G. (2007). Limited cone-beam CT and intraoral radiography for the diagnosis of periapical pathology. *Oral Surg. Oral Med. Oral Pathol. Oral Radiol. Endod.* 103: 114–119.

Low, K.M., Dula, K., Burgin, W., and von Arx, T. (2008). Comparison of periapical radiography and limited cone-beam tomography in posterior maxillary teeth referred for apical surgery. *J. Endod.* 34: 557–562.

Montagner, F., Gomes, B.P., and Kumar, P.S. (2010). Molecular fingerprinting reveals the presence of unique communities associated with paired samples of root canals and acute apical abscesses. *J. Endod.* 36: 1475–1479.

Nixdorf, D.R., Moana-Filho, E.J., Law, A.S. et al. (2010a). Frequency of nonodontogenic pain after endodontic therapy: a systematic review and meta-analysis. *J. Endod.* 36: 1494–1498.

Nixdorf, D.R., Moana-Filho, E.J., Law, A.S. et al. (2010b). Frequency of persistent tooth pain after root canal therapy: a systematic review and meta-analysis. *J. Endod.* 36: 224–230.

Paheco, M.A., Teixeira, F.B., Hargreaves, K.M., and Diogenes, A. (2011). Prevalence of mechanical allodynia in endodontic patients. *J. Endod.* 37: e24.

Patel, S., Dawood, A., Mannocci, F. et al. (2009). Detection of periapical bone defects in human jaws using cone beam computed tomography and intraoral radiography. *Int. Endod. J.* 42: 507–515.

Petersson, K., Soderstrom, C., Kiani-Anaraki, M., and Levy, G. (1999). Evaluation of the ability of thermal and electrical tests to register pulp vitality. *Endod. Dent. Traumatol.* 15: 127–131.

Pileggi, R., Dumsha, T.C., and Myslinksi, N.R. (1996). The reliability of electric pulp test after concussion injury. *Endod. Dent. Traumatol.* 12: 16–19.

Ray, H.A. and Trope, M. (1995). Periapical status of endodontically treated teeth in relation to the technical quality of the root filling and the coronal restoration. *Int. Endod. J.* 28: 12–18.

Salehrabi, R. and Rotstein, I. (2010). Epidemiologic evaluation of the outcomes of orthograde endodontic retreatment. *J. Endod.* 36: 790–792.

Scarfe, W.C., Czerniejewski, V.J., Farman, A.G. et al. (1999). In vivo accuracy and reliability of color-coded image enhancements for the assessment of periradicular lesion dimensions. *Oral Surg. Oral Med. Oral Pathol. Oral Radiol. Endod.* 88: 603–611.

Siqueira, J.F. Jr., (2003). Microbial causes of endodontic flare-ups. *Int. Endod. J.* 36: 453–463.

Sundqvist, G. (1992). Ecology of the root canal flora. *J. Endod.* 18: 427–430.

Taylor, P.E. and Byers, M.R. (1990). An immunocytochemical study of the morphological reaction of nerves containing calcitonin gene-related peptide to microabscess formation and healing in rat molars. *Arch. Oral Biol.* 35: 629–638.

Weisleder, R., Yamauchi, S., Caplan, D.J. et al. (2009). The validity of pulp testing: a clinical study. *J. Am. Dent. Assoc.* 140: 1013–1017.

13

Prosthodontic Restoration

Diagnosis and Treatment Planning

13.1 Documenting Patient Health Histories

Optimal prosthodontic restorative treatment for a dental patient can be provided only after the clinician has obtained and reviewed the medical, social, and dental histories of the patient and documented them in the patient's dental record. A patient's needs, desires, and attitudes concerning prosthodontic restoration of their oral cavity (Figures 13.1–13.8) for form, function, and esthetics should also be interpreted by the clinician and documented in the patient's dental record (Jahangiri et al. 2011). A truthful assessment and documentation of a patient's personality, psychological state, and expectations is of paramount importance to achieve favorable prosthodontic outcomes (see Figure 13.9).

Figures 13.1–13.5 show a completely edentulous male patient who exhibits normal anterior–posterior residual ridge relations intraorally, but has excessive loss of vertical dimension and a prognathic facial profile with old dentures in place. The patient expressed dissatisfaction with his appearance when wearing dentures saying that they made him look "ape-like." Unfortunately, the patient allowed this negative personal image of himself to affect his ability to interact socially withdrawing from friends and family members. Figures 13.6–13.8 show the same patient who now exhibits an orthognathic facial profile after a significant increase in the vertical dimension of occlusion

Physical Evaluation and Treatment Planning in Dental Practice, Second Edition.
Géza T. Terézhalmy, Michaell A. Huber, Lily T. García and Ronald L. Occhionero.
© 2021 John Wiley & Sons, Inc. Published 2021 by John Wiley & Sons, Inc.
Companion Website: www.wiley.com/go/terezhalmy/physical

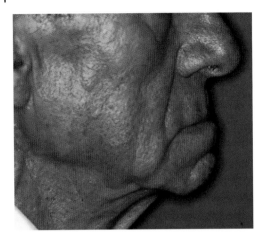

Figure 13.1 Pre-treatment lateral facial view of complete denture patient with excessive loss of vertical dimension of occlusion and prognathic profile.

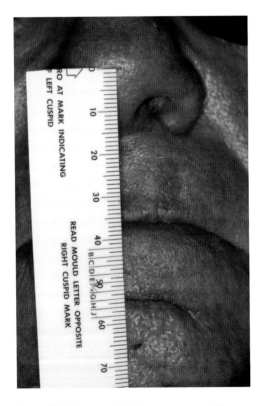

Figure 13.2 Extraoral facial measurement of vertical dimension of patient in Figure 13.1 with old complete dentures in maximum intercuspation (66 mm).

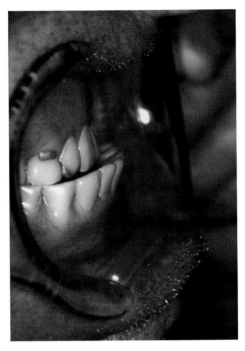

Figure 13.3 Completely edentulous patient shown in Figure 13.1 with old dentures in maximum intercuspation showing Class III anterior tooth and maxillomandibular denture relations.

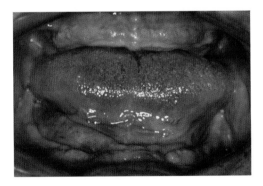

Figure 13.4 Intraoral frontal view of completely edentulous patient in Figure 13.1 showing normal ridge relations with mandible at physiologic rest position.

and prosthodontic restorative treatment to Class I ridge and occlusal relations with new maxillary and mandibular complete dentures. The restoration of the patient's lower face height and characterization of the acrylic resin denture teeth allowed the patient to feel

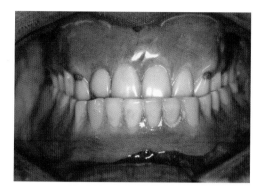

Figure 13.5 Intraoral frontal view of patient with old dentures in maximum intercuspation showing significant posterior tooth wear, and Class III anterior tooth and bilateral posterior cross bite relations.

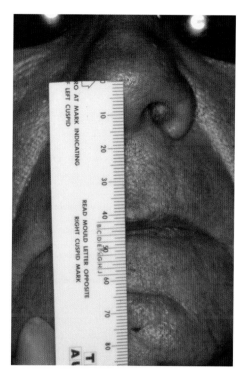

Figure 13.7 Extraoral facial measurement of vertical dimension of patient in Figure 13.1 with new complete dentures in maximum intercuspation (75 mm).

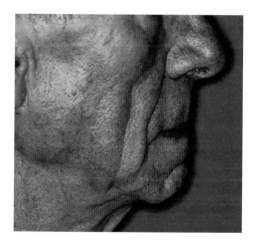

Figure 13.6 Post-treatment lateral facial view of complete denture patient with vertical dimension of occlusion restored with new complete dentures.

much better about his personal appearance and dramatically improved his outlook on life allowing him once again to socialize and connect with others.

13.2 Documenting Clinical, Radiographic, and Photographic Findings

In order to properly evaluate a dental patient for prosthodontic treatment, very thorough clinical and radiographic examinations of all

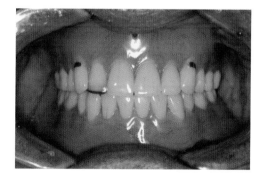

Figure 13.8 Intraoral frontal view of new complete dentures showing elimination of Class III anterior tooth and bilateral posterior crossbite relations due to proper restoration of vertical dimension of occlusion.

soft and hard tissues, existing teeth, occlusal relations, and edentulous areas should be completed and all pathologic and non-pathologic problems documented and charted in the patient's dental record. The prosthodontic

Interview of Removable Prosthodontic Patients

1. Gender? _____

2. Age? _____

3. Chief Dental Complaint? _____

4. Why do you want removable dental prostheses? _____

5. When and why were your missing teeth extracted? _____

6. If you are wearing removable dental prostheses, how old are they? _____

7. What problems are you having with your present removable dental prostheses? _____

8. What do you like most about your present removable dental prostheses? _____

9. What do you like least about your present removable dental prostheses? _____

10. Evaluation of patient's present removable dental prostheses:

	Patient's Opinion		Clinical Observation	
	Acceptable	Unacceptable	Acceptable	Unacceptable
a. Esthetics	☐	☐	☐	☐
b. Phonetics	☐	☐	☐	☐
c. Vertical Dimension	☐	☐	☐	☐
d. Retention	☐	☐	☐	☐
e. Stability	☐	☐	☐	☐
f. Comfort	☐	☐	☐	☐
g. Chewing Efficiency	☐	☐	☐	☐
h. Posterior Tooth Form	☐ Anatomic		☐ Non-anatomic	

Figure 13.9 Written interview form to aid in the evaluation of a patient's personality, psychological state, and expectations regarding removable prostheses.

evaluation form for partially and completely edentulous patients shown in Figure 13.10 can provide an organized way to approach these clinical activities.

In addition to radiographs, utilization of intraoral and extraoral photographs can document the patient's facial form, face height, supporting teeth, edentulous areas, occlusion, and dental conditions that will help the clinician arrive at a correct diagnosis and treatment plan. Critical information can also be gathered at the initial assessment of the patient requiring prosthodontic restorations by making diagnostic impressions and maxillomandibular records. In this manner, the diagnostic casts can allow for extraoral visualization of tooth alignment and positions, ridge form, interarch and interocclusal relationships of the patient's dentition and edentulous areas and be used to treatment plan fixed and removable prosthodontic restorations and survey and design removable partial dentures. As seen in Figures 13.11–13.16, the patient's functional and esthetic demands, as well as financial

Clinical Evaluation of Partially and Completely Edentulous Patients

Prosthodontic Diagnostic Index	I Favorable	II Moderately Compromised	III Substantially Compromised	IV Severely Compromised
PART 1. Oral Examination	☐/☐	Maxillary/Mandibular		
Mucosal Thickness	☐/☐ Thin	☐/☐ Very Thin	☐/☐ Thick	☐/☐ Flabby
Residual Ridge Undercuts	☐/☐ None	☐/☐ 2 mm	☐/☐ 2-4 mm	☐/☐ > 4 mm
Tori/Exostoses	☐/☐ None	☐/☐ Small	☐/☐ Large	☐/☐ Very Large
Genial Tubercles	☐ Normal			☐ Large
Frenula Attachments	☐/☐ > 12 mm	☐/☐ 6-12 mm	☐/☐ 3-6 mm	☐/☐ < 3mm
Floor of Mouth Depth	☐ > 12 mm	☐ 3-6 mm	☐ < 3 mm	☐ No Space
Tongue Position	☐ Normal	☐ Squared	☐ Broad and Retruded	☐ Severely Retruded
Retromylohyoid Space	☐ > 12 mm	☐ 6-12 mm	☐ 3-6 mm	☐ < 3 mm
Mylohyoid Muscle Attachments	☐ > 12 mm	☐ 6-12 mm	☐ 3-6 mm	☐ < 3 mm
Soft Palate - Angle/Width	☐ < 45°/6-12 mm	☐ 45-70°/3-6 mm	☐ > 70°/< 3 mm	
Gag Reflex	☐ Normal	☐ Mildly Sensitive	☐ Hypersensitive	☐ Medication Needed
Muscle Tone	☐ Light	☐ Moderate	☐ Heavy	
Saliva	☐ Normal	☐ Abundant	☐ Xerostomia	
Mandibular Movement	☐ Normal	☐ Moderate Limits	☐ Substantial Limits	☐ Severe Limits

PART 2. Arch Configurations/Maxillomandibular Relationships

	I	II	III	IV
Kennedy Classification	☐/☐ Class IV	☐/☐ Class III	☐/☐ Class II	☐/☐ Class I
Modification Spaces		☐ Yes	☐ Yes	☐ Yes
Arch Size	☐/☐ Large	☐/☐ Medium	☐/☐ Small	☐ Significant Differences
Maxillary Ridge and Palate Form	☐ Square	☐ Tapered	☐ Flat	☐ Highly Resorbed
Mandibular Ridge Height	☐/☐ > 12 mm	☐/☐ 6-12 mm	☐/☐ 3-6 mm	☐/☐ < 3 mm
Interarch Distance	☐/☐ 25-35 mm	☐/☐ 20-25 mm	☐/☐ 15-20 mm	☐/☐ < 15 mm
Ridge Relationship	☐ Orthognathic	☐ Prognathic	☐ Retrognathic	
Ridge Parallelism	☐/☐ Parallel	☐/☐ Divergent		

PART 3. Pretreatment Considerations

Psychological Classification	☐ Philosophical	☐ Exacting	☐ Hysterical	☐ Indifferent
Radiographic Evaluation	☐ Normal	☐ Abnormal		
Comments:				

PART 4. Esthetic Considerations

Pre-extraction Records	☐ Casts	☐ Photographs	☐ Description	
Facial Form	☐ Square	☐ Tapered	☐ Ovoid	
Complexion	☐ Light	☐ Medium	☐ Dark	
Personality	☐ Delicate	☐ Medium	☐ Vigorous	

PART 5. Preprosthetic Soft and Hard Tissue Treatment Considerations

Tissue Treatment	☐ None Indicated	☐ Maxillary	☐ Mandibular	
Surgical Treatment	☐ None Indicated	☐ Maxillary	☐ Mandibular	
Condition and Procedure Needed:				

PART 6. Prosthodontic Diagnostic Index (PDI) and Prognosis

PDI (circle one of the four)   Favorable   I   II   III   IV   Unfavorable

Prognosis   Uncomplicated, Low Risk ⟶ Complex, High Risk

Comments for Referral:
(for PDI III or IV)

Figure 13.10 Prosthodontic diagnosis form used for pretreatment evaluation of partially and completely edentulous patients.

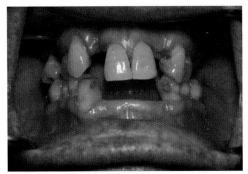

Figure 13.11 Partially edentulous patient with missing mandibular anterior teeth and no right side canine guidance due to loss of long span fixed partial denture #22–27.

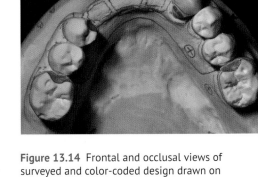

Figure 13.14 Frontal and occlusal views of surveyed and color-coded design drawn on mandibular diagnostic cast for rotational path RPD.

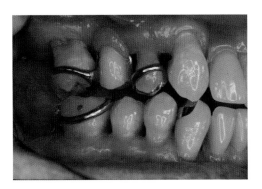

Figure 13.12 Patient with survey crown #27 and mandibular Class IV rotational path RPD restoring right side canine guidance and missing anterior teeth.

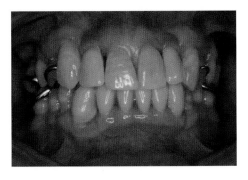

Figure 13.15 Frontal view of completed maxillary and mandibular RPDs.

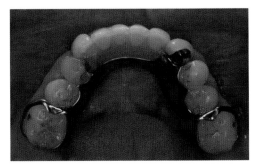

Figure 13.16 Occlusal view of mandibular rotational path RPD.

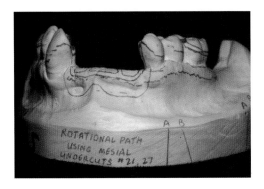

Figure 13.13 Frontal and occlusal views of surveyed and color-coded design drawn on mandibular diagnostic cast for rotational path RPD.

constraints, often times result in a choice of removable prostheses rather than fixed partial dentures or implant-supported prostheses for restoration of long span edentulous spaces.

A prerequisite to diagnosis and treatment planning different prosthodontic treatment

Appendix J-1

Removable Partial Denture Design Examination

Student Name_____Student Code_____Date_____

Faculty Evaluation

Pass Error

Patient History
____ ____   Records and Correctly Interprets Medical, Social, and Dental History
____ ____   Recognizes Need for and Obtains Consultations and Tests

Head and Neck Examination
____ ____   Evaluates All Soft and Hard Tissues
____ ____   Evaluates Existing Teeth, Edentulous Areas, and Dental Conditions
____ ____   Evaluates Occlusion and Tempromandibular Function
____ ____   Evaluates Tooth Alignment and Spacing

Radiographic Examination
____ ____   Prescribes and Takes Appropriate Radiographs
____ ____   Evaluates Radiographs Correctly

Diagnosis and Treatment Planning
____ ____   Establishes Appropriate Need for Distal Extension Removable Partial Denture
____ ____   Discusses Diagnosis/Prognosis/Risk vs. Benefits/Alternatives
____ ____   Develops Properly Sequenced Comprehensive Treatment Plan
____ ____   Educates Patient Regarding Appointments/Costs for Treatment

Survey and Design
____ ____   Accurate Diagnostic Casts and Jaw Relation Records Obtained
____ ____   Diagnostic Casts Mounted Properly in Appropriate Articulator
____ ____   Color-coded Design Drawn Neatly and Accurately on Cast
____ ____   Path of Insertion/Withdrawal and Tilt of Cast Correctly Identified by Tripod Marks
____ ____   Survey Lines Drawn on All Teeth Contacted by Metal Framework
____ ____   Guiding Planes and Areas of Axial Recontouring Identified
____ ____   Sufficient Occlusal Clearance Present or Occlusal Reduction Identified
____ ____   Rests/Rest Seats and Indirect Retainers Properly Located and Drawn Correctly
____ ____   Major Connector Properly Selected and Drawn Correctly
____ ____   Appropriate Abutment Teeth and Clasp Assemblies Selected for the Class of RPD
____ ____   Clasps Correctly Related to Survey Lines and Hard and Soft Tissue Undercuts
____ ____   Amount of Undercut Located and Marked Correctly in Red on Abutment Teeth
____ ____   Acrylic Resin Denture Base Coverage Properly Extended
____ ____   Metal Retention Features and Distal Extension Cast Stops Drawn Correctly
____ ____   Appropriate Replacement Teeth Selected and Properly Drawn

        [   ]   **Final Numeric Grade**

                                      _____
                                          Faculty Signature

A (4.00-3.50) = No errors needing correction.
B (3.49-3.00) = Minor errors, some improvement indicated.
C (2.99-2.00) = Moderate errors, definite improvement indicated.
D (1.99-1.00) = Major errors, major improvement indicated.
F   (< 1.00) = Unacceptable, remediation required.

Figure 13.17 Evaluation form to assess dental students for their diagnosis and treatment planning of removable partial dentures.

options and a key to the success of any dental treatment is a well-organized and well-performed data-gathering process (Hollender et al. 2003). For example, as an aid to determine if conventional removable prosthodontic therapy would be better for a partially edentulous patient than fixed or implant prosthodontic therapy, a standardized form can help "put it all together" for dental students and licensed practitioners as they diagnose, treatment plan, and survey and design a removable partial denture (Figure 13.17).

The comprehensive examination of a patient in need of prosthodontic restoration should include the clinician's extraoral, intraoral, and periodontal findings; interpretation of radiographs; and consultations with dental specialists. A problem-focused systematic approach that employs a Subjective, Objective, Assessment, Plan (SOAP) format for chart entries will insure that proper assessments and documentation are completed in a logical, legal, and timely manner (Terezhalmy et al. 2009). The following SOAP progress notes with **blue and italicized** headings is an example of how to properly document the evaluation, diagnosis, and treatment planning for the partially edentulous patient in Figures 13.18–13.22.

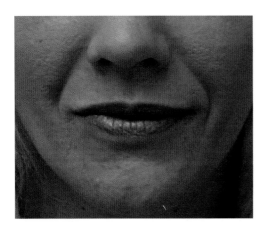

Figure 13.18 Extraoral frontal view of partially edentulous patient.

SUBJECTIVE (S):

Chief Complaint: 34-year old Caucasian female wants her painful upper teeth removed today.

Meds: none.

ADE: NKDA; NKADE (Adverse Drug Experiences: No Known Drug Allergies; No Known Adverse Drug Experiences)

PMHx: Childbirth × 4.

PDentHx: Multiple extractions of carious posterior teeth. Patient states that she cannot afford extensive alloy and/or composite restorations, root canals, crowns, or implants.

FamHx: Mother had breast cancer.

SocHx: Denies use of alcohol, reports pack/day smoking habit.

OBJECTIVE (O):

Vital Signs: BP – 130/75.

Clinical Findings: Multiple missing teeth and grossly decayed teeth # 6, 7, 8, 9, 10, 11, 15, 21, 22.

Radiographs: Panoramic radiograph taken three months previous to appointment (Figure 13.1) shows teeth #3, 4, 5, 14, 15, 21, 22 present. Periodontal problems and healing extraction sites noted in maxillary and mandibular arches.

Photographs: Intraoral, extraoral frontal, and occlusal digital images recorded after healing of extraction sites.

Diagnostic Casts: Color-coded survey and design completed for Kennedy Class I mandibular bilateral distal extension Removable Partial Dentures (RPD). I-bar retentive clasps and cingulum rests selected based on fit, function, and esthetics.

13.3 Designing Prosthodontic Treatment Plans

Treatment planning for a prosthodontic patient can be viewed as the development of a series of dental procedures that are necessary to maintain health or to restore a diseased dentition

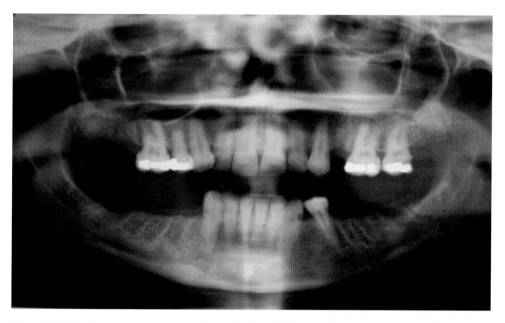

Figure 13.19 Pretreatment panoramic radiograph of partially edentulous patient in Figure 13.18.

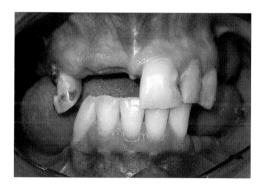

Figure 13.20 Intraoral frontal view of partially edentulous patient in Figure 13.18.

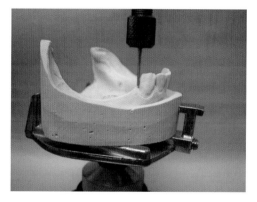

Figure 13.21 Survey of mandibular diagnostic cast for RPD.

to a state of health. In order to accomplish these goals, clinicians should develop detailed dental discipline oriented treatment plans for every patient undergoing comprehensive prosthodontic care. It is also important that a systematic approach is utilized to complete all necessary dental procedures in the fewest number of patient visits.

With that in mind, clinicians should establish goals for treatment planning a prosthodontic patient based on (i) addressing the patient's chief complaint; (ii) eliminating disease; (iii) restoring function; (iv) restoring esthetics; (v) preventing future disease; and (vi) providing cost-effective care.

The actual treatment planning process for fixed and/or removable prosthodontic procedures should involve using a problem list as a guide, integrating risk assessment, addressing each problem, determining priorities for treatment, examining the relationship between problems, establishing a prognosis, and presenting alternatives to the patient.

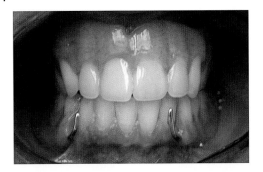

Figure 13.22 Intraoral frontal view of immediate removable prostheses.

Develop a Problem List and Diagnostic Summary

After the initial patient assessment and clinical, radiographic, and photographic findings are well documented, then a problem list should be developed to help aid in diagnosis, treatment planning, and prognostic interpretation for prosthodontic treatments. The assessments (A) and treatment plan options (P) provided to the patient in Figure 13.19 should be entered in the patient's dental record, following the SOAP format, after entry of the Subjective information (S) and Objective findings (O).

ASSESSMENT (A):

Problem List: See Figures 13.18, 13.20, and 13.21 for clinical, radiographic, and photographic findings to document patient's dental conditions by teeth, tooth surfaces, and edentulous spaces.

Diagnostic Summary: List and summarize problems by medical and dental disciplines – Systemic; Oral Pathology; Preventive; Occlusion/TMJ; Periodontics; Oral and Maxillofacial Surgery; Endodontics; Operative Dentistry; Fixed Prosthodontics; Implant Prosthodontics; Removable Prosthodontics and Orthodontics.

Assessment: Extract symptomatic teeth #7, 8, and 15 immediately due to pain and retain teeth # 6, 9, 10, and 11 to maintain vertical dimension of occlusion for maxillomandibular relations for fabrication of maxillary and mandibular removable prostheses in accordance with accepted treatment plan.

PLAN (P):

Treatment Plan options for the restoration of form, function, and esthetics should take in to account the patient's expectations, dental IQ, financial constraints, and compliance with maintenance protocols for fixed and removable prostheses. The patient should be informed of the prognosis and the risks and benefits of optional therapy and no therapy, in other words, "No treatment" as an option would be included in this section.

Option #1 – Maxillary and Mandibular Immediate Complete Dentures with extraction of all remaining teeth at time of delivery of prostheses. Good to Fair Prognosis.

Option #2 – Maxillary Immediate Complete Denture opposing Mandibular Removable Partial Denture (RPD). Extract #21 and 22 and fabricate mandibular metal RPD and restore #23-F and #27-F with composite resin to establish retentive undercuts for I-bar clasp and restore #22-L and #27-L for cingulum rest seats for vertical support of metal framework. Extract remaining maxillary teeth at time of simultaneous delivery of maxillary immediate complete denture and mandibular bilateral distal extension RPD. Excellent to Good Prognosis.

Patient chose Option #2 based on her desire to keep some mandibular teeth for function and esthetic reasons, the minimal cost for composite resin restorations on RPD abutment teeth compared to surveyed crowns, and both final prostheses are removable.

Use a Prosthodontic Diagnostic Index for Referral

Based on the education, training, experience, and practice location of some clinicians, dental patients that require complex treatment may need referral to a prosthodontist. Upon completion of Figures 13.9 and 13.10, it would be appropriate to discuss with the patient that referral to a specialist for prosthodontic restorative care is indicated due to the complexity of the proposed dental treatment, a high-risk prognosis, and the availability of specialty care.

The American College of Prosthodontists (ACP) developed Prosthodontic Diagnostic Index (PDI) classification systems for completely edentulous, partially edentulous, and completely dentate patients based on diagnostic findings and the severity of their pretreatment dental conditions (McGarry et al. 1999; McGarry et al. 2002; McGarry et al. 2004). The guidelines in each of the ACP classification systems were designed and are intended to help diagnose and determine appropriate treatments for patients seeking dental care.

As an example, four categories are defined in the ACP PDI for partially edentulous patients, Class I to Class IV, with Class I representing a simple, uncomplicated clinical situation (favorable prognosis) and class IV representing a highly complex clinical situation (unfavorable prognosis). Each class of partially edentulous patients is differentiated by specific diagnostic criteria.

Benefits of the PDI classification systems for clinicians include:

(1) Improved treatment planning.
(2) Improved professional communication.
(3) Insurance reimbursement commensurate with complexity of care.
(4) Improved screening tool for dental school admission clinics.
(5) Standardized criteria for outcomes assessment and research.
(6) Enhanced diagnostic consistency.
(7) Simplified aid in the decision to refer a patient.

It should also be noted that the PDI classification and diagnosis for the partially edentulous patient is independent of the proposed treatment meaning that the index is not limited to only conventional RPDs, but may include fixed and/or implant-supported removable partial denture prostheses (Figures 13.23 and

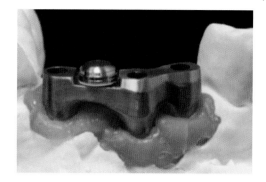

Figure 13.23 Precision-milled metal framework with locator attachment for retention of implant-assisted maxillary Class IV RPD.

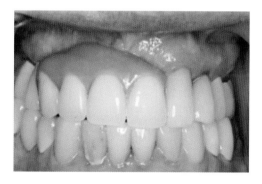

Figure 13.24 Wax try-in of removable partial overdenture in Figure 13.23 to assess fit, function, phonetics, and esthetics.

13.24). Proper prosthodontic diagnosis allows for anticipating and acknowledging the complexity of treatment options and it provides the best possible dental care for the patient.

The following diagnostic criteria are designed to help in treatment planning partially edentulous patients:

• Location and extent of edentulous areas.
• Abutment tooth condition.
• Occlusal scheme.
• Residual ridge.
• Conditions creating a guarded prognosis.

Some of the indications for referral of partially edentulous patients to a prosthodontist for restorative care include:

(1) Changes to the occlusal plane.
(2) Changes to the occlusal vertical dimension.

(3) Multiple adjunctive procedures are necessary.

(4) Very high esthetic concerns.

(5) Refractory patient (stubborn or unmanageable – not yielding or resistant to treatment).

Based on anatomical, functional, systemic, and psychological conditions of a patient, the PDI would classify the following **partially edentulous patients** as Class I, II, III, or IV:

Class I Single arch missing two maxillary or four incisors, and/or missing two posterior teeth. No pre-prosthetic surgery needed. Class I molar/skeletal relations (stable maximum intercuspation position). Adequate residual ridge bone height, soft tissue support, and attached mucosa (Figures 13.25 and 13.26).

Class II Both arches missing two maxillary or four mandibular incisors, or missing two

or more teeth plus a canine. Abutment teeth unable to retain coronal restorations; require local adjunctive therapy that may include periodontics, endodontics, and/or orthodontics. Class I molar/skeletal relations but requires equilibration and/or enameloplasty. Residual ridge displays a loss of vertical and horizontal hard and soft tissue support (Figures 13.27 and 13.28).

Class III Missing three or more adjacent teeth in any arch. Abutment teeth are not able to support intracoronal or extracoronal restorations and require extensive adjunctive therapy, which may include periodontics, endodontics, and/or orthodontics. Class II or Class III molar/skeletal relations, malocclusion, but no need to alter occlusal vertical dimension. Extensive loss of hard and soft tissue of

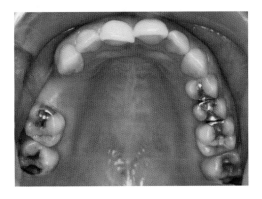

Figure 13.25 PDI Class I partially edentulous patient.

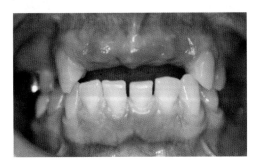

Figure 13.26 PDI Class I partially edentulous patient.

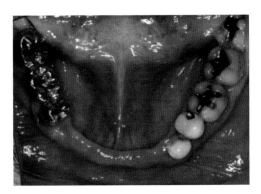

Figure 13.27 PDI Class II partially edentulous patient.

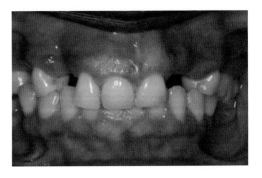

Figure 13.28 PDI Class II partially edentulous patient.

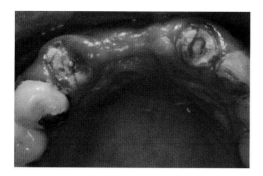

Figure 13.29 PDI Class III partially edentulous patient.

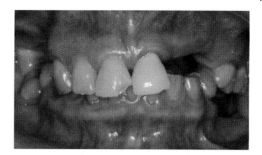

Figure 13.31 PDI Class IV partially edentulous patient.

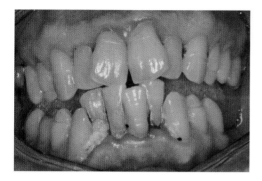

Figure 13.30 PDI Class III partially edentulous patient.

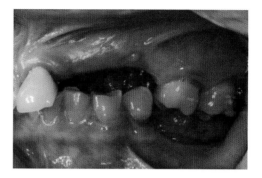

Figure 13.32 PDI Class IV partially edentulous patient.

residual ridge requires pre-prosthetic surgery (Figures 13.29 and 13.30).

Class IV Long span with multiple missing teeth in both arches resulting in extruded teeth. Severely compromised or missing strategic abutment teeth in four or more sextants. Need to re-establish entire occlusion with alteration of occlusal vertical dimension. Deficient hard and soft tissue support requires pre-prosthetic surgery. Systemic, functional, and/or psychological impairments creating a guarded prognosis (Figures 13.31 and 13.32).

Survey and Design Removable Partial Dentures for the Partially Edentulous Patient

In order to enhance communication with the patient and the dental laboratory, the definitive metal and acrylic resin components

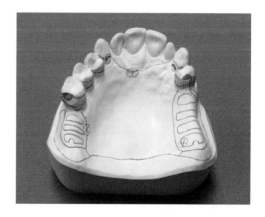

Figure 13.33 Color-coded design drawn on diagnostic cast for a maxillary distal extension RPD.

and tooth alterations for a definitive removable partial denture can be drawn on the surveyed diagnostic cast using a color-coded design (Figures 13.33 and 13.34). The dentist should also draw a design on the laboratory work authorization form that coincides with

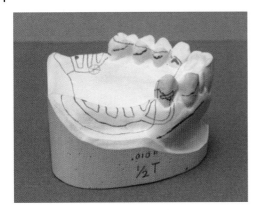

Figure 13.34 ½ T-bar clasp assembly drawn on maxillary left premolar to retain and support left side of a maxillary distal extension RPD.

the written description of the RPD and its components. The color-coded diagnostic cast can be used chairside by the dentist as a "blueprint" for the preparation of abutment teeth for guide planes, retentive undercuts, rest seats, and occlusal clearance.

Mounted diagnostic casts and the survey and design of removable partial dentures should be an integral part of the physical evaluation, diagnosis, and treatment planning process for the partially edentulous patient (Phoenix et al. 2003). When utilized, these adjunctive diagnostic procedures can help improve the prognosis and outcome of the prosthodontic treatment for the complex multidisciplinary phased-treatment patient such as this patient

who needed extensive endodontic and oral surgical procedures before prosthodontic rehabilitation with a maxillary complete overdenture and a mandibular Class I removable partial overdenture (Figures 13.35–13.41).

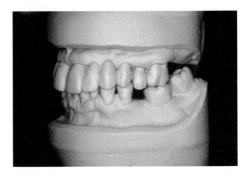

Figure 13.36 Pre-treatment left lateral view of mounted diagnostic casts.

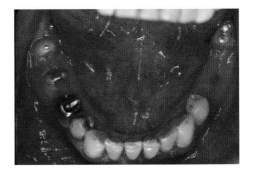

Figure 13.37 Occlusal view of abutment teeth for support of mandibular removable partial overdenture.

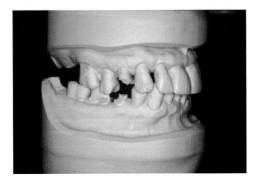

Figure 13.35 Pre-treatment right lateral view of mounted diagnostic casts.

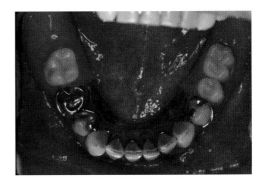

Figure 13.38 Post-treatment occlusal view of mandibular partial overdenture.

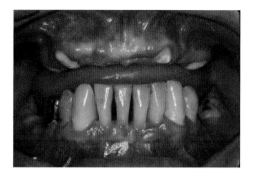

Figure 13.39 Frontal view of abutment teeth for maxillary complete overdenture.

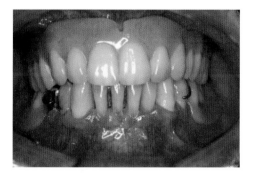

Figure 13.40 Post-treatment view of maxillary complete overdenture opposing mandibular bilateral distal extension removable partial overdenture.

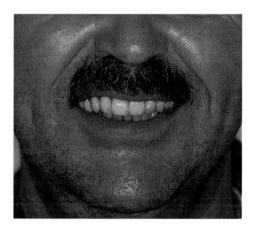

Figure 13.41 Post-treatment frontal view of patient wearing maxillary complete overdenture and mandibular partial overdenture.

Fabricate Radiographic Stent for Implants for the Partially and Completely Edentulous Patient

In addition to designing an RPD for a partially edentulous patient, it may also be necessary to fabricate a radiographic stent to determine if dental implants are a viable treatment option. The radiographic stent is fabricated on the patient's diagnostic cast. The patient wears the radiographic stent when a cone beam computerized tomogram (CBCT) is made to determine if adequate bone is available for placement of implants based on the form, function, and esthetics of the replacement teeth (Figures 13.42–13.44).

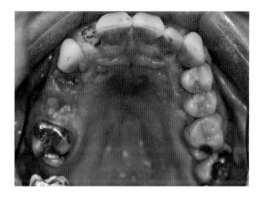

Figure 13.42 Occlusal view of a partially edentulous patient.

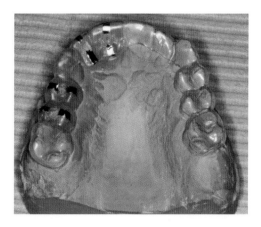

Figure 13.43 Maxillary diagnostic cast of patient in Figure 13.42 with radiographic stent fabricated for CBCT.

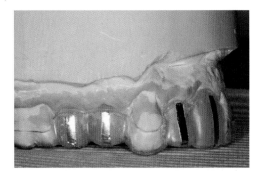

Figure 13.44 Lateral view of radiographic stent showing aluminum foil placed mesiodistally for each tooth to be restored with an implant.

Clinicians will often find that the use of a panoramic radiograph for treatment planning dental implants is limited as it can only be viewed in one dimension (Figure 13.45). Computerized tomography provides a three-dimensional view of the partially edentulous area for treatment planning dental implants (Rose et al. 2004). It is important to center the radiographic marker (strip of aluminum foil) mesiodistally in the edentulous space for each tooth that will be restored with an implant crown. The marker allows for the CBCT to be sectioned so the surgeon

and restorative dentist can accurately measure the bucco-lingual dimension and height of bone available for the implant fixture based on where the implant crown will be positioned for esthetics and function (Figures 13.46–13.49).

Discuss Prognosis and Alternative Treatments with Patient

For ethical and legal reasons, it is essential that the patient be informed of the different prosthodontic options for dental treatment and also provided an estimate of the overall cost, prognosis, and anticipated longevity/viability for each alternative therapy (Ozar and Sokol 2002). Clinicians should offer at least two treatment plan options to the patient before both dentist and patient agree upon the final treatment. The options may include only fixed, removable, or implant options or a combination of these types of prostheses, especially if missing teeth are to be replaced. One of the proposed plans could be the ideal treatment plan and the other an alternate treatment plan, with both focused on what is "best" for the patient. A copy of the itemized and signed final treatment plan should be given

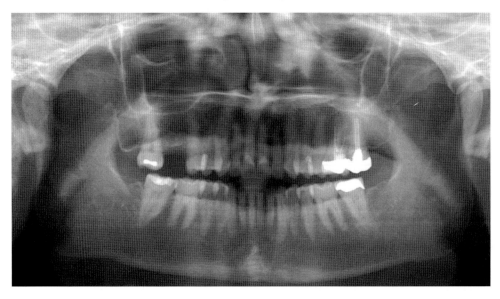

Figure 13.45 Panoramic radiograph of patient missing upper right 1st molar treatment planned for a single tooth implant.

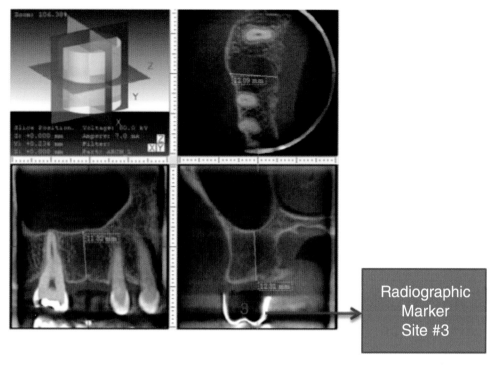

Figure 13.46 CBCT image in lower right shows outline of radiographic marker placed mesiodistally on tooth #3 in radiographic stent. CBCT images show different views of width and height of bone available for implant placement in extraction site #3.

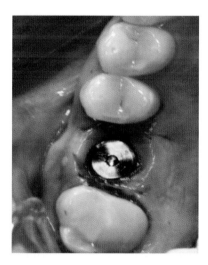

Figure 13.47 Intraoral occlusal view of healing abutment on implant at #3 site.

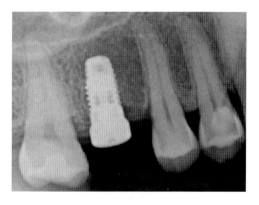

Figure 13.48 Periapical radiograph of implant fixture surgically placed at #3 site.

to the patient and the original kept on file in the dentist's office for insurance purposes and medico-legal reasons. The option to do "no treatment" should also be presented with the benefits of treatment and the risks of no treatment thoroughly explained to the patient (Terezhalmy et al. 2009).

The clinician must also determine if the results of the proposed prosthodontic therapy is important and applicable to the patient. In order to provide a clinically significant therapy

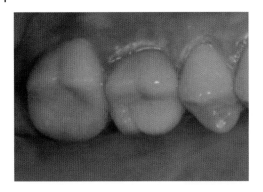

Figure 13.49 Final complete crown for restoration of implant at #3 site.

and provide the patient with a prognosis, one should distinguish the importance and meaning of results of therapy reported in the dental literature so the patient can make an informed decision. The prognosis for a specific therapy must go beyond "statistics" and take into account the patient's preferences, values, and circumstances in combination with the clinician's experience and judgment. The key to providing the "best" prosthodontic treatment is to be able to translate research findings into practice to help the patient and clinician make informed dental care decisions (Forrest et al. 2009).

Patients are often treatment planned with the understanding that certain therapies will have better long-term outcomes than others. Prosthodontics is a treatment-oriented specialty and has traditionally provided dental treatment for patients with two activities: replace defective and/or missing teeth and restore dental arches to an "ideal" occlusion. Unfortunately, in certain situations, these outcomes may be at odds with patient preferences. Other outcomes, not advocated by traditional clinicians, should be considered when making prosthodontic treatment decisions. Certain pathologies, such as caries and periodontal disease may have significant outcomes for the success of prosthodontic therapies, including loss of tooth structure, pocket formation, mobility, abscess formation, and tooth loss. Other outcomes of significant relevance to partially and completely edentulous patients

include elimination of pain, difficulty with mastication, esthetics, and quality of life.

Prosthodontics has traditionally recommended proactive treatment to avoid poor outcomes, such as crowning teeth with cracked enamel or large amalgam restorations and replacing all missing teeth. *The question for the dentist to consider is: Which of these outcomes is clinically relevant and how likely are these outcomes with or without intervention?* Making a prediction of outcome (prognosis) becomes an important clinical skill. The astute clinician should recognize that decisions to intervene are crucial and in some cases may be *less* desirable to patients (Newman et al. 2006).

Design a Properly Sequenced Comprehensive Treatment Plan

There are five phases of dental treatment that should be recognized as necessary to properly sequence a comprehensive treatment plan for a patient (Terezhalmy et al. 2009). Phase I is emergency treatment to alleviate pain, bleeding, or swelling. Phase II is the removal and control of pathologic conditions that need periodontal, endodontic, surgical, and/or operative dentistry therapy. Phase III is the prosthodontic repair or replacement of non-pathologic dental conditions, such as severely worn, fractured, and/or missing teeth. Phase IV is the re-assessment of pathologic and non-pathologic conditions once all dental therapies have been completed. And, finally, Phase V is maintenance dental therapy and periodic recall evaluations to assess the outcomes of treatment.

As an example of a properly sequenced comprehensive treatment plan, a clinician would take into account that a grossly carious molar tooth cannot be planned for endodontic therapy and subsequently repaired with a core build-up and a complete coverage crown if the tooth is non-restorable or has a guarded to hopeless periodontal prognosis. Although not an emergency situation, extraction of the tooth is indicated and the "best" option for the patient would be a fixed, removable, or implant

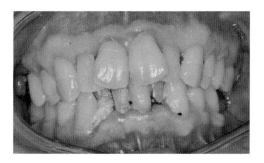

Figure 13.50 Partially edentulous patient with extensive dental problems.

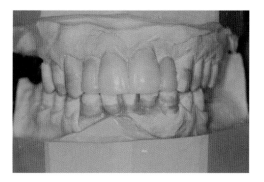

Figure 13.51 Wax-up to aid in the diagnosis and treatment planning of interdisciplinary dental care for patient in Figure 13.50.

prosthesis offered as Phase III treatment after Phase II surgical therapy.

Diagnostic wax-ups of the proposed restorations should also be completed and shown to the more complex patient when discussing the need for a properly sequenced comprehensive treatment plan that involves interdisciplinary care and referral to specialists (Figures 13.50 and 13.51).

Educate Patient Regarding Appointment Sequence

The first appointment after a prosthodontic treatment plan has been finalized should start with trying to resolve the patient's chief complaint, such as a decayed, fractured, or mobile tooth. Unfortunately, on many occasions, the clinician will find it necessary to focus on resolving other dental conditions, such as active periodontal disease, carious

lesions, or destructive parafunctional habits that the patient may not find important to address before they receive their "new" crowns or prosthesis. For this reason, it is incumbent upon the dentist to educate the patient from the very beginning of dental therapy about the proper "sequence" of appointments based upon a phased approach to dental treatment.

The five different "phases" of dental treatment that can assist the clinician in sequencing dental appointments are:

Phase I: Emergency treatment.
Phase II: Removal of disease (gingivitis, periodontitis, caries, pulpal and periapical pathology, oral surgery, etc.)
Phase III: Replacement and final restoration of teeth (fixed, removable, and implant-supported prostheses).
Phase IV: Re-assessment
Phase V: Recall and maintenance.

The following complex patient treatment plan is an example of the different "steps" for replacement and final restoration of teeth that can assist the clinician in sequencing dental appointments based on the delivery of major disciplines of prosthodontic care. When the final treatment plan is presented to the patient, the clinician should always discuss the type of restorations, restorative materials, fixed and removable prostheses, esthetic expectations, complications, limitations, and oral hygiene requirements (Figures 13.52–13.60).

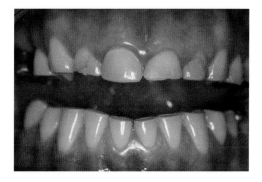

Figure 13.52 Pre-treatment intraoral view of partially edentulous patient with severe wear of natural dentition.

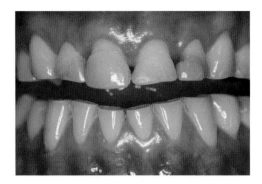

Figure 13.53 Post-surgical intraoral view of patient showing crown lengthened maxillary anterior teeth.

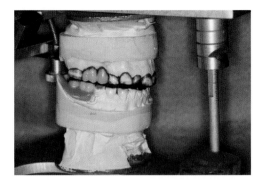

Figure 13.56 Diagnostic mounting and wax-up for complete mouth reconstruction. Custom incisal guide table insures anterior guidance designed in wax-up will be transferred to the final maxillary and mandibular metal-ceramic anterior crowns.

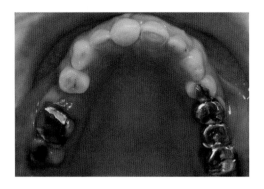

Figure 13.54 Maxillary occlusal view of patient with erosion of lingual surfaces of anterior teeth due to acidic insult and fractured right first molar.

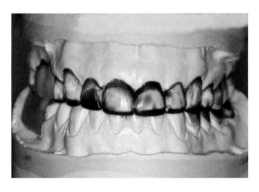

Figure 13.57 Pre-treatment frontal view of diagnostic wax-ups showing short clinical crown lengths on maxillary anterior teeth and need for periodontal crown lengthening.

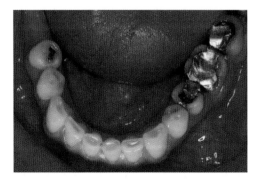

Figure 13.55 Mandibular occlusal view of patient with missing right molars and severe wear of teeth due to bruxism.

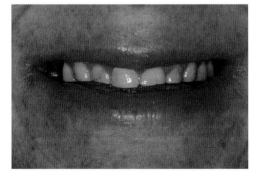

Figure 13.58 Pre-treatment extraoral view of patient before periodontal crown lengthening of maxillary anterior teeth.

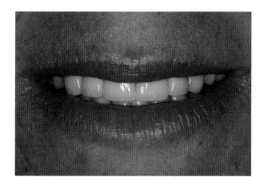

Figure 13.59 Post-treatment extraoral view of patient after full mouth reconstruction.

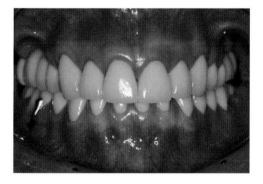

Figure 13.60 Post-treatment intraoral view of patient after full mouth reconstruction with maxillary crowns, maxillary fixed partial dentures, mandibular surveyed crowns, and mandibular unilateral distal extension RPD.

Treatment Plan and Appointment Sequence for Prosthodontic Reconstruction of a Complex Patient

1. Preventive procedures to improve oral hygiene and periodontal condition, including scaling, root planning, prophylaxis, and oral hygiene instruction.
2. Referral for psychiatric and dietary counseling based on enamel loss and a medical history of anorexia.
3. Occlusal evaluation, including diagnostic casts, facebow transfer, maxillomandibular records, articulation of casts, and diagnostic wax patterns.
4. Survey and design of a mandibular unilateral distal extension RPD.
5. Referral to oral surgeon for extraction of severely fractured, non-restorable maxillary right first molar.
6. Referral to periodontist for maxillary anterior tooth crown lengthening.
7. Replacement of defective amalgams and/or composite resins to establish sound foundations for complete crowns and fixed partial dentures.
8. Construction of an occlusal splint to stabilize anterior teeth after crown lengthening, increase patient's vertical dimension of occlusion (VDO), and evaluate mutually protected occlusal scheme.
9. Preparation of teeth for complete coverage crowns and fixed partial denture (FPD) and wear of full mouth provisional restorations.
10. Re-evaluation in four to six weeks of new VDO and mutually protected occlusal scheme, and molar extraction site healing.
11. Master impression of all prepared teeth for fabrication of permanent crowns and FPDs.
12. Fabrication, try-in, adjustment of occlusion, and cementation of maxillary metal-ceramic crowns and FPDs and mandibular surveyed crowns.
13. Master impression of mandibular arch with new surveyed crowns for unilateral distal extension RPD.
14. Framework try-in, altered cast impression, wax try-in, and delivery of metal-based unilateral distal extension mandibular RPD.
15. Fabrication of hard acrylic maxillary occlusal guard for nocturnal bruxism.
16. Deliver occlusal guard, provide wear and care instructions for fixed and removable prostheses, and review oral hygiene instructions.
17. Re-evaluation, recall, and periodontal maintenance appointments scheduled at three-month intervals.

Educate Patient Regarding Costs of Treatment

As mentioned earlier, the success or failure of prosthodontic clinical procedures often depends upon the assessment of a patient's personality, as well as, risk management of their dental problems. It is not uncommon for prosthodontic care and treatment of a patient in a dental office to take multiple visits at great expense to the patient. Some patients may even have certain expectations for the delivery of dental care and should be informed that during the course of treatment unexpected complications or new conditions may arise that may result in higher costs. Before initiating any prosthodontic procedures, it is important to educate the patient regarding the appropriate sequence of visits, the necessity for and cost of consultations and specialty care, the cost of each appointment and the total cost for the treatment planned, and the time needed for each appointment to properly manage _all_ of their dental conditions.

At times, a patient with dental disease that has been stabilized with Phase II treatment may have their prosthodontic care produced in "stages" whereby not all of the fixed, removable, and/or implant prostheses in the treatment plan are fabricated at the same time. This allows for financially challenged patients to afford and pay for parts of the prosthodontic treatment plan over an extended period of time (Nesbit 2007). For example, a partially edentulous patient that needs multiple surveyed crowns and maxillary and mandibular RPD can be offered a sequenced treatment plan to do the surveyed crowns in one year and the RPDs in the next year.

In some situations, not only will diagnostic criteria, but also patient modifiers, in addition to financial constraints require alternative treatment planning that result in lower cost to the patient. For example, a definitive metal-base removable partial denture may have to be treatment planned to replace 3 missing teeth from the upper right 2nd molar to the upper right canine because of the patient's heavy wear due to bruxism, high caries risk, and/or the length of span of a fixed partial denture. If implants are not affordable to the patient, the patient is a poorly controlled diabetic, or a chronic smoker, then a maxillary Kennedy Class III tooth borne RPD may be a relatively inexpensive compromise and provide acceptable esthetics, phonetics, and function for this patient (Nesbit et al. 2007).

Case 13.1 Diagnostic Summary and Treatment Planning for a Patient

The diagnostic summary documents the problem list and diagnosis of your clinical and radiographic examination of your patient. In addition it also documents the following items:

1. Explanation of treatment plan options.
2. Risks and benefits of all options.
3. Patient's choice of treatment plan choice.
4. Documentation of patient's acceptance of treatment plan.
5. Comments made by the patient regarding treatment plan alterations.
6. Your recommendations if alterations are made (especially if they are contrary to treatment options recommended).
7. Assistance with continuity of care for your patients. As patients are treated and possibly relocate, it documents the reasoning for a specific treatment plan.

The diagnostic summary can be written in a **SOAP** format. It includes:

1. **Subjective** and **objective** findings.
2. **Assessment** and problem list categorized by dental disciplines.
3. Documentation of treatment **plan** and options explained to the patient.
4. Explanation of risks and benefits for all treatment plans and options.

5. Patient's choice of treatment and that all questions regarding treatment, including its risks and benefits are fully understood by the patient, and that the patient had all questions answered.

The following is the recommended format of a **Diagnostic Summary** for the complex patient in Figures 13.61–13.65:

S: Chief Complaint (in patient's own words). Review Medications, Adverse Drug Experiences, Medical History, Dental History, Family History, and Social History.

What should you know about the patient's medical, dental, family, and social history? Why is it important for you as a clinician to have this information? Answer: *NEVER TREAT A STRANGER!*

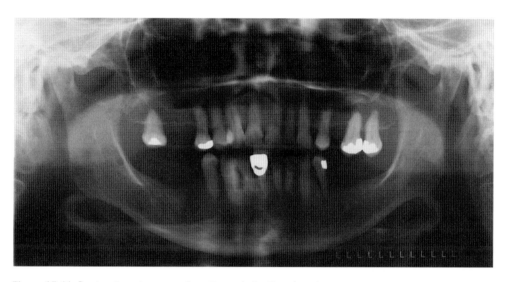

Figure 13.61 Pre-treatment panoramic radiograph for Case 1 patient.

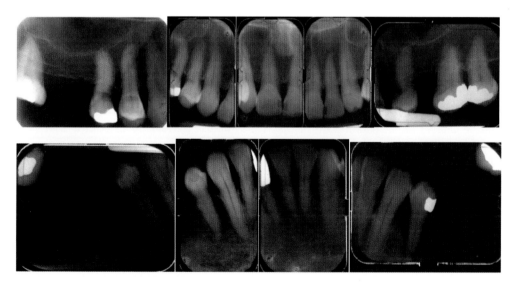

Figure 13.62 Pre-treatment periapical radiographs for Case 1 patient.

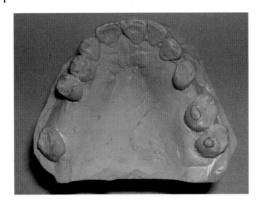

Figure 13.63 Maxillary diagnostic cast for Case 1 patient.

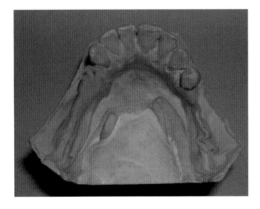

Figure 13.64 Mandibular diagnostic cast for Case 1 patient.

O: Record vital signs. List the significant extraoral and intraoral findings including pathologic and non-pathologic conditions, existing restorations, and prostheses. All clinical, radiographic, and periodontal findings should be charted on an odontogram in the patient's dental health record. This can be completed as part of a patient's electronic health record (EHR) or completed on a form that is maintained in a patient's paper chart.

What clinical findings should be recorded to diagnose periodontal disease? When should definitive periodontal therapy be initiated for a patient? Answer: *Probing depths, gingival margin level, mucogingival junction level, bleeding on probing/purulence, furcation involvements, tooth mobility, supragingival plaque, supragingival and subgingival calculus. Phase II: Removal of dental disease (gingivitis, periodontitis, caries, pulpal and periapical pathology, oral surgery, etc.) completed before Phase III: Prosthodontic replacement and restoration of teeth.*

A: List and summarize problems by dental disciplines. Problems listed in sequential order: **(1, 2, 3, etc.).**

Systemic: List medical problems that could influence your proposed treatment. Provide summary of patient's medications, past medical history, past dental history, social history, and family history. Provide ASA risk status and dental management considerations.

Example: Type II Diabetes – degree of blood sugar control with oral insulin medications varies weekly, thus delayed healing may be experienced; allergic to Penicillin and latex. ASA II. Patient cleared for routine dental care with modifications based on blood sugar levels at time of treatment. Do not prescribe Penicillin. Use nitrile gloves and avoid patient contact with latex dental products.

Oral Pathology: Summarize any head or neck lesions and provide a differential diagnosis if possible.

Example: Small, irregular areas of dekeratinization of filiform papillae on dorsal surface of tongue. (1) Appearance is consistent with benign migratory glossitis (geographic tongue). Observation indicated.

Preventive: Summarize level of risk based upon caries, cancer risk, and nutritional assessments.

Example: Xerostomia associated with poor control of diabetes (or due to prescription medications) and chewing of mint lozenges places patient at moderate risk for cervical caries. (2)

Occlusion/TMJ: Summarize TMJ assessment and occlusal problems.

Example: Class III occlusion – noncontributory. Also can list canine or group function guidance, if any loss of vertical dimension due to occlusal attrition, and any symptoms with TMJs.

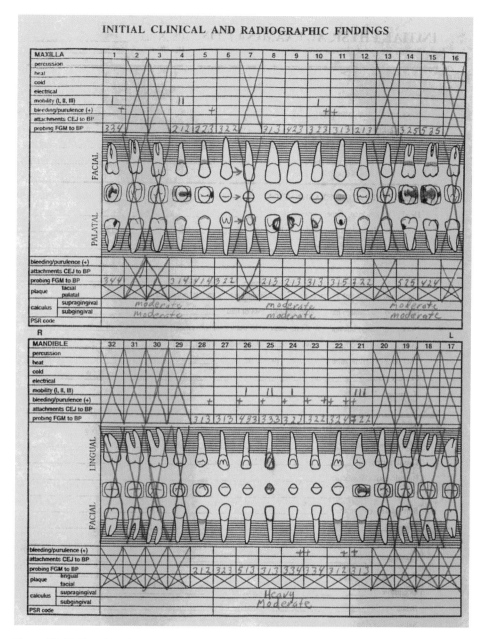

Figure 13.65 Charting of clinical, radiographic, and periodontal findings on odontogram in paper-based chart.

Periodontics: Summarize assessment of gingivitis and periodontitis.

Example: Chronic generalized moderate periodontitis all quadrants with moderate to heavy supragingival and subgingival calculus. (3) Localized severe periodontitis with Class III

mobility #21. Prognosis #4, 14, and 15 is guarded with #15 supra-erupted beyond occlusal plane. (4) #21 has hopeless prognosis. (5)

Oral and Maxillofacial Surgery: Summarize problems for tooth and soft and/or hard tissue removal.

Example: #15 supraerupted below occlusal plane affects placement of mandibular distal extension RPD. (4) #21 localized severe periodontitis, Class III mobility, and hopeless periodontal prognosis. (5)

Endodontics: Summarize pulpal and periapical problems.

Example: *Non-contributory.*

Operative Dentistry: Summarize character of caries and defective restorations.

Example: Caries #1-L (6) #4-D incipient (7) #5-M (8) #8-M recurrent (9) #9-M recurrent (10) #11-M (11) #14-M (12) #15-M and D (13) Cervical erosion #4-F (14) #5-F (15) #14-F (16) #15-F (17) #21-F (18) #22-F (19) and #28-F (20)

Fixed Prosthodontics: Summarize problems necessitating crown and bridge treatment.

Example: #4 needs MOD core build-up necessitating PFM survey crown (21) and #14 has large amalgam build-up necessitating PFM survey crown. (21)

Implant Prosthodontics: Summarize problems and rationales for implant treatment.

Example: Maxillary and mandibular implant placement options discussed, but removable prosthetic treatment is less expensive option due to financial constraints of patient.

Removable Prosthodontics: Describe problems and rationale for removable prosthetic treatment.

Example: Missing #2, 3, 7 (space closed), 13, and 16, maxillary arch needs tooth supported RPD (21) Missing #17, 18, 19, 20, 29, 30, 31, and 32, mandibular arch needs bilateral distal extension RPD. (22)

Orthodontics: Summarize problem and rationale for orthodontic treatment.

Example: #7 missing but space closed. #15 supra-erupted to be extracted. Non-contributory.

P: Explanation of treatment options, risks and benefits discussed, patient accepted treatment plan (by description) or patient rejects portion of treatment, reviewed risks and benefits of accepted treatment or no treatment with patient, patient had all questions answered. Final treatment plan signed and dated by patient.

Treatment Plan – By Description

A sequential numbering system in the Problem List in the A portion of the SOAP format can be used to document the phase, tooth/surfaces, diagnosis, procedure code, and treatment planned for the patient.

Additional problem numbers can be added sequentially among or after those listed as in the example below. It should be noted that dental discipline treatment was "phased" for this patient based on clinical, radiographic, and photographic findings and the diagnoses of both pathologic and non-pathologic conditions. See Table 13.1 and Figure 13.66.

13.4 Summary

This chapter provides a review of traditional clinical concepts for the diagnosis and treatment planning of fixed, removable, and implant prosthodontic procedures. Although published "indices" for prosthodontic diagnosis have been presented and should be followed, it is noteworthy that excellent clinical care for completely dentate and partially edentulous patients may be achieved with classic treatment approaches as well as new evidence-based therapies. It is hoped that the diagnosis and treatment planning guidelines and principles presented in this chapter will improve the fit, function, and esthetics of dental prostheses provided by clinicians and insure the best possible sequencing and quality of restorative care for simple, as well as, complex patients.

Table 13.1 List identifying problem, phase, tooth/surfaces, diagnosis, and procedure code for the dental treatment planned for this patient.

Problem	Phase	Tooth/Surfaces	Diagnosis	Procedure Code	Treatment Description
1	2	Tongue	Glossitis		Monitor benign condition
2	2	All	Caries Risk	1204	Fluoride application
2	2	All	Caries Risk	1303	Oral hygiene instruction
3	2	UR	Mod Perio	4341	SCRP
3	2	UL	Mod Perio	4341	SCRP
3	2	LL	Mod Perio	4341	SCRP
3	2	LR	Mod Perio	4341	SCRP
4	2	15	Supra-erupted	7110	Extraction
5	2	21	Hopeless Perio	7110	Extraction
6	2	1-L	L Caries	2140	Amalgam, 1 surface
7	2	4-MOD	D Caries	2950	Amalgam, Core build-up
8	2	5-MO	M Caries	2150	Amalgam, 2 surface
9	2	8-ML	M Caries	2331	Resin, 2 surface anterior
10	2	9-ML	M Caries	2331	Resin, 2 surface anterior
11	2	11-L	L Caries	2330	Resin, 1 surface anterior
12	2	14-MOD	M Caries	2950	Amalgam, Core build-up
13					No treatment, see Problem 4.
14		4-F	Cervical Erosion	2385	Resin, 1 surface posterior
15	2	5-F	Cervical Erosion	2385	Resin, 1 surface posterior
16					No treatment, see Problem 21
17					No treatment, see Problem 4
18					No treatment, see Problem 5
19	2	22-F	Cervical Erosion	2330	Resin, 1 surface anterior
20	2	28-F	Cervical Erosion	2385	Resin, 1 surface posterior
21	3	4	RPD Abutment	2750	PFM Survey Crown
21	3	14	RPD Abutment	2750	PFM Survey Crown
21	3	Max Arch		5213	RPD, maxillary Class III
22	3	Mand Arch		5214	RPD, mandibular Class I
3	4				Perio Reassessment
All	4				Case Reassessment
All	5				Recall

Prosthodontic restorative treatment is identified as Phase 3 in the sequential planning of delivery of care.

RECOMMENDATIONS FOR NEW REMOVABLE PARTIAL DENTURE(S)

1. Surgical _____
2. Periodontal _____
3. Operative _____
4. Fixed bridge restorations _____
5. Endodontics _____ 6. Orthodontics _____
7. Tentative survey:
   a. Classification: I _____ II _____ III _____ IV _____ Modifications: _____
   b. Tissue undercuts: yes _____ no _____ Location _____
   c. Type major connector:
      Maxillary: A-P _____ U _____ Strap _____ Plate _____
      Mandibular: Bar _____ Lingual plate _____
8. Type of teeth: anatomical _____ non-anatomical _____ resin _____ porcelain _____
9. Indicate occlusal corrections: _____
   _____

10. Tentative abutment requirements:

Tooth No.	Recontour Indicated	Type Restoration	Type Direct Retainer	Location Aux. Rests	Other

11. Outline tentative design in pencil.

PRELIMINARY DESIGN

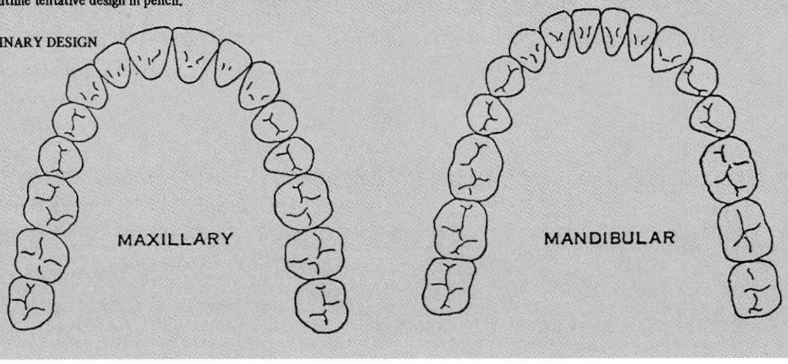

MAXILLARY   MANDIBULAR

Figure 13.66 Recommendation form with preliminary designs for RPDs summarizes the diagnosis and planning of Phase I and II dental discipline treatment needed before Phase III fixed and removable prosthodontics treatment.

References

Forrest, J.L., Miller, S.A., Overman, P.R., and Newman, M.G. (2009). *Evidence-Based Decision Making*, 127–132. Philadelphia: Lippincott Williams & Wilkins.

Hollender, L.G., Arcuri, M.R., and Lang, B.R. (2003). Chapter 3 diagnosis and treatment planning. In: *Osseointegration in Dentistry: An Overview*, 2e (eds. P. Worthington, B.R. Lang and J.E. Rubenstein), 19–29. Chicago: Quintessence Publishing Co., 86–87.

Jahangiri, L., Moghadam, M., Choi, M., and Ferguson, M. (2011). *Case 1 Treatment of an Edentulous Patient with Conventional Denture Prostheses. In: Clinical Cases in Prosthodontics*, 9–14. Singapore: Blackwell Publishing Ltd.

McGarry, T.J., Nimmo, A., Skiba, J.F. et al. (1999). Classification system for complete edentulism. *J. Prosthodont.* 8: 27–39.

McGarry, T.J., Nimmo, A., Skiba, J.F. et al. (2002). Classification system for partial edentulism. *J. Prosthodont.* 11: 181–193.

McGarry, T.J., Nimmo, A., Skiba, J.F. et al. (2004). Classification system for completely dentate patients. *J. Prosthodont.* 13: 73–82.

Nesbit, S.P. (2007). The motivationally or financially impaired patient. In: *Treatment Planning in Dentistry*, 2e (eds. S.J. Stefanac and S.P. Nesbit), 442–443. Philadelphia: Mosby, Inc. and 453.

Nesbit, S.P., Kanjirath, and Stefanac, S.J. (2007). The definitive phase of treatment. In: *Treatment Planning in Dentistry*, 2e (eds. S.J. Stefanac and S.P. Nesbit), 200–209. Philadelphia: Mosby, Inc.

Newman, M.G., Takei, H.H., and Klokkevold, P.R. (2006). *Carranza's Clinical Periodontology*, 10e, 38–39. St. Louis: WB Saunders.

Ozar, D.T. and Sokol, D.J. (2002). *Dental Ethics at Chairside. Professional Principles and Practical Applications*, 2e, 57. Washington: Georgetown University Press, 291.

Phoenix, R.D., Cagna, D.R., and DeFreest, C.F. (2003). *Stewart's Clinical Removable Partial Prosthodontics*, 3e, 127. Chicago: Quintessence Pub Co., Inc.

Rose, L.F., Mealey, B.L., Genco, R.J., and Cohen, D.W. (2004). *Periodontics: Medicine, Surgery, and Implants*, 623–624. St. Louis: Mosby Inc.

Terezhalmy, G.T., Huber, M.A., and Jones, A.C. (2009). *Physical Evaluation in Dental Practice*, 8–9. Wiley Blackwell.

Terezhalmy, G.T., Huber, M.A., and Jones, A.C. (2009). *Physical Evaluation in Dental Practice*, 233. Wiley Blackwell.

Terezhalmy, G.T., Huber, M.A., and Jones, A.C. (2009). *Physical Evaluation in Dental Practice*, 229–232. Wiley Blackwell.

14

Exam, Diagnosis and Treatment Planning in Pediatric Patients

The goal of treatment planning in pediatric patients is not only to deliver high quality care and promote good oral health, but also to give young patients a pleasant dental experience, thus cultivating their positive attitude toward dental care throughout lifetime. Treatment planning in children is unique for several reasons. First of all, from infant to adolescence, a child goes through dynamic changes cognitively, emotionally, and socially, as well as in dental and craniofacial development. Therefore, a treatment plan should take these developmental changes into consideration. Second, treatment planning in children is dictated by a child's ability to cooperate with the treatment and the behavior management techniques available to the dentist. Finally, in addition to communication with the patient, clear communication with the patient's parent is a must. Parental and family support is required for a successful treatment planning. A good treatment plan can only be achieved after a comprehensive history review, a thorough examination and accurate diagnosis.

14.1 The Complete History and Examination

Thorough examination and data collecting regarding a patient's condition is mandatory at every child's first visit to the dentist. A systemic approach is necessary to collect data to reach an accurate diagnosis. A complete examination of the pediatric dental patient should include assessment of the following:

- Chief complaint.
- Medical and dental history.
- General growth and development.
- Clinical examination, including extraoral examination, intraoral examination.
- Radiographic examination and other diagnostic tools.
- Caries risk assessment.
- Behavior assessment.

At the first visit, the child and his or her parents form their first impression about the attitudes of the dentist and the dental team

Physical Evaluation and Treatment Planning in Dental Practice, Second Edition.
Géza T. Terézhalmy, Michaell A. Huber, Lily T. García and Ronald L. Occhionero.
© 2021 John Wiley & Sons, Inc. Published 2021 by John Wiley & Sons, Inc.
Companion Website: www.wiley.com/go/terezhalmy/physical

toward the treatment of the child. Therefore, it is important that the dental team provides them with a warm and supportive environment and the examination is done in a friendly and relaxed atmosphere. On the other hand, this first visit is a great opportunity for the dentist to form an impression of the general background of the child and the family, their concerns, their expectations and their attitudes toward dentistry. In a pediatric dental setting, it is common that the parent is the one speaking on behalf of the child, thus it is easy for the dentist to overlook the child and his/her concerns. The dentist should keep in mind that communicating directly with the child is an important step toward gaining his/her trust, which is critical for the success of any treatment indicated; this is especially true for school-aged children and teenagers. Meanwhile, talking directly to the child may also help the dentist to identify cases of child abuse in the case of trauma.

1) Chief complaint or history of current disease

   The chief complaint is the main symptom or reason for which the patient or parent seeks treatment. The most common chief complaints in a pediatric dental office include "toothache," "cavities," "chipped tooth," "loose tooth" and "double-layer teeth." The dentist needs to address the chief complaint by collecting and evaluating all relevant information regardless of whether the problem requires intervention or not. For example, when a patient presents with a "toothache", further investigation on the history and characteristics of the pain provides valuable information on pulp status assessment, thus leading to appropriate treatment planning. Sometimes, a comprehensive diagnosis of all of the patient's problems or potential problems may need to be postponed until more urgent conditions or chief complaints are addressed and resolved. For example, a patient with acute odontogenic infection needs immediate treatment. A chief complaint reported by the parent may not be the reflection of that of the child. For example, the parent's attitude towards the child's malocclusion may not be shared by the child. The dentist needs to understand that the child's perspective on the matter may have a considerable effect on the potential success of any future treatment.

2) The history (medical history, dental history and family and social history)

   The basic elements of a complete history are listed in Table 14.1.

   • Medical history

   The parent or guardian is usually the historian for the child. A general health history form can be used to determine the child's health background and also brings the oral and dental problems into a broader perspective of total patient care. The elements of a comprehensive medical history are included in Table 14.1. Figure 14.1 is the health history form used in the pediatric dental clinic at The University of Texas Health Science Center at San Antonio (UTHSCA); a brief review of all the systems is included. The parent or the guardian can complete this standard form; however, a good interview should never be omitted from an examination visit, and it is more efficient for the trained dental assistant to ask the questions in an informal interview style and then to present the findings to the dentist. In this manner, before the dentist examines the child, he or she is informed regarding the child's general health and is aware of the need for obtaining additional information from the parent or the child's physician if indicated.

   Congenital or acquired diseases may cause or predispose to oral problems (e.g. craniofacial syndromes, diabetes), or may have effects on the delivery of treatment of oral disease in the child (e.g. hematological disorders, congenital heart diseases). In most cases, a short

Table 14.1 Basic elements of a complete history.

Main category	Components
Personal data	• Patient's name, gender, age and address • Parent's name • Financial responsibility
Chief complaints (history of current illness)	• Symptoms (characteristics, duration, triggering factors, etc.) • History of pain if caries, toothache or other pain • History of injury if trauma (what, when, where and how, immediate management, etc.)
Medical history	• Pregnancy history (duration, mother's health, use of medication) • Delivery history (complications, birth weight, prematurity) • Neonatal period (birth weight, respiratory problems, feeding problems, neonatal teeth) • Child's health (childhood diseases, somatic development, psychomotor development, and previous medication use) • Medication (previous used, current using, adverse or allergic reaction) • Surgical history (use of general anesthesia) • History of hospitalizations • Review of all systems (cardiac, respiratory, etc.) • Sleeping disturbances
Dental history	• Past dental experience (treatment received and acceptance to the treatment) • Oral habits (pacifier, thumb sucking, bruxism) • Fluoride exposure (topical and systemic) • Oral hygiene (home care routine) • Dietary habits or feeding habits (type, amount and frequency of sugary snacks, breastfeeding habits and duration, bottle use, content and duration) • History of dental trauma • Age of first tooth eruption
Family history	• Number of children in the family • Housing condition • Parent's occupations • Child's attendance and performance at schools • History of genetic disease • Caries history of siblings and caregiver

and noncontributory history is common in children. Occasionally, when the parents report an acute or chronic systemic disease or anomaly, the dentist should conduct the history interview and consult the child's physician to learn the status of the condition, the current therapy and the long-range prognosis. When a child patient with severe systemic disease needs extensive dental treatment, oral rehabilitation in a hospital setting under general anesthesia after the physician consultation may be appropriate. Sometimes, the American Society of Anesthesiologists (ASA) physical status classification (Table 14.2) is used to classify the patient's baseline health status. This information is particularly useful when we consider a patient's candidacy for in-office sedation. Patients who are in ASA class I and II are usually considered appropriate candidates for in-office sedation; while children in ASA III and IV require additional consideration due to increased risk of experiencing adverse sedation events resulting from their underlying medical conditions. Consultation from specialists and/or

MEDICAL HISTORY

☐ Yes ☐ No Is your child being treated by a physician?
☐ Yes ☐ No Has your child ever been hospitalized?
If yes, for what, when? _____
☐ Yes ☐ No Has your child has ever received general anesthesia?
If yes, were there any complications? _____
☐ Yes ☐ No Has any family member had complication during general anesthesia? If yes, explain _____
☐ Yes ☐ No Is your child allergic to any medications?
If yes what? _____
☐ Yes ☐ No Is your child taking any medications at this time?
If yes, what? _____

Child's Physician/Pediatrician

Dr _____

Physician's Phone# _____

Physician's Address _____

Date of Last Visit _____

Purpose of Last Visit _____

Has this child ever been diagonsed with any of the following conditions?

Yes	No		Yes	No		Yes	No	
☐	☐	Anemia	☐	☐	Eye Problems	☐	☐	Otitis (Ear Infection)
☐	☐	Arthritis	☐	☐	Hearing Loss	☐	☐	Pneumonia
☐	☐	Asthma	☐	☐	Heart Murmur	☐	☐	Pregnancy
☐	☐	Brain Injury	☐	☐	Hepatitis	☐	☐	Rheumatic Fever
☐	☐	Bleeding Problems	☐	☐	HIV (AIDS)	☐	☐	Scarlet Fever
☐	☐	Cancer	☐	☐	Hyperactivity	☐	☐	Sickle Cell Anemia
☐	☐	Cerebral Palsy	☐	☐	Jaundice	☐	☐	Spina Bifida
☐	☐	Convulsions/Seizures	☐	☐	Leukemia	☐	☐	Syndrome _____
☐	☐	Cystic Fibrosis	☐	☐	Measles	☐	☐	Whooping Cough
☐	☐	Developmentally Delayed	☐	☐	Mental Retardation	☐	☐	Other: _____
☐	☐	Diabetes	☐	☐	Orthopedic Problems	☐	☐	Immunization Up to Date

DENTAL HISTORY

Yes	No		Yes	No	
☐	☐	Does your child brush regularly?	☐	☐	Has your child been seen by a dentist before?
☐	☐	Is your drinking water fluoridated?	☐	☐	Has your child had any accidents involving his/her teeth?
☐	☐	Does your child use:	☐	☐	Does your child have a dental condition that seems to
☐	☐	Fluoride vitamins?	☐	☐	"run in the family (hereditary)" If so, please indicate:
☐	☐	Fluoride rinse/gel?			
☐	☐	Fluoride toothpaste?	☐	☐	Is there anything you would like to discuss personally with the dentist who examines your child?

How do you expect your child to react to dental treatment?
☐ Very well   ☐ Moderately well   ☐ Not well   Why _____

If your child had any pets, hobbies, or special interest, please list: _____

_____ _____ _____
Signature   Date   Reviewer

Office Use Only
MEDICAL HISTORY ALERT

Medical History, Update Summary _____
Date   Reviewer

Medical History, Update Summary _____
Date   Reviewer

Medical History, Update Summary _____
Date   Reviewer

Figure 14.1 Patient history form used at UTHSCSA Pediatric Dental Clinics (Source: Courtesy of Department of Developmental Dentistry, University of Texas Health Science Center San Antonio).

an anesthesiologist is necessary for safe management of these patients.

The dental team should also be alert to identifying potentially communicable infectious conditions that may threaten the health of the patient and others. It is prudent to postpone elective non-emergency dental care for a patient who shows signs or symptoms of acute infectious disease until the patient recovers.

Known drug allergies should be recorded in a conspicuous location on the chart as an alert so that the information is

Table 14.2 ASA physical status classification.

Class	Description
I	A normally healthy patient
II	A patient with mild systemic disease
III	A patient with severe systemic disease
IV	A patient with severe systemic disease that is a constant threat to life
V	A moribund patient who is not expected to survive without the operation

available when in needed. Attention should be paid when parents may confuse nausea with a true allergic reaction. Sometimes, the dentist needs to address the issues directly with a physician to obtain accurate information.

Before the examination, a summary of the health status of the child should be documented in the examination form to ensure review and highlight important information. This summary serves as a convenient reminder to the dental team, also to verify that the dentist has reviewed the history and made an assessment on its impact on treatment.

- Dental history
The elements of a dental history are listed in Table 14.1. The patient's dental history should be comprehensive and included in the history form as well (Figure 14.1). This should cover past dental problems and previous care, previous and current fluoride exposure, current oral hygiene practice, dietary habits, feeding practice, previous and current non-nutritive sucking habits, history of dental trauma and an eruption-developmental profile. A developmental model has been used in collecting dental history to provide the dentist an age-specific set of findings that can be converted to preventive instruction in the anticipatory guidance counseling. For example, the questions regarding bottle use and weaning are important during an infant exam;

however, they become "non-applicable" when a child has outgrown these questions. Additional information needs to be obtained when a parent reports a previous history of restorative treatment. Knowledge on the previous use of local anesthesia, sedation, and rubber dam isolation, as well as the child's response and acceptance toward past dental treatments is valuable to the dental team, since it allows the dentist to make a more accurate assessment on how well the child is likely to cooperate with future treatment. Factors of importance for identifying etiology of current diseases (erosion, oral habits) and future dental health (oral hygiene and diet at home) should be also discussed in dental history. Obtaining dental history also reveals the parent's attitude toward dental health, which affects the family's compliance toward dental treatment; therefore, sometimes it is appropriate and realistic to modify a treatment plan to accommodate the family's expectation without compromising the quality of the care.

- Family history and social history
Familial history may also be relevant to the patient's oral condition and may provide important diagnostic information in some hereditary disorders, such as oligodontia, amelogenesis imperfecta (AI), dentinogenesis imperfecta and ectodermal dysplasia. Knowledge on the child's family socioeconomic status and immigrant status is also relevant, since parents/caregivers/patients of low socioeconomic status and with a background of recent immigration are known risk factors for dental caries (Vargas et al. 1998; Nunn et al. 2009).

Information regarding the child's social and psychological development is important, since the child's learning, behavioral or communication problems at home, school or other social settings may result in behavioral problems at the dental office due to the child's inability to communicate effectively with the dentist and follow instructions. This inability may be a result of a learning disorder, therefore the child's learning process should be inquired about; for example, asking a school-aged child his or her performance at school will be appropriate. However, sometimes this information is difficult to obtain, particularly when the parents are aware of the problems but are reluctant to discuss them. Under these circumstances, it is better for the dentist to conduct the interview. When the parents meet the dentist privately, they are more likely to discuss the child's problems openly.

3) General appraisal on growth and development

This first step of the examination is usually achieved in the waiting room or similar nonthreatening environment. It usually includes the assessment of patient's stature, physical appearance, vital signs and gross signs of disease. To effectively assess a child's general growth and development, a dentist need to be familiar with the physical and behavioral developmental milestones of children from different age groups which are discussed in detail in various textbooks. Vital signs are collected at the appointments, to not only identify any abnormalities, but also to fulfill our medicolegal role of providing baseline health data for an emergency situation. Accurate vital signs of blood pressure, pulse and respiration rate can only be obtained when the child is calm and relaxed; therefore taking such vital signs can be deferred until the child has become more comfortable with the environment, but these important data must be collected prior to the administration of any drugs. Weight should be measured and recorded in a chart for future use when drug calculation and administration is required. Height, with weight and BMI index, can be used as an index of

physical development. General appraisal usually serves as the initial contact between the dental team and the child patient; the interaction between the two provides an excellent opportunity to observe the child's behavior and assess the potential cooperation of the child.

4) Clinical exam

A comprehensive clinical examination should include a head and neck examination, extraoral facial examination and intraoral examination. The examination form used at pediatric dental clinics of UTHSCSA is shown in Figure 14.2. The clinical examination, whether the initial examination or a recall examination, should be all inclusive. The dentist needs to be a sharp observer, who can gather useful information while getting acquainted with a patient even before the patient is seated in the dental chair. Also, a chairside examination provides another good opportunity for the dentist to observe behavior and assess potential cooperation, as well as for the child to develop confidence and trust in the dentist. By the end of an examination visit, the rapport between the child and the dentist should have been established. Age appropriate technique should be used during examination. For example, during an infant exam, a dental chair is unnecessary and the least preferred approach. A knee-to-knee position should be used for infant examination (Figure 14.3), the details of which will be discussed later in this chapter.

I. Examination of head and neck

A systemic approach is recommended. Assessment of each anatomical structure for integrity, function, development, and pathology should be included. The elements of this part of the examination, possible abnormal findings and etiology are listed in Table 14.3. The dentist should be familiar with the normal, to be able to identify the variations that may

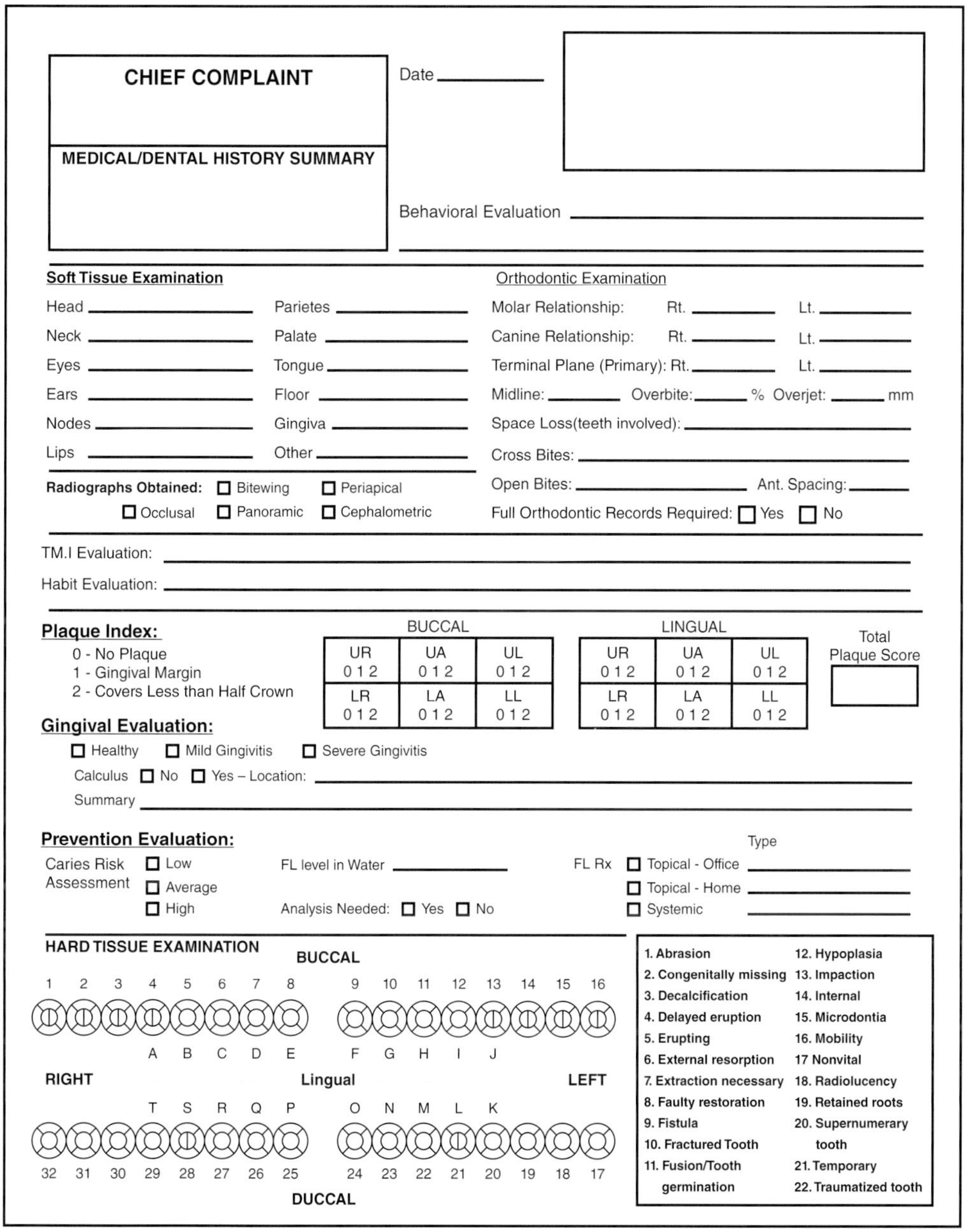

CHIEF COMPLAINT

Date _____

MEDICAL/DENTAL HISTORY SUMMARY

Behavioral Evaluation _____

Soft Tissue Examination

Head _____   Parietes _____
Neck _____   Palate _____
Eyes _____   Tongue _____
Ears _____   Floor _____
Nodes _____   Gingiva _____
Lips _____   Other _____

Radiographs Obtained: ☐ Bitewing ☐ Periapical
☐ Occlusal ☐ Panoramic ☐ Cephalometric

Orthodontic Examination

Molar Relationship: Rt. _____   Lt. _____
Canine Relationship: Rt. _____   Lt. _____
Terminal Plane (Primary): Rt. _____   Lt. _____
Midline: _____ Overbite: _____ % Overjet: _____ mm
Space Loss(teeth involved): _____
Cross Bites: _____
Open Bites: _____ Ant. Spacing: _____
Full Orthodontic Records Required: ☐ Yes ☐ No

TM.I Evaluation: _____

Habit Evaluation: _____

Plaque Index:
  0 - No Plaque
  1 - Gingival Margin
  2 - Covers Less than Half Crown

Gingival Evaluation:
  ☐ Healthy ☐ Mild Gingivitis ☐ Severe Gingivitis
  Calculus ☐ No ☐ Yes – Location: _____
  Summary _____

BUCCAL			LINGUAL			Total Plaque Score
UR	UA	UL	UR	UA	UL	
0 1 2	0 1 2	0 1 2	0 1 2	0 1 2	0 1 2	
LR	LA	LL	LR	LA	LL	
0 1 2	0 1 2	0 1 2	0 1 2	0 1 2	0 1 2	

Prevention Evaluation:

Caries Risk Assessment ☐ Low ☐ Average ☐ High

FL level in Water _____
Analysis Needed: ☐ Yes ☐ No

Type
FL Rx ☐ Topical - Office _____
☐ Topical - Home _____
☐ Systemic _____

HARD TISSUE EXAMINATION

BUCCAL

1 2 3 4 5 6 7 8   9 10 11 12 13 14 15 16

A B C D E   F G H I J

RIGHT   Lingual   LEFT

T S R Q P   O N M L K

32 31 30 29 28 27 26 25   24 23 22 21 20 19 18 17

DUCCAL

1. Abrasion
2. Congenitally missing
3. Decalcification
4. Delayed eruption
5. Erupting
6. External resorption
7. Extraction necessary
8. Faulty restoration
9. Fistula
10. Fractured Tooth
11. Fusion/Tooth germination
12. Hypoplasia
13. Impaction
14. Internal
15. Microdontia
16. Mobility
17 Nonvital
18. Radiolucency
19. Retained roots
20. Supernumerary tooth
21. Temporary
22. Traumatized tooth

Figure 14.2 UTHSCSA Pediatric dental examination form (Source: Courtesy of Department of Developmental Dentistry, University of Texas Health Science Center San Antonio).

indicate any problem. A detailed facial examination describing skeletal and dental relationships in three spatial planes: anteroposterior, vertical, and transverse is discussed in the orthodontic evaluation chapter (Chapter 15).

II. Intraoral examination

A systemic approach is recommended in order to avoid omission of any important conditions. It is easy for the dentist to look first for the obvious carious lesion, thus the following order is commonly

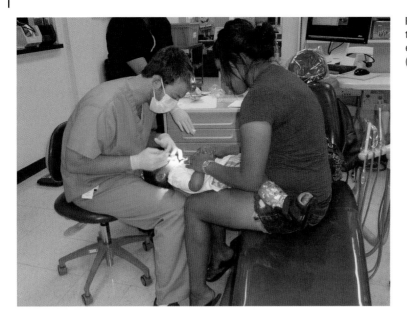

Figure 14.3 The technique of infant examination (knee-to-knee exam).

used: soft tissues, periodontal tissues, occlusion, and teeth.

i. Soft tissues

The elements and order of this part of the examination, of possible abnormal findings and etiology are listed in Table 14.4. The Mallampati score (Table 14.5) is used to predict the ease of intubation by the anesthesiologist. It is based on the visibility of the base of the uvula, faucial pillars (the arches in front of and behind the tonsils) and soft palate (Mallampati et al. 1985). A high Mallampati score (class 3 or 4) is associated with more difficult intubation as well as a higher incidence of sleep apnea (Nuckton et al. 2006). Similarly, the size of the tonsils is assessed using Brodsky grading system based on tonsillar airway obstruction (Table 14.6). Adenotonsillar enlargement is the major etiology factor of obstructive sleep apnea in otherwise healthy children (Nixon and Brouillette 2005). High score on parietes examination combined with a history of snoring and sleep apnea put an individual patient at higher risk for adverse complications when sedation or general anesthesia is considered for effective patient management.

ii. Periodontal tissues

It is rare to find periodontal pocketing in the primary dentition. A complete periodontal examination of all teeth for pocketing or attachment loss is not necessary in children unless there is an associated medical condition or radiographic signs of bone loss. Systemic probing can usually be postponed until teenage years. However, gingival tissue should be examined for inflammation and bleeding to detect gingivitis. The level of oral hygiene should be assessed by a scoring system. The existence and location of the staining and calculus need to be documented. Localized gingival recession can sometimes be seen in children with traumatic occlusion; the location and amount of recession should be noted.

Table 14.3 The elements of head and neck examination, common abnormality and possible etiology.

Structure	Things to examine	Abnormality and examples of possible etiology
Skull	Symmetry	Asymmetry/craniofacial anomaly/craniosynostosis
	Size	
Hair	Quality	Dryness/malnutrition, ectodermal dysplasia
	Quantity	Baldness/chemotherapy, ectodermal dysplasia, self-mutilation
	Color	Lice or other infestation/unsanitary home conditions or neglect
Eyes	Vision	Abnormal movement and reaction to light/cranial nerve damage
	Position and orientation	
	Movement	Variation in orientation/genetic malformation syndrome
	Reaction to light	
Ears	Hearing	Malformations/genetic syndrome (e.g. Treacher Collins)
	Integrity and structure of external ear and auditory canal	Hearing loss/trauma, developmental disability
Nose	Size and shape	Malformation/genetic anomaly (e.g. ectodermal dysplasia)
	location	Malposition/genetic malformation syndrome (e.g. median facial cleft)
	Function	Discharge/upper respiratory tract infection(URI), asthma, allergy
Lips	Integrity	Clefting/genetic clefting syndrome, cleft lip and or palate
	Closure	Poor closure and incompetence/malocclusion
	Symmetry	Asymmetry/cranial nerve damage, Bell's palsy
	Lesions	Ulcerations/herpes infection
Face	Symmetry	Asymmetry swelling/cellulitis
		bilateral swelling/mumps
Skin/ Scalp	Moisture	Dryness/dehydration, dermatitis, ectodermal dysplasia
	Color	Redness/cellulitis, allergic reaction
	Texture	Edema/cellulitis, renal disease
	Lesions	Laceration, bruises/trauma, abuse
	Temperature	Ulceration/infectious disease, abuse
		Increase temperature/cellulitis or other infections
TMJ	Symmetry	Deviation/trauma, TMJD
	Movement	Limitation/trauma, TMJD, arthritis
	Pain	Crepitus, pain/TMJD
	Range of motion	
Lymph nodes	Size	Enlarged but mobile/infection
	Mobility	Enlarged and fixation/neoplasia
	Location	Lower face and jaw/common, indicative of infection
		Neck and clavicular region/rare, indicative of more serious ailments.
Thyroid	Size	Enlarged/goiter, tumor

Table 14.4 The elements of soft tissue intraoral examination, common abnormality and possible etiology.

Structure	Things to examine	Common abnormality and examples of possible etiology
Inside of lips	Color	Pallor/anemia
	Swelling	Swelling/mucocle, hematoma
	Lesions	Ulceration/herpes or other infections, trauma, aphthous
Buccal mucosa	Color	Pallor/anemia
	Lesion	Ulceration/aphthous, herpes or other infections,
	Swelling	cheek biting trauma, abuse
		Swelling/salivary gland infection, mumps
Alveolar sulci	Swelling	Swelling/odontogenic infections, dental alveolar abscess
	Integrity	
		Fistula/chronic odontogenic infection
	Lesions	
		Ulceration/herpes, other infections, trauma
Palates	Integrity	Cleft/congenital defect, genetic syndromes
	Lesions	Ulceration/herpes, herpangina, mononucleosis,
	Function	abuse
		Petechiae/sexual abuse
		Deviation/cranial nerve damage
Tonsils and pharynx	Size of the tonsils	Enlarged tonsils/tonsillitis, upper respiratory tract infection (URI)
	color	
		Redness/ tonsillitis, URI
Tongue	Color	Redness/glossitis, geographical tongue
	Movement	Deviation/cranial nerve damage
	Lesions	Ulceration/aphthous, herpes, trauma
	Integrity	
		Laceration/trauma
		Piercing
Floor of the mouth	Swelling	Swelling/ranula, salivary stone, hematoma by trauma
	Color	
	Lesions	Redness/hematoma by trauma
	Salivary function	Ulceration/aphthous ulceration, abuse
Frenal attachments	Position	Abnormal position may have periodontal or speech complications

iii. Occlusion

A brief examination of occlusion should be included in the routine exam (Figure 14.2). The details of a comprehensive orthodontic evaluation are discussed in Chapter 15. Crowding, misaligned teeth, midline shift, mandibular deviations are easy to identify. Some simple occlusal discrepancies should be recognized and treated early, for example functional posterior crossbites. Non-nutritive digit sucking habits should also be documented and intervention at appropriate age should be considered.

iv. Teeth

The elements of examination of the teeth are listed in Table 14.7. Careful inspection, good lighting, and

Table 14.5 Mallampati score.

Class	Description
1	Full visibility of tonsils, uvula and soft palate
2	Visibility of hard and soft palate, upper portion of tonsils and uvula
3	Soft and hard palate and base of the uvula are visible
4	Only hard palate visible

Table 14.6 Brodsky grading system.

Grading	Description
0	Tonsils inside the tonsillar fossa with no air way obstruction
1+	Tonsils slightly out of the tonsillar fossa occupy ≤25% of the oropharyngeal width
2+	Tonsils occupy 26–50% of the oropharyngeal width
3+	Tonsils occupy 51–75% of the oropharyngeal width
4+	Tonsils occupy >75% of the oropharyngeal width

clean and dry teeth are required for accurate diagnosis of initial caries lesions and minor changes in color and mineralization disturbances.

5) Radiographic exam and other supplemental diagnostic tools

In many cases, radiographic examination is essential for diagnosis, treatment planning and surveillance on certain changes and pathologies related to teeth and jaws. However, a radiographic examination should not be done based on a patient's age; it should only be done when its diagnostic value has been established by a dentist through a prior history review and clinical examination. In other words, an X-ray should only be taken when its diagnostic yield influences treatment planning, resulting in a more appropriate treatment considered more beneficial to the patient. There are

Table 14.7 Examination of the teeth.

Things to examine	Selected findings
Number	Hypodontia/oligodonitia
	Supernumerary tooth
Position	Rotation
	Infraocclusion
	Ectopic eruption
Eruption status	Partial eruption
	Impaction
Eruption patterns	Asymmetrical eruption pattern
	Delayed eruption
Morphology	Microdontia
	Dens evaginatus
Surface structure	Erosion
	Attrition
	Fracture
	Fluorosis
	Enamel hypoplasia/hypomineralization
	Amelogenesis imperfecta
Color	Grey – tetracycline staining
	Pink – post-trauma intra pulpal bleeding
	Grey – pulp necrosis
	White – decalcification, fluorosis
	Amber translucence – dentinogenesis imperfecta
Cavitated caries lesions	Size
	Color
	Depth
Existing restorations	Overhang
	Marginal breakdown
	Recurrent decay
Mobility	Increased mobility/exfoliation, advanced pulpal pathology
	Decreased mobility/ankylosis
Percussion sensitivity	Positive/food impaction, advanced pulpal pathology

several common indications for taking radiographies in children and adolescents:

- Diagnosis of caries and its sequelae.
- Diagnosis of trauma to teeth and supporting tissue.

- Detection of developmental and acquired dental anomalies.
- Detection of bony pathology.
- Aid the treatment planning prior to orthodontic treatment.
- Aid the treatment planning prior to oral surgery.

The recommendations for radiographs in pediatric dental patients are summarized in Table 14.8, modified from those given by the American Academy of Pediatric Dentistry (AAPD). The intervals between bitewings are dictated by the child's dental developmental stage and individual caries risk assessment. The most commonly used intraoral radiographs are bitewing, periapical, and anterior occlusal films, while the most commonly used extraoral radiographs include panoramic radiographs, lateral cephalogram and cone beam computed tomography (CBCT). The selected radiographs for above mentioned indications are summarized in Table 14.9.

Obtaining a "good" intraoral X-ray can be challenging for some young patients. Taking radiography is one of the first "treatments" a child may receive in a dental office. The experience should be as pleasant as possible so that it can provide the dental team an opportunity to observe the child's response and shape the child's behavior through this "moderately" threatening dental experience. There are some suggestions and tips for obtaining good intraoral radiographs in young children:

- Explain the procedure by using "tell–show–do" technique. Demonstrate the procedure on the child's doll or stuffed animal, the parent or older siblings without actual radiation exposure (Figure 14.4).
- If a film or digital sensor holder is used, before placing the film in the holder intraorally, practice with the holder without the film. If the child can close the mouth and bite on the bitepiece satisfactorily, then mount the film in the holder and place them carefully in the mouth.
- Recruit parental help. If the child can't sit on the chair alone, he or she can be placed on the lap of a parent with the child' head leaning against the parent's chest and the parent's hand placed on the child's forehead to stabilize the child and minimize the risk of patient movement during exposure (Figure 14.5).
- Use a film or sensor size which can be tolerated by the child, size 0 or 1 films should be used for bitewings and periapicals in preschoolers. Size 2 films should be used for occlusals in primary dentition, while size 4 films should be used for occlusals during mixed dentition.
- The whole process should be well-organized to favor quick exposure and less discomfort. The film should be placed in the mouth after the child is well-seated and the X-ray beam is correctly positioned to minimize discomfort.
- Gagging can be minimized by empathy, distraction, and a well-organized procedure. In cases of extreme gagging, use of local anesthetic or nitrous oxide sedation can be considered.
- The easiest film should be taken first, usually meaning the maxillary anterior occlusal film.
- If a child does not tolerate the procedure after repeated tries, give positive reinforcement, praise his/her effort and defer the radiographic exam to next visit in a non-emergency situation.

Sometimes, a radiograph with diagnostic quality cannot be obtained in spite of good effort from both the child and the dental team or because of the child's limited ability to cooperate due to young age, medical condition or disability. In the cases of unsuccessful radiographic exam, the diagnostic value expected from the radiographs should be reevaluated. In a non-emergency situation, if there are no clinical signs of dental disease, deferral of the radiographic

Table 14.8 Radiographic protocol for pediatric dentistry.

Stage of development (Age by years)	Considerations	Radiographs	Rationale
Primary dentition (3–5)	Open contacts No apparent abnormalities	None	Can examine proximal by visualization or probing
	Closed contacts No apparent abnormalities	2 bitewings	Cannot examine proximals clinically
	Extensive caries and/or suspected pathology	2 bitewings and selected PAs	Additional diagnostic information
Anterior eruption phase (5 to 7)	Incisor eruptions imminent or in progress	Augment above with anterior occlusal films – primary teeth use size 2 film – permanent teeth use size 4 film	Evaluate for pathology and timing of eruption
Mixed dentition (7 to 12)	No apparent abnormalities	2 bitewings plus panoramic file or 8-film survey	Evaluate proximal, dental development and eruption sequence
	Extensive caries and/or suspected pathology	Augment with selected PAs	Additional diagnostic information
Early permanent dentition	No apparent abnormalities	2–4 bitewings plus panoramic film or 12-film survey	Evaluate proximal, dental development and screening exam
	Extensive caries and/or suspected pathology	Augment with selected PAs	Additional diagnostic information
AT RECALL EXAMINATIONS			
Primary dentition and mixed dentition	– Caries risk – Incipient interproximal lesions on previous X-rays – Restorative treatment since last recall	– 2 bitewings and selected PAs of teeth that had pulp treatment and/or SSCs done at 6–12 month intervals if closed contact, with clinical caries or increased caries risk – 2 bitewings at 12–24 month intervals if closed contact, no clinical caries and no increased caries risk	– Compare bitewings form last set to evaluate the progression of the incipient lesions – PAs to check furcation or periapical lesions
Early permanent dentition	– Caries risk – Incipient interproximal lesions on previous X-rays – Restorative treatment since last recall	– 2–4 bitewings and selected PAs of teeth that had previous pulp treatment at 6–12 month interval if closed contact, with clinical caries or increased caries risk – 2 or 4 bitewings at 18–36 month intervals if no clinical caries and no increased caries risk	– Compare bitewings form last set to evaluate the progression of the incipient lesions – PAs to check periapical lesions

Table 14.9 Indications for radiographs, selected films and their diagnostic values.

Indications	Selected films and things to watch
Caries and its sequelae	Bitewings – Interproximal and occlusal caries at posterior region, pulp involvement, furcation radiolucent area
	Periapicals – pulp involvement, furcal and periapical radiolucent area, internal and external root resorption
	Anterior occlusals – interproximal caries at anterior region, pulp involvement, periapical radiolucent area
Trauma to teeth and supporting tissue	Anterior occlusals – luxation, displacement, Root fracture, alveolar bone fracture
	Periapical – see occlusals, multiple exposure with different angles on each involved tooth to detect fracture line
	Panoramics – jaw fractures, condyle fracture
	Soft tissue intraoral films – localization of foreign body imbedded in soft tissue
	Extraoral lateral projection – determine the position and direction of displaced
	CT and CBCT – additional diagnostic information in severe cases
Developmental and acquired dental anomalies	Periapicals – localized
	Panoramic – localized or generalized
	CBCT or CT – additional diagnostic information needed
Bony pathology	Periapicals – localized
	Panoramic – localized or generalized
	CBCT or CT – additional diagnostic information needed
Treatment planning prior to orthodontics	Panoramic (see details in Chapter 15)
	Lateral cephalometric
	CBCT
Treatment planning prior to oral surgery	Periapicals – localization of the operative object, in relation to important neighboring structures.
	Panoramic – localization of the operative object, in relation to important neighboring structures.
	CBCT or CT – additional diagnostic information needed

examination to a later time is acceptable. While in an emergency situation or there are clear clinical signs of dental disease, sometimes it is necessary to refer the patient to a specialist to have the radiographic examination done with advanced behavior management techniques, such as sedation. Some special supplemental diagnostic tools provide information that may influence treatment planning. A pulp vitality test is required following trauma to the permanent dentition, but it is unreliable and less valuable in the primary dentition and young permanent teeth. A thermal test can be used in permanent teeth to assess pulp vitality, but has limited diagnostic value in primary teeth. In young children, these tests may not be fully understood; sometimes the pain and discomfort triggered by these tests may result in loss of the child's confidence and disruptive behavior during future treatment. A false positive is not uncommon from an anxious child. Sometimes, diet analysis, salivary flow, salivary buffering capacity and salivary streptococcus mutant levels need to be investigated for an accurate caries risk assessment. On rare occasions, blood tests

Figure 14.4 Use a stuffed animal as a model to demonstrate radiographic examination.

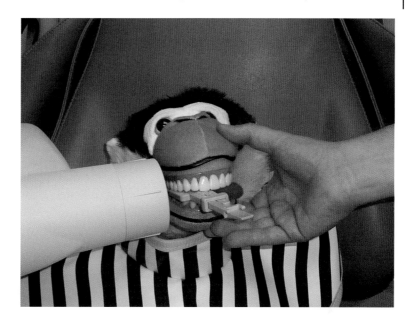

Figure 14.5 Use parental assistance in radiographic examination.

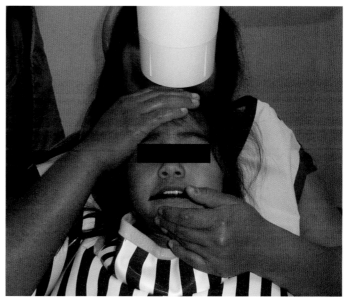

may be performed to rule out systemic conditions contributing to oral pathological findings.

6) Caries risk assessment

Caries risk assessment is the determination of the likelihood of the incidence of caries or the likelihood in changes of caries activity already established (Reich et al. 1999). Caries risk assessment needs to be performed at every examination visit (initial and recall) and can only be done after careful history taking and a comprehensive examination. Current caries risk assessment models involve a combination of factors including diet, fluoride exposure, a susceptible host, and microflora that interplay with a variety of social, cultural, and behavioral factors (Featherston 2004).

Using a caries risk assessment tool, the dentist is able to identify the high-risk individual and provides timely intervention to prevent caries or white spot lesions becoming cavitations. The caries risk assessment tools for different age groups developed by AAPD should be used to classify the child's risk for caries (Figures 14.6 and 14.7).

7) Behavior assessment

One of the goals of pediatric dentistry is to guide the children through their dental experiences and promote positive dental attitudes and improve his/her dental health in the future. Therefore, accurate assessment of the child's behavior, ability to cooperate and communicate; and adjusting the behavior management accordingly are essential for the success of any dental treatment. An examination visit provides a moderately threatening environment for behavior assessment, as well as development of behavioral interactions between dentist and the child. The factors influencing a child's dental behaviors include his/her cognitive development, temperament, reaction to strangers, parental anxiety, fear, previous dental or medical experience and awareness of dental problems. For example, research has shown a significant correlation between maternal anxiety and a child's cooperative behavior at the first dental visit, especially in children younger than four years old. A child who has had a positive previous medical or dental experience is more like to be cooperative with the dentist. Previous surgical experiences have been shown to have negative effect on the behavior at the first dental visit. When a child believes that a dental problem exists, regardless of the seriousness of the condition, there is a tendency toward negative behavior on the first dental visit. With this knowledge in mind, related information to assist

Factors	High risk	Moderate risk	Low risk
Risk factors, social/biological			
Mother/primary caregiver has active dental caries	Yes		
Parent/caregiver has life-time of poverty, low health literacy	Yes		
Child has frequent exposure (>3 times/day) between-meal sugar-containing snacks or beverages per day	Yes		
Child uses bottle or non-spill cup containing natural or added sugar frequently, between meals and/or at bedtime	Yes		
Child is a recent immigrant		Yes	
Child has special health care needs		Yes	
Protective factors			
Child receives optimally-fluoridated drinking water or fluoride supplements			Yes
Child has teeth brushed daily with fluoridated toothpaste			Yes
Child receives topical fluoride from health professional			Yes
Child has dental home/regular dental care			Yes
Clinical findings			
Child has non-cavitated (incipient/white spot) caries or enamel defects	Yes		
Child has visible cavities or fillings or missing teeth due to caries	Yes		
Child has visible plaque on teeth	Yes		

Circling those conditions that apply to a specific patient helps the practitioner and parent understand the factors that contribute to or protect from caries. Risk assessment categorization of low, moderate, or high is based on preponderance of factors for the individual. However, clinical judgment may justify the use of one factor (e.g., frequent exposure to sugar-containing snacks or beverages, more than one decayed missing filled surfaces [dmfs]) in determining overall risk.

Overall assessment of the child's dental caries risk: High ☐   Moderate ☐   Low ☐

Figure 14.6 Caries-risk assessment form for 0–5 years old by AAPD (Source: Ramos-Gomez FJ, Crall J, Gansky SA, Slayton RL, Featherstone JDB (2007). Caries risk assessment appropriate for the age 1 visit (infants and toddlers). J Calif Dent Assoc 35 (10): 687–702. Adapted with permission from the California Dental Association).

Factors	High risk	Moderate risk	Low risk
Risk factors, social/biological			
Patient has life-time of poverty, low health literacy	Yes		
Patient has frequent exposure (>3 times/day) between-meal sugar-containing snacks or beverages per day	Yes		
Child is a recent immigrant		Yes	
Patient has special health care needs		Yes	
Protective factors			
Patient receives optimally-fluoridated drinking water			Yes
Patient brushes teeth daily with fluoridated toothpaste			Yes
Patient receives topical fluoride from health professional			Yes
Patient has dental home/regular dental care			Yes
Clinical findings			
Patient has ≥1 interproximal caries lesions	Yes		
Patient has active non-cavitated (white spot) caries lesions or enamel defects	Yes		
Patient has low salivary flow	Yes		
Patient has defective restorations		Yes	
Patient wears an intraoral appliance		Yes	

Circling those conditions that apply to a specific patient helps the practitioner and patient/parent understand the factors that contribute to or protect from caries. Risk assessment categorization of low, moderate, or high is based on preponderance of factors for the individual. However, clinical judgment may justify the use of one factor (e.g., interproximal lesions, low salivary flow) in determining overall risk.

Overall assessment of the dental caries risk: High ☐ Moderate ☐ Low ☐

Figure 14.7 Caries-risk assessment form for >6 years old by AAPD (Source: Featherstone JBD, Domejean-Orliaguet S, Jenson L, et al. (2007). Caries risk assessment in practice for age 6 through adult. J Calif Dent Assoc 35 (10): 703–13. Adapted with permission from the California Dental Association).

behavior assessment should be gathered by observation of the child's interaction with the parent, the dentist and the dental team, also by questioning the child's parent during history interview.

Several systems have been developed for classifying the behavior of children in the dental environment. The most commonly used two systems are summarized in Table 14.10. The use of these behavior scale systems provides a means for recording behaviors and assisting the dentist in managing behaviors. However, it should be noted that use the scale alone does not communicate sufficient clinical information especially regarding uncooperative children, therefore, a short description of the clinical behavior following the scale grading can be useful, such as "hands up, cried at fluoride varnish." A child's behavior during examination is taken into account to be a predictor of his/her behavior during future treatment. However, since no single assessment tool is completely accurate and reliable, and a child's behavior is influenced by multiple physical, social, emotional, and intellectual factors, as well as temperament and attitude, it is critical that dentists master a wide range of behavior guidance techniques to meet the needs of the individual child and be flexible in their implementation.

8) Interval of examination

The most common interval of examination is six months. However, more frequent examinations may be required for some patients. The patients who are a high caries risk, who have special health needs, or who are extremely fearful, can be considered for more frequent examination visits. The purposes of this strategy are reevaluation of caries or disease risk, reinforcement of preventive activities at home, reevaluation of the patient's health status, and desensitization by repetitive exposure to dental procedures to allay fear and anxiety.

Table 14.10 Two of the most commonly used systems classifying the behavior of children in the dental environment.

Wright's clinical classification	
Cooperative	Reasonably relaxed, minimal apprehension, may be enthusiastic, can be treated by a straightforward, behavior-shaping approach. When guidelines for behavior are established, they perform within the framework provided.
Lacking in cooperative ability	Very young children with whom communication cannot be established and of whom comprehension cannot be expected
	Children with specific debilitating or disabling conditions which prohibits cooperation in the usual manner
Potentially cooperative	Children who have the ability to perform cooperatively, their behavior can be modified to become cooperative
	Can be defiant, timid, uncontrolled, tense-cooperative or whining
Frankl behavioral rating scale	
1 – Definitely negative	Refusal of treatment, forceful crying, fearfulness, or any other overt evidence of extreme negativism
2 – Negative	Reluctance to accept treatment, uncooperativeness, some evidence of negative attitude but not pronounced (sullen, withdraw)
3 + Positive	Acceptance of treatment, cautious behavior at times, willingness to comply with the dentist, at times with reservation, but patient follows the dentist's directions cooperatively
4 ++ Definitely positive	Good rapport with the dentist, interest in the dental procedures, laughter and enjoyment

14.2 Diagnosis

A series of diagnoses or a problem list should be extracted from the patient history, clinical and radiographic examination and supportive data collected from your complete examination. Diagnosis by definition is an act of identifying a disease from its signs and symptoms. Thus the ability to recognize the existence of an abnormal state will be the first and most important step. In the pediatric population, abnormalities in need of active management and those that only need to be identified and monitored should be separated. For example, a carious primary molar in a seven-year-old needs treatment, while a carious incisor with increased mobility just needs surveillance since it is near exfoliation. Determining the cause of the abnormality is essential in the management of certain diseases. For example,

identifying the cause of early childhood caries (ECC) and implementing preventive measurement, warrants the likelihood of successful outcome of the treatment in both the short and long term; on the other hand, amelogenesis imperfecta is a genetic condition with guarded prognosis.

A comprehensive diagnosis or problem list should include the following elements:

- Caries or disease risk including contributing factors.
- Soft tissue diagnosis including periodontal status, soft tissue trauma, trauma of periodontal tissue and soft tissue lesion.
- Hard tissue diagnosis including dental caries, developmental defects, dental trauma of hard tissue, malocclusion.
- Pulp diagnosis if deep caries.
- Behavior assessment on potential cooperation.

Table 14.11 Pulp diagnosis of primary dentition.

Diagnostic tools	Diagnosis	
History of pain	Normal pulp or reversible pulpitis	Irreversible pulpitis or necrotic pulp
	Thermal or chemical triggered	Spontaneous
	Intermittent and transitory	Prolonged stimulated pain
	Can be relieved by OTC analgesic	Nocturnal
Soft tissue	Normal	Inflamed, parulis, abscess, fistula
Mobility (comparing with contralateral tooth)	Physiological	Pathological
Percussion	Negative	Positive
Radiographic findings	Intact continuous PDL space	Widened and/or discontinuous PDL space
	Intact pericapical and furcation bone	
	No internal root resorption	Furcation and/or periapical radiolucencies
	No pathological external root resorption	Progressive internal resorption
		Pathological external root resorption
		Dystrophic intrapulpal calcification
Findings during treatment	Red color bleeding	Dark red or pulp bleeding
	Hemostasis achieved within five minutes	Excessive bleeding

Dental caries experienced among toddlers and preschoolers is alarmingly high in the United States. ECC, a term adapted by AAPD for this condition, reflects its multifactoral etiology. By definition, the disease of ECC is the presence of one or more decayed (non-cavitated or cavitated lesions), missing (due to caries), or filled tooth surfaces in any primary tooth in a child under the age of six. Moreover, in children younger than three years of age, any sign of smooth surface caries is indicative of severe early childhood caries (S-ECC). From ages 3 through 5, one or more cavitated, missing, or filled smooth surfaces in primary maxillary anterior teeth or a decayed, missing, or filled score of ≥ 4 (age 3), ≥ 5 (age 4), or ≥ 6 (age 5) surfaces also constitutes S-ECC (Drury et al. 1999). A child with a diagnosis of ECC or S-ECC will most likely to experience new caries lesions in both the primary dentition and permanent dentition, therefore, in addition to restorative treatment of the carious teeth, personalized preventive strategies should be included into his/her treatment planning. When carious lesions advance deep into dentin, pulp inflammation can be developed even without experiencing any clinical symptoms. Assessment of pulp status of the teeth with deep caries is required in the selection of teeth for different types of pulp therapy. Clinical and radiographic assessment for pulp diagnosis in primary dentition is summarized in Table 14.11. Diagnosis of most soft tissue and hard tissue anomalies in pediatric population is similar to that of the general population and has been discussed extensively in textbooks.

14.3 Treatment Planning

An appropriate treatment plan should be reached after the above-mentioned information collecting and problem listing. In pediatric patients, the treatment plan should facilitate the child to develop a positive attitude toward dental care and ensure the child enters adulthood with good oral health. Therefore, treatment planning for young children may be slightly different from that of adults; compromise sometimes needs to be made to gain a child's trust and to motivate the parents towards prevention. In addition to emergency care (if indicated), a preventive and operative treatment plan, and a behavior management or modification plan is crucial for the success of any treatment plan in children.

A variety of factors must be considered prior to the development of the treatment plan. They include the child's caries risk, general health, ability to cooperate, dental development, as well as the family's level of compliance, parental finances and attitude toward dental care. For example, in a preschooler with high caries risk, the choice of a stainless steel crown over multi-surface restoration should be recommended to avoid surfaces left exposed to recurrent decay. Another example is that extraction is chosen over pulp treatment in an immunosuppressed patient, especially when the vitality of the pulp is in question. For most patients, no single treatment plan is ideal. After considering all factors, a recommended plan along with reasonable alternative plans, and the risks and benefits to be derived from each plan should be discussed with the dentist, the parent and sometimes, the patient.

I. Components of a treatment plan

    i. Emergency care plan

        It is a priority of any treatment plan to manage emergencies, such as odontogenic infection and dental trauma. In cases of acute infection, extraction of involved teeth is usually the treatment of choice. However, it is a less than ideal introduction of dental care for young children which may have a disruptive effect on their behavior towards future dental care. In cases of dental trauma, usually it is necessary to carry out immediate treatment, such

as pulp capping, temporary restoration, reposition, and splinting to relieve pain and ensure better prognosis of involved teeth. It is quite often that emergency care is delivered prior to a comprehensive exam and long-term treatment planning. It is reasonable to delay the comprehensive treatment planning until the acute problems have resolved, since it is better to assess a child's potential in cooperation and the parent's ability in compliance when the child is not in pain and the parent is not under stress.

    ii. Preventive treatment plan

        In the modern view of caries management, preventive care is the most important aspect of treatment planning for young children. It is an ongoing part of any child's dental care, and should be constantly reinforced and modified as the child develops and their behavior and perceptions change (Welbury 2001). Tailoring preventive care based on an individual's caries risk is fundamental to effective caries management. A child's caries risk can change over time due to changes in home care, diet, oral microflora or physical condition. Maximal effects of caries assessment can only be achieved by performing it regularly and frequently, at least at recall examination visits every six months. The interval for frequency of professional preventive services, such as prophylaxis and topical fluoride treatment, should be based on risk for caries and periodontal disease. Children at moderate caries risk should receive these treatments at least every six months, while those with high caries risk should receive them more frequently (every three to six months). Anticipatory guidance is complementary to risk assessment and has become an integral part of each visit. Anticipatory guidance is defined as proactive

Table 14.12 Dietary fluoride supplementation schedule.

Age	< 0.3 ppm F ion	0.3–0.6 ppm F ion	>0.6 ppm F ion
Birth–6 months	0	0	0
6 months–3 years	0.25 mg	0	0
3–6 years	0.50 mg	0.25 mg	0
6 years up to at least 16 years	1.00 mg	0.50 mg	0

Case 1

8-year-old residing in an area with <0.3 ppm F ion

Rx: Sodium fluoride tabs (1 mg F ion/tablet)

Disp: 120 tabs

Sig: before bedtime after a thorough brushing, chew one tablet, swish and swallow

- Sodium fluoride tablets are supplied in 0.25 mg, 0.50 mg, 1 mg F ion/tablet

Case 2

4-year-old residing in an area with <0.3 ppm F ion

Rx: Sodium fluoride oral drops (0.5 mg F ion/ml)

Disp: 60 ml

Sig: Place 1 ml in any liquid, swish and drink once daily

- Sodium fluoride oral drop supplied in 0.25 mg F ion/drop and 0.5 mg F ion/ml.

counseling of parents and patients about developmental changes that will occur in the interval between health supervision visits that include information about daily caretaking specific to that upcoming interval (Pinkham et al. 2005). In a pediatric dental visit, topics to be included in anticipatory guidance discussion are oral development, oral hygiene, diet and nutrition, fluoride exposure, non-nutritive habits, injury prevention and speech/language development, which cover the major concerns related to caries, periodontal disease, trauma, and malocclusion. In older patients, counseling on substance abuse and oral piercing should be incorporated in anticipatory guidance. The advice given during anticipatory guidance counseling should be realistic, age-appropriate, and tailored to each individual case. Other preventive measurements include fluoride supplementation and sealants. Fluoride supplement should be considered when fluoride exposure is not optimal. The guidelines for fluoride supplementation recommended by the AAPD, the American Academy of Periodontology (AAP), American Dental Association (ADA) and endorsed by CDC and samples of prescription are shown in Table 14.12. The need for sealant placement should be assessed at the periodic exam; at-risk pits and fissures should be sealed as soon as possible. Recommendations for pediatric oral health assessment, preventive services, and anticipatory guidance/counseling from AAPD are seen in Figure 14.8.

It is known that surgical intervention alone does not stop caries progression. Modern management of dental caries is more conservative and more focused on individualized treatment based on a child's age, caries risk, and level of patient/parent cooperation and compliance. AAPD has developed

Recommendations for Pediatric Oral Health Assessment, Preventive Services, and Anticipatory Guidance/Counseling

Since each child is unique, these recommendations are designed for the care of children who have no contributing medical conditions and are developing normally. These recommendations will need to be modified for children with special health care needs or if disease or trauma manifests variations from normal. The American Academy of Pediatric Dentistry (AAPD) emphasizes the importance of very early professional intervention and the continuity of care based on the individualized needs of the child. Refer to the text of this guideline for supporting information and references.

AMERICAN ACADEMY OF PEDIATRIC DENTISTRY	6 TO 12 MONTHS	12 TO 24 MONTHS	2 TO 6 YEARS	6 TO 12 YEARS	12 YEARS AND OLDER
Clinical oral examination [1]	•	•	•	•	•
Assess oral growth and development [2]	•	•	•	•	•
Caries-risk assessment [3]	•	•	•	•	•
Radiographic assessment [4]	•	•	•	•	•
Prophylaxis and topical fluoride [3,4]	•	•	•	•	•
Fluoride supplementation [5]	•	•	•	•	•
Anticipatory guidance/counseling [6]	•	•	•	•	•
Oral hygiene counseling [7]	Parent	Parent	Patient/parent	Patient/parent	Patient
Dietary counseling [8]	•	•	•	•	•
Injury prevention counseling [9]	•	•	•	•	•
Counseling for nonnutritive habits [10]	•	•	•	•	•
Counseling for speech/language development			•		
Substance abuse counseling				•	•
Counseling for intraoral/perioral piercing				•	•
Assessment and treatment of developing malocclusion			•	•	•
Assessment for pit and fissure sealants [11]				•	•
Assessment and/or removal of third molars					•
Transition to adult dental care					•

1. First examination at the eruption of the first tooth and no later than 12 months. Repeat every 6 months or as indicated by child's risk status/susceptibility to disease. Includes assessment of pathology and injuries.
2. By clinical examination.
3. Must be repeated regularly and frequently to maximize effectiveness.
4. Timing, selection, and frequency determined by child's history, clinical findings, and susceptibility to oral disease.
5. Consider when systemic fluoride exposure is suboptimal. Up to at least 16 years.
6. Appropriate discussion and counseling should be an integral part of each visit for care.
7. Initially, responsibility of parent; as child matures, jointly with parent; then, when indicated, only child.

8. At every appointment; initially discuss appropriate feeding practices, then the role of refined carbohydrates and frequency of snacking in caries development and childhood obesity.
9. Initially play objects, pacifiers, car seats; when learning to walk; then with sports and routine playing, including the importance of mouthguards.
10. At first, discuss the need for additional sucking: digits vs pacifiers; then the need to wean from the habit before malocclusion or skeletal dysplasia occurs. For school-aged children and adolescent patients, counsel regarding any existing habits such as fingernail biting, clenching, or bruxism.
11. For caries-susceptible primary molars, permanent molars, premolars, and anterior teeth with deep pits and fissures; placed as soon as possible after eruption.

Figure 14.8 Recommendations for pediatric dental oral health assessment, preventive services, and anticipatory guidance/counseling (Source: Recommendations for Pediatric Oral Health Assessment, Preventive Services, and Anticipatory Guidance/Counseling. © 2011, American Academy of Pediatric Dentistry).

caries management protocols for different age groups based on clinical trials, systemic reviews and expert recommendations to guide the dentists to determine an individual patient's type and frequency of diagnostic, preventive and restorative care. Examples of caries management protocols suggested by AAPD will be seen and discussed later in this chapter.

iii. Operative treatment plan

The operative treatment plan should be realistic and takes the restorability, the lifespan and the importance in dental development of the tooth into consideration. A child's dental development dictates the decision of extraction versus restoration of the primary teeth during mixed dentition. A carious primary molar near exfoliation should be extracted instead of being restored. A carious primary second molar should be maintained in the arch if possible prior to the eruption of permanent first molar. Aesthetic concerns should also be addressed. However, it is not advisable to restore maxillary incisors prior to restoration of posterior teeth based solely on parents' esthetic concerns since it is likely that the parents may not bring the patient back for subsequent visits after their main concerns have been addressed; this scenario is particularly true when the family's interest in preserving primary teeth is limited.

Caries risk of the patient should always be considered when a decision on type of restorations is to be made. In high caries-risk children, definitive treatment of primary teeth with SSCs is better over time than multisurface intracoronal restorations, especially in children under the age of four (Holland et al. 1986; Randall 2002). The use of SSCs is also highly recommended in children who receive treatment

under sedation or general anesthesia, since these children are usually with increased caries risk, limited ability of cooperation, or developmental or medical disability. SSCs usually last longer and therefore decrease the frequency of sedation or general anesthesia (Seale 2002).

A good treatment plan should be designed in a way so that the child's teeth can be restored in the shortest possible time period. The approach used by most pediatric dentists is the practice of quadrant dentistry. This approach makes maximum use of the time available, reduces the number of visits, and local analgesia is often used which is usually economically beneficial to the parents. Using this method, a whole quadrant of the dentition is isolated under a rubber dam and up to four teeth can be treated in a single visit which usually can be completed within 45 minutes by an experienced pediatric dentist. Quadrant dentistry is designed to make the appointment short to accommodate the short attention span of younger children. Another approach called side dentistry has also been used when a child is under sedation, or has limited needs for operative treatment, or is mature enough to tolerate longer appointments. In side dentistry, two quadrants from one side of the mouth are treated. When practicing side dentistry in younger children under sedation, care must be taken to prevent overdose of local anesthetic agents (Table 14.13).

The sequence of the operative treatments should be also included in the treatment planning. When treating a child who has not experienced operative dentistry in the past, it is common to start the introduction to operative dentistry with the simplest restoration and the easiest local analgesia. By doing

Table 14.13 Commonly used local anesthetics in pediatric dentistry.

Anesthetic	Maximum dosage		Maximum total dosage (mg)	Dosage per cartridge (mg)		Vasoconstrictor per cartridge (µg)	
	mg/kg	mg/lb		1.7 ml	1.8 ml	1.7 ml	1.8 ml
Lidocaine	4.4	2.0	300				
2%				34	36		
2% + 1 : 50 000 epinephrine				34	36	34	36
2% + 1 : 100 000 epinephrine				34	36	17	18
Articaine	7.0	3.2	500				
4% + 1 : 100 000 epinephrine				68	72	17	18
Mepivacane	4.4	2.0	300				
3% plain				51	54		
2% + 1 : 100 000 epinephrine				34	36	17	18
2% + 1 : 20 000 levonordefrin				34	36	85	90

a simple restoration at the first operative visit using basic behavior management techniques of "tell–show–do" and positive reinforcement, the child becomes acquainted with the sensations associated with topical and local analgesia, rubber dam placement, and rotary instruments. Successful completion of the first restoration will build the child's confidence and trust in the dentist; also it will establish rapport and communication between the child and the dentist. Local anesthesia is important for a successful operative visit. A maxillary quadrant should be treated first due to easy and less painful injection of maxillary infiltration. The maxillary anterior region is usually treated last due to the painful injection and to avoid compliance issues mentioned above. It is advisable to avoid extraction in the first operative visit if possible to ease the child into clinical dentistry. If a patient presents with many asymptomatic large carious lesions, interim restorations with glass ionomer after gross excavation without local anesthesia can be performed at the initial visit to slow down caries progression and avoid pain induced by food impaction. Then the treatment of these teeth can be incorporated into a quadrant or side dentistry treatment planning. The use of glass ionomer as temporary restoration for caries control has been shown to be valuable in assessing pulp vitality of those teeth with signs of reversible pulpitis (Vij et al. 2004).

iv. Orthodontic treatment plan

Space maintenance or other orthodontic care should only be considered when all restorative treatment is complete and the patient and parent demonstrate that they are able to maintain good oral health. The details of orthodontic treatment planning in pediatric patients are discussed in Chapter 15.

v. Behavior management plan

A positive attitude and acceptance toward dental care throughout life is influenced by a person's dental experience during childhood. In pediatric dentistry, the main goal of any treatment plan is to find the most efficient way of completing all the necessary restoration in the fewest number of visits, but at the same time managing the child's behavior in such a way that all dental care is readily accepted (Curzon et al. 1996). The ability to lead the child through a pleasant dental experience is a fundamental skill for a pediatric dentist or a dentist who is treating the pediatric population. In most cases, a dentist should be able to manage the child's behavior and provide dental care at the highest standard by using basic behavior management techniques. However, when a child is "impossible to control" and resistant to treatment, the dentist may have to refer the child to another dentist, preferably a specialist pediatric dentist, where advanced behavior guidance techniques, such as protective stabilization, sedation, and general anesthesia, are available. The interaction and communication between a child and a dentist is unique, therefore there should not be rigid rules regarding the use of different behavior guidance techniques. Behavior guidance is more of an art than a science. To master the art of behavior guidance, one needs constant practice and reevaluation, effective communication skills and a keen eye for observation.

Behavior assessment should be done and documented based on the behavior rating scale during an initial exam visit. A behavior management plan should be included in the comprehensive treatment planning especially when operative treatment needs are indicated. The key of the behavior management plan should be preventing behavior problems to achieve a positive experience for both the child and the parent. Most commonly used basic traditional behavior guidance techniques, such as communication, euphemisms, tell–show–do, positive reinforcement, distraction, voice control and non-verbal communication, are usually incorporated in every visit and can be used in any patient. Details of these techniques are explained in several textbooks and AAPD guidelines and some practical tips for basic behavior management are summarized as below:

- When communicating, the dentist should speak directly to the child and maintain eye contact.
- When giving instructions to a child, the dentist should use language in terms that they can understand and be concise.
- Age appropriate euphemisms should be used to create a more relaxed environment.
- Tell–show–do is the key for behavior shaping. The dentist should explain the procedure to be performed and the sensations that the child should expect to child to build trust and confidence.
- Following directions and appropriate behavior should be positively reinforced by praising, which makes the child more likely to repeat the behavior.
- Inappropriate behavior should be calmly discouraged or ignored, which reduce the likelihood of similar behavior in the future.
- Voice control is a controlled alteration of voice volume, tone, or pace to influence and direct the patient's behavior (AAPD). Its usage should be explained to the parents to avoid misunderstanding due to its possible aversive effect.

- Distraction can be done by singing, story-telling by the dentist or the dental assistant, or utilizing the state-of-art equipment, such as TV over the dental chair.
- Modeling can be considered when a sibling shows appropriate behavior.
- A set of rules should be established and reinforced during the appointment so that the child understands the limits of acceptable behavior.
- A calm, confident dentist with a positive attitude gives the child a sense of security which increases the likelihood of positive behavior.
- The organization and readiness for each visit presents a professional image of the dental team to the patient and the parents.
- Scheduling younger patients for operative appointment in the morning is usually beneficial since they are more likely to be attentive and behave better earlier during the day.

In many cases, nitrous oxide/oxygen inhalation is included in behavior management plans to reduce anxiety, enhance effective communication, increase tolerance for longer operative appointments and reduce gagging. Nitrous oxide is fast-acting and non-invasive and usually very well accepted by both the child and the parent. However, it cannot be used in the patients who cannot tolerate a nasal hood or breathe through the nose due to age, lack of cooperation ability or disability, or certain medical conditions, such as middle ear infections. Detailed information concerning the indications, contraindications, and additional clinical considerations may be found in many textbooks and AAPD guidelines.

The presence or absence of the parent during treatment has been a controversial topic for years among practitioners and parents. Parental presence can be beneficial and is encouraged when the patient is very young (up to four years old) or is disabled. Under these circumstances, the parent can be a great asset in supporting and communicating with the child. However, when patients grow older and mature, it is becoming increasingly important to establish a more direct dentist–child instead of dentist–parent relationship. The advocates supporting parental absence believe that parental presence may create a barrier in developing a rapport between the dentist and the child, may distract the child's attention from the dentist, may distract the dentist's attention from the child, and may make the dentist less relaxed. However, there are the benefits of parental presence, such as witnessing the dentist's positive approach, witnessing the child's behavior and rapid feedback and gaining informed consent from the parents when needed. The dentist should be aware that the parent's desire to be present during treatment has changed drastically in recent years and he/she should consider parent's desire and wishes while taking into account the benefits and drawbacks resulting from the decision. It is important that the dentist develops an office policy on this topic and discusses it openly with the parent prior to the treatment. More and more dentists allow parental presence during treatment with the agreement that the parent acts as a silent observer who is willing to extend effective support when asked and to leave when their behavior is interfering with treatment.

The commonly used advanced behavior guidance techniques include protective stabilization, sedation, and general anesthesia. Appropriate use of these techniques requires additional training through a residency program or an extensive continuing education course. Protective stabilization is an aversive behavior management technique, and its usage has been a topic of concern. The dentist needs to keep in mind that protective stabilization can only be used to ensure the safety of patient, the parent and the dental team, to perform urgent and limited exam or treatment in a uncooperative patient due to lack of maturity or mental or physical disability, or to reduce untoward movement during sedation. Patient stabilization should never be done in a cooperative patient or a potentially cooperative patient for non-urgent care requiring lengthy appointments. The tightness and duration of the stabilization must be monitored to avoid restricting circulation or respiration. An informed consent must be obtained and documented prior to use of this technique. The use of sedation and general anesthesia is not covered in this chapter.

Adequate pain control using local anesthesia is important to allow the completion of an operative appointment within a reasonable amount of time. Most children can tolerate a long appointment as long as sufficient anesthesia is achieved. It is highly recommended that topical anesthesia gel to the mucous membrane be used prior to the injection. The most commonly used topical anesthetic agent is 20% benzocaine, which is available in the form of gel and is pleasant tasting with different flavors to choose from. It is advisable to have two or more different flavors available in the office, thus the choice of which flavor to use can be made by the child. By giving the power of making this decision to the child, he/she can feel a sense of control and participation. The most commonly

used injectable local anesthetic agents are listed in Table 14.13. The details of the different techniques for local analgesia in children have been described in many textbooks. The overall approach in local anesthesia injection in children is the careful explanation throughout the process in language the child can understand. The simple language and euphemisms, such as "put the tooth to sleep with magic sleepy juice," "you will feel a little pinch like a mosquito bite," is appropriate to use. Use of warmed analgesic agents and slow administration of the injections are also helpful in easing the discomfort associated with injection. Traditional behavior management techniques such as distraction and positive reinforcement should also be used during the injection. Local anesthesia is one of the most critical moments during the dental appointment. Successful management of the child patient during this process is essential in earning the child's trust and establishing rapport. Self-induced postoperative soft tissue injury is not uncommon in young children; behavioral precautions, such as do not bite or suck on lip/cheek, should be discussed. The child may associate the pain and discomfort triggered by this type of injury with the dental appointment, thus showing avoidance behaviors at the subsequent visits.

II. Parental discussion

A treatment plan cannot be completed successfully without parental understanding and support. It is important that the full details of the complete treatment plan be discussed with the parents, including the choice of the restorations; especially when aesthetics concerns are involved, the use of local anesthetic agents, the use of nitrous oxide, the proposed preventive measurement at home, as well as the number of visits needed and the duration of time period needed. This conversation helps the parent to understand the intent of the treatment plan, and also facilitates the dentist to understand the parental expectations and concerns. A parent is more likely to accept a treatment plan which addresses his/her concerns; however, unrealistic expectations from the parents should not be ignored by the dentist as well. Healthy and effective communication between the dentist and the parent based on mutual understanding is critical for risk management and informed consent. In the area of patient management, when certain aversive behavior management techniques are required, such as physical restraint by the parent or a papoose board, or voice control, an informed consent is necessary and should be documented in the patient's record.

14.4 Risk Based, Age Appropriate Diagnosis and Treatment Planning

I. From 0 to 3 years old.

In 1986, the AAPD adopted a position on infant oral health recommending that the first dental visit occur within six months of the eruption of the first primary tooth. In 2006, the AAPD adopted the concept of dental home, recommending that establishment of a dental home begins no later than 12 months of age.

Infant oral health visits are preventive dentistry at its best. It is a unique opportunity for the dentist to start the infant patient from a state free of acquired disease and conditions and keep him/her there. One of the main goals of infant oral health visit is identification and elimination of risk factors before the disease occurs, so that the disease process can be prevented. The dentist should realize that maintaining total oral health is an ongoing process. The

establishment of the dental home at the infant oral health visit is the first step to ensure an ongoing relationship between the dentist and the patient, so that all aspects of oral healthcare can be delivered in a comprehensive, continuously accessible, coordinated, and family-centered way (AAPD).

In the infant's first dental visit, in addition to a general health history, a focused risk-based history aimed at predisposing factors for dental conditions should be included. An infant oral health questionnaire recommended by Texas Department of State Health Services is shown in Figure 14.9. In this form, not only the risks for infectious diseases, such as caries, but also the risks for other preventable dental conditions, such as traumatic injury and orthodontic problems, are also discussed. The risk elements are divided into several categories, including general health, diet and nutrition, fluoride exposure, oral habits, injury prevention, oral development, and oral hygiene.

The oral examination in an infant is different from a typical child oral examination. Usually, the use of dental chair is not required and is not preferred. The preferred exam technique is called knee-to-knee examination (Figure 14.3) in which the parent and the dentist sit facing each other with their knees touching. In this position, the infant is initially held facing the parent, then reclined onto the lap of the dentist. The parent has the infant's leg wrapping around his/her torso, tucks the infant's feet in place with his/her elbows, and holds the infant's hands while the dentist stabilizes the infant's head and looks down for exam. Using this position, the parent is actively involved in the examination acting as an immobilizer, and also has the perfect view of the oral cavity. The dentist should use this opportunity to teach the parent about the infant's oral development and health status, and

Child's Name ———————————————————————— Date ——————

Child's Age ————————————— Child's Date of Birth ———————————

HEALTH HISTORY   Yes   No
Did the birth mother have any problems during pregnancy?   ☐   ☐
Was your child premature?   ☐   ☐
Was your child's birth weight low?   ☐   ☐
Were there any complications at birth?   ☐   ☐
Has your child been ill?   ☐   ☐
Is your child on any medications?   ☐   ☐

DIET AND NUTRITION
Is/was your child breastfed?   ☐   ☐
Does your child sleep with a bottle?   ☐   ☐
Does your child drink from a cup?   ☐   ☐
Does your child walk around drinking from a bottle or cup?   ☐   ☐
Is your child on a special diet?   ☐   ☐
How many times does your child snack each day? _____
How many bottles does your child have each day? _____

FLUORIDE ADEQUACY
Do you know the fluoride level of your water?   ☐   ☐
Do you have well water?   ☐   ☐
Do you use bottled water?   ☐   ☐
Do you use a water conditioner or filtration system?   ☐   ☐
       If yes, please list _____
Do you use fluoride toothpaste for your child?   ☐   ☐

ORAL HABITS
Does your child use a pacifier?   ☐   ☐
Does your child suck a thumb or fingers?   ☐   ☐
Does your child grind his/her teeth day or night?   ☐   ☐

INJURY PREVENTION
Is your child walking?   ☐   ☐
Is your home childproofed?   ☐   ☐
Do you use a car seat for your child?   ☐   ☐
Has your child had an injury to his/her mouth or face?   ☐   ☐

ORAL DEVELOPMENT
Does your child have any teeth?   ☐   ☐
Child's age (in months) when the first tooth came in? _____
Has your child had teething problems?   ☐   ☐
Have you noticed any problems with your child's mouth or teeth? ☐   ☐
Does your child complain of mouth pain?   ☐   ☐
Have any of your children ever had cavities?   ☐   ☐
Have you or your children ever had a bed dental experience?   ☐   ☐

ORAL HYGIENE
Do you clean your child's gums/teeth?   ☐   ☐
Do you use a toothbrush to clean your child's teeth?   ☐   ☐
Do you use toothpaste to clean your child's teeth?   ☐   ☐

Figure 14.9 First dental home oral health questionnaire recommended by Texas Department of State Health Services (Source: Oral Health and the Dental Risk Assessment Questionnaires, Texas Department of State Health Service).

demonstrate oral hygiene. In an infant examination, a healthy oral cavity should be seen in most cases, however, the dentist should be observant about the oral hygiene, the quality of the teeth in terms of hypoplasia and the dental development. The child may cry during the examination. The parent should be informed that it is a normal reaction and useful since his/her mouth is wide open while crying.

A risk profile should be developed based on the risk-focused history taking and a thorough oral examination. Infants with increased risk for caries can be identified using this tool prior to the development of the caries. This group of infants should be subjected to more intense and aggressive preventive and restorative treatment.

Anticipatory guidance is an essential part of the infant oral health visit. It is the complement to risk assessment and covers the six areas of topics mentioned earlier. Dental anticipatory guidance recommended by the Texas Department of State Health Services for infants and children from birth to one year old, and one to three years old are shown in Figures 14.10 and 14.11. The recommendations should be made based on the individual risk assessment to promote the protective factors and eliminate the risk factors. Once a recommendation is made, the dentist should ensure its implementation by reevaluating the issue at an appropriate interval or at the next recall visit.

In spite of preventive measures, dental caries in primary dentition is on the rise. It is not uncommon to discover white spot lesions or even cavitated caries lesion during an infant examination. Example of caries management protocol for one to two-year-olds recommended by AAPD is shown in Figure 14.12. More frequent recall and professional topical fluoride treatment are recommended for high-risk children (every three to six months). Fluoride varnish is usually appropriate for this

age group because its application takes less time, creates less patient discomfort and is well accepted by the children. Fluoridated toothpaste is recommended for this age group if the child is at moderate or high caries risk. A "smear" amount for children younger than two years of age and a "pea-sized" amount for children age two to five years are considered appropriate and may decrease risk of fluorosis. In a compliant household, fluoride supplements can be prescribed based on the guidelines (Table 14.12); however, the fluoride level of the drinking water, and other dietary sources of fluoride (drinking water from day care, beverages, infant formula, etc.) should be carefully evaluated before doing so to avoid intake of excess fluoride. Most white lesions or incipient lesions are managed and monitored by these conservative interventions.

When managing carious lesions in children of this age group, an operative treatment plan can be challenging for many dentists due to the patient's very young age and limited capacity in cooperating for dental treatment in an office setting. In addition to professionally applied topical fluoride treatment, there are several techniques that can be used as temporary measures in managing caries in this age group, such as disking/slicing and ITR (interim therapeutic restoration). Disking/slicing is a technique originally used for relieving crowding in a mixed dentition by reducing the mesial-distal dimension of a primary tooth using a high speed diamond bur. When interproximal incipient lesions are detected at the anterior region with closed contact, disking/slicing can be used to remove the small caries lesion and open the contact to facilitate effective cleaning with a toothbrush and application of topical fluoride on the affected area. This procedure can be done quickly in a knee-to-knee position

DENTAL ANTICIPATORY GUIDANCE

BIRTH – 1 YEAR OLD	
Take Home Messages • Cavities are preventable • Infectious disease • Transmitted to the baby from parents/caregivers	Parents/Caregivers can ensure good oral health for their baby by: ❖ Making healthy food, snack, and drink choices on a daily basis ❖ Cleaning your baby's mouth and the appropriate use of fluoride on a daily basis as directed by your dentist ❖ Regular visits at your dental home starting at 6 months of age
Oral Health and Home Care • Avoid sharing of bottles, cups, pacifiers, and toys to reduce bacteria transmission	❖ Begin wiping the mouth with a soft cloth or brushing with a soft toothbrush twice a day as soon as the first tooth comes into the mouth ❖ Use a very small amount (smear) of fluoride toothpaste ❖ Parents/caregivers need to maintain their own oral health through regular dental visits and treatment, if needed, to reduce the spread of bacteria to their baby that causes tooth decay ❖ Parents/caregivers need to avoid sharing utensils and cups with their baby to reduce the spread of bacteria that causes tooth decay ❖ Parents/caregivers need to check the baby's front and back teeth for white, brown or black spots (signs of tooth decay) ❖ Parents/caregivers need to become familiar with the appearance of the baby's mouth
Development of the Mouth and Teeth	❖ Discuss primary (baby) tooth eruption patterns ❖ Emphasize the importance of baby teeth for chewing, speaking, jaw development and self-esteem ❖ Discuss teething and ways to soothe sore gums, such as chewing on teething rings and washcloths
Oral Habits	❖ Encourage breastfeeding ❖ Advise parents/caregivers that removing the child from the breast or bottle after feeding and wiping baby's gums and teeth with a damp washcloth or brushing the teeth reduces the risk of Early Childhood Caries (ECC) ❖ Review pacifier use
Diet, Nutrition and Food Choices	❖ Remind parents/caregivers never to put baby to bed with a bottle with anything other than water in it or allow feeding "at will" ❖ Emphasize that it is the frequency of exposures, not the amount of sugar and carbohydrates that affects the susceptibility to cavities ❖ Encourage using a cup by 1 year of age ❖ Encourage offering healthy snacks and drinks to their baby
Fluoride Needs	❖ Discuss the family's source of drinking water (bottled versus tap water, filtered versus non-filtered, reverse osmosis, etc.) ❖ Review total fluoride exposure from all sources (water, foods, toothpaste, etc.) ❖ Encourage drinking fluoridated water (tap or bottled) ❖ Consider fluoride needs (e.g. fluoride toothpaste, fluoride varnish, fluoride supplements)
Injury Prevention	❖ Review child-proofing of home including electrical cord safety and poison control ❖ Emphasize use of properly secured car seat ❖ Encourage caregivers to keep emergency numbers handy
Antimicrobials, Medications, and Oral Health	❖ Consider use of antimicrobials as appropriate to prevent tooth decay ❖ Remind parents/caregivers that oral medicines contain sweeteners that can cause tooth decay and to wipe the baby's mouth with a soft, damp washcloth after giving medicines

Figure 14.10 Dental anticipatory guidance for children of birth to one-year-old, recommended by Texas Department of State Health Services (Source: Dental Anticipatory Guidance [E08–12876]; Used with permission from Texas Department of State Health Service).

and under physical restraint with parental permission.

ITR is used when caries control is necessary to restore and prevent further decalcification and caries in young children, uncooperative patients, special-needs patients or when placement of traditional dental restorations is not feasible and has to be postponed (Deery 2005). The ITR procedure is done by grossly removing caries using hand instruments or slow speed rotary instruments, then restoring the tooth with an adhesive restorative material, such as glass ionomer cement.

1 - 3 YEARS OLD	
Take Home Messages • **Cavities are preventable** • **Infectious disease** • **Transmitted to the toddler from parents/caregivers**	**Parents/Caregivers can ensure good oral health for their toddler by:** ❖ Making healthy food, snack, and drink choices on a daily basis ❖ Cleaning your toddler's mouth and the appropriate use of fluoride on a daily basis as directed by your dentist ❖ Regular visits at your dental home starting at 6 months of age
Oral Health and Home Care • **Avoid sharing of spoons, cups, pacifiers, and toys to reduce bacteria transmission**	❖ Remind parents/caregivers of the need to continue regular dental visits for their toddler in the dental home based on updated risk assessment ❖ Review the parents'/caregivers' role in brushing the toddler's teeth and gums especially at bedtime; discuss toothbrush and toothpaste selection ❖ Use a very small amount (smear) of fluoride toothpaste ❖ Review with the parents/caregivers the need to maintain their own oral health to reduce the spread of bacteria to their toddler that causes tooth decay ❖ Parents/caregivers need to avoid sharing utensils and cups with their toddler to reduce the spread of bacteria that causes tooth decay ❖ Parents/caregivers need to check their toddler's front and back teeth for white, brown or black spots (signs of cavities) and the rest of the mouth for swelling, bleeding, and/or changes ❖ Parents/caregivers need to be familiar with the appearance of the toddler's mouth
Development of the Mouth and Teeth	❖ Discuss primary (baby) tooth eruption patterns for toddlers ❖ Emphasize the importance of baby teeth for chewing, speaking, jaw development and self-esteem ❖ Discuss teething and ways to soothe sore gums, such as chewing on cool teething rings and washcloths or teething gels used appropriately
Oral Habits	❖ Review pacifier use ❖ Begin weaning of non-nutritive sucking habits by two years of age
Diet, Nutrition and Food Choices	❖ Discuss healthy nutritional choices for diet and oral health and encourage offering healthy foods, snacks and drinks to their toddler ❖ Emphasize that it is the <u>frequency</u> of exposures, not the <u>amount</u> of sugar that affects the susceptibility to cavities ❖ Do not use sippy cup like a bottle; make sure the toddler is no longer using a bottle
Fluoride Needs	❖ Discuss the family's source of drinking water (bottled versus tap water, filtered versus non-filtered, reverse osmosis, etc.) ❖ Review total fluoride exposure from all sources (water, foods, toothpaste, etc.); encourage drinking fluoridated water (tap or bottled) ❖ Discuss the potential of fluorosis in areas of high natural fluoride content ❖ Consider fluoride needs (e.g. fluoride toothpaste, fluoride varnish, fluoride supplements)
Injury Prevention • **No running with objects in the mouth (toothbrushes, pencils, etc.)**	❖ Review child-proofing of home including electrical cord safety and poison control ❖ Emphasize use of properly secured car seat ❖ Emphasize use of helmets when toddler is riding tricycle or in seat of adult bike ❖ Encourage caregivers to keep emergency numbers handy
Antimicrobials, Medications and Oral Health	❖ Consider use of antimicrobials as appropriate to prevent tooth decay ❖ Remind parents/caregivers that oral medicines contain sweeteners that can cause tooth decay and to wipe the toddler's mouth with a soft, moist washcloth or brush the toddler's teeth after giving medicines

Figure 14.11 Dental anticipatory guidance for children of one to three years old, recommended by Texas Department of State Health Services (Source: Dental Anticipatory Guidance [E08–12876]; Used with permission from Texas Department of State Health Service).

Studies showed that ITR can reduce the levels of cariogenic oral bacteria in the oral cavity (Wambier et al. 2007). Using fluoride-releasing glass ionomer as restorative material is also beneficial for caries management. When using ITR, the parent should be informed of the temporary nature of these restorations and that the follow-up care using topical fluoride and maintaining good oral hygiene are mandatory and important for successful outcomes. Research has shown that ITR is most successful when applied to one surface or small 2-surface restorations (Ersin et al. 2006). Failed restorations are usually seen in cases of inadequate

Risk Category	Diagnostics	Interventions			Restorative
		Fluoride	Dietary Counseling	Sealants	
Low risk	– Recall every six to 12 months – Radiographs every 12 to 24 months	– Drink optimally fluoridated water – Twice daily brushing with fluoridated toothpaste	Yes	Yes	– Surveillance
Moderate risk	– Recall every six months – Radiographs every six to 12 months	– Drink optimally fluoridated water – Twice daily brushing with fluoridated toothpaste – Fluoride supplements – Professional topical treatment every six months	Yes	Yes	– Active surveillance of non-cavitated (white spot) caries lesions – Restore of cavitated or enlarging caries lesions
High risk	– Recall every three months – Radiographs every six months	– Drink optimally fluoridated water – Twice daily brushing with fluoridated toothpaste – Professional topical treatment every three months – Silver diamine fluoride on cavitated lesions	Yes	Yes	– Active surveillance of non-cavitated (white spot) caries lesions – Restore of cavitated or enlarging caries lesions

Figure 14.12 Example of a caries management pathways for 0–5 years old (Source: Copyright © 2020 American Academy of Pediatric Dentistry and reprinted with their permission. The Reference Manual of Pediatric Dentistry 2020:243–247. Available at: https://www.aapd.org/research/oral-healthpolicies--recommendations/caries-risk-assessment-and-management-forinfants-children-and-adolescents/).

cavity preparation, lack of retention and insufficient bulk (Mandari et al. 2003). ITRs should be replaced with traditional restorations when the child is old enough to cooperate with dental treatment or when advance behavior management techniques, such as sedation and general anesthesia, are appropriate and available for patient management.

Most traditional behavior management techniques based on effective communication have limited use in this age group due to their lack of psychological or emotional maturity. Protective stabilization can be utilized with parental consent when an urgent and short procedure needs to be done safely. If a child in this age group has multiple cavitated lesions and needs extensive treatment, definitive restorations placed using advanced behavior management techniques, such as sedation or general anesthesia, should be considered as valid treatment options to override the patient's lack of or limited capacity of cooperation and protect his/her developing psyche. Empirically, general

anesthesia becomes a more cost-effective option when a child needs more than three operative appointments under sedation to finish a treatment plan. General anesthesia provides an optimal environment for high quality dental care and is sometimes necessary especially when all other techniques fail to manage the patient. The details of advanced behavior management techniques can be found in textbooks and are not in the scope of this chapter for reasons mentioned earlier.

In terms of different types of definitive restorations, when multisurface restoration are indicated in these high-risk patients, SSCs should be chosen over class II amalgams and resins due to their higher success rate (Holland et al. 1986). SSCs can be used to restore anterior teeth as well; however, when esthetics are a concern, open-faced SSCs with resin composite facing can be used. Currently, several brands of primary SSCs with tooth-colored veneers are commercially available. Although gaining popularity, the shortcomings of these veneered SSCs include that they are difficult or impossible to adjust for adaption and prone to fracture or loss of facing. Composite resin strip crowns are usually not recommended for the high-risk patient in this age group. Full coverage restoration should be strongly considered in children who require sedation or anesthesia (Seale 2002). A summary and comparison of different options on treatment approach are shown in Table 14.14.

In some cases, severely decayed primary teeth may have to be extracted due to unrestorability or odontogenic infection. The most commonly extracted teeth in this age group are maxillary incisors since they are the most affected teeth by ECC. Clinical experiences and research have shown that early extraction of primary incisors has little effect on masticatory function, speech development and space maintenance. Therefore no treatment on replacing missing primary incisors is appropriate unless aesthetic concerns are raised by parents. If a primary molar is lost prematurely due to severe decay during this age group, an appropriate space maintainer should be considered if the patient is able to tolerate the treatment, can maintain good oral health, and the family has demonstrated adequate compliance to dental care. It is ideal for a space maintainer to be placed within the first six months after extraction; however, often space maintenance has to be deferred in these patients due to their lack of maturity. The details on different choices of space maintainer are discussed in Chapter 15.

II. 3–6 years old

The children in this age group are going through dramatic changes bodily, dentally, as well as cognitively, emotionally, and socially. During this period, the child's dentition is relatively stable in complete primary dentition with root maturation by three years of age. However, permanent dentition is continuously developing and permanent first molars are approaching their eruption. Towards the end of this time period, root resorption of primary incisors can be observed during radiographic examination. At this age group, the child becomes more verbally equipped with a bigger vocabulary, has a longer attention span, gains control over impulses, is able to handle separation from parents and is susceptible to praise.

Although earlier dental examinations have been advocated by AAPD, it is still common that the examination of a three-year-old new patient is his/her first dental experience. New place, new people and new things introduced during a dental examination can be difficult to handle for some patients. Tell–show–do is the most commonly used approach during an examination and well-accepted by most parent and patients. This technique

Table 14.14 Comparison of different restorative treatment regiments for children of 0–3 years old.

	ITR	Sedation	GA
Risk	Low	Increased	Increased
Time	Long-term follow-ups	Multiple visits	One-time visit, limited follow-ups
Esthetics	Questionable	Good	Best
Cost	Lower	Hundreds/visit	Thousands
Success rate	Varies	Varies	Highest
Advanced training needed	No	Yes	Yes

involves the explanation, demonstration, and completion of each step during the examination. The examination should start with a "just fingers" inspection. If this step is well-accepted by the child, it is possible for the dentist to gain trust and cooperation for the use of dental instruments, such as mirror and explorer. The mirror should be introduced first due to its non-threating and familiar appearance. Most children in this group can successfully complete a dental examination by using the above-mentioned approach. However, some of them can still be uncooperative. For these patients, the dentist needs to make a decision on how to manage the behavior. Parental assisted knee-to-knee examination can be performed. A routine examination can be deferred or can be completed in a step-by-step manner over multiple appointments to relieve the child's fear and anxiety by desensitization. Protective stabilization should only be used with parental consent when an emergency exam is needed or the patient's ability for cooperation is limited and has little chance to improve in the future due to medical or mental disability. Risk assessment and anticipatory guidance still are essential parts of the examination visit. Caries risk assessment for 0–5 year-olds recommended by AAPD is shown in Figure 14.6. Recommendations for oral health assessment, preventive services, and anticipatory guidance are shown in Figure 14.8. Dental anticipatory guidance recommendations made by the Texas Department of State Health Services for this age group are shown in Figure 14.13. Assessment of developing occlusion and a systemic facial examination should be incorporated in the routine examination visit, the details of which are discussed in Chapter 15. Prophylaxis can be done using a toothbrush or rotary instrument. Again, starting prophylaxis using things

familiar to the child, such as a toothbrush, is beneficial in building confidence and trust in the young patient. Sometimes, rubber-cup prophylaxis is introduced in the examination visit to evaluate the patient's response and acceptance toward the sensations associated with rotary instruments, which provides useful behavior information for the dentist, especially when operative treatment is planned for this patient. However, attention should be paid to minimize loss of the fluoride-rich layer of enamel by using least abrasive paste with light pressure. Fluoride varnish is still the most commonly used professionally applied topical fluoride for these children, while topical fluoride in gel or foam formulation can be used in the older children in this age group. Towards the last 6–12 months of this time period, eruption of the permanent first molars may occur, the caries-susceptibility of the deep pits and fissures should be evaluated, and the need for sealant placement should be assessed at each periodic visit.

Example of a caries management protocol for three to five-year-olds is shown in Figure 14.14. Using 0.5% fluoride with caution brushing is recommended for patients with increased caries risk due to reduced risk of accidental fluoride ingestion in this age group. When considering the restorative treatment plan for patients in this age group, the basic principle in choosing the type of restoration remains the same. Empirically, if a patient who is four year old or younger has four or more interproximal caries, full coverage restorations such as SSCs should be highly recommended to restore these teeth over intracoronal multisurface restorations due to their superior long-term prognosis, even the carious lesions are small. During the later stage of this time period, whether or not to restore a carious lesion in primary incisors may be dictated by the extent of the root resorption. If exfoliation of the

3 – 5 YEARS OLD	
Take Home Messages • **Cavities are preventable** • **Infectious disease** • **Transmitted to the child from parents/caregivers**	**Parents/Caregivers can ensure good oral health for their child by:** ❖ Making healthy food, snack, and drink choices on a daily basis ❖ Cleaning your child's mouth and the appropriate use of fluoride on a daily basis as directed by your dentist ❖ Regular visits at your dental home starting at 6 months of age
Oral Health and Home Care	❖ Remind parents/caregivers of the need to continue regular dental visits for their child in the dental home based on an updated risk assessment ❖ Review the parents/caregivers continuing role in brushing the child's teeth especially at bedtime ❖ Discuss toothbrush and toothpaste selection and use of a very small amount (pea-sized drop) of fluoride toothpaste ❖ Review with the parents/caregivers the need to maintain their own oral health through regular dental visits and treatment, if needed, to reduce the spread of bacteria to their child that causes tooth decay ❖ Parents/caregivers need to avoid sharing with their child things that have been in the their own mouths ❖ Parents/caregivers need to check their child's front and back teeth for white, brown or black spots (signs of tooth decay) ❖ Encourage parents/caregivers to become familiar with the appearance of the child's mouth ❖ Encourage parents/caregivers to consider dental sealants for primary (baby) and permanent (adult) teeth as indicated
Development of the Mouth and Teeth	❖ Discuss permanent tooth eruption patterns for children ❖ Emphasize the importance of primary and permanent teeth for chewing, speaking, jaw development and self-esteem ❖ Discuss the eruption of the first permanent molars and remind parents/caregivers that a baby tooth will not be lost when this occurs
Oral Habits	❖ Discuss consequences of digit sucking and prolonged non-nutritive sucking (e.g. pacifier) and begin professional intervention if necessary ❖ Discuss consequences of the eating, drinking or sucking on acidic foods such as lemons, limes, sodas, pickles, and acidic powders
Diet, Nutrition and Food Choices	❖ Discuss and encourage healthy choices for diet including snacks and drinks ❖ Emphasize that it is the frequency of exposures, not the amount of sugar that affects the susceptibility to cavities ❖ Emphasize that the child should be completely weaned from bottle/sippy cup and drinking exclusively from a regular cup
Fluoride Needs	❖ Discuss the family's source of drinking water (bottled versus tap water, filtered versus non-filtered, reverse osmosis, etc.) ❖ Review total fluoride exposure from all sources (water, foods, toothpaste, etc.); encourage drinking fluoridated water (tap or bottled) ❖ Discuss the potential of fluorosis in areas of high natural fluoride content ❖ Consider fluoride needs (e.g. fluoride toothpaste, fluoride varnish, fluoride supplements)
Injury Prevention	❖ Review home safety and poison control ❖ Emphasize use of helmets when child is riding tri/bicycle or in seat of adult bike ❖ Emphasize use of mouth guards in sports ❖ Encourage caregivers to keep emergency numbers handy
Antimicrobials, Medications and Oral Health	❖ Consider use of antimicrobials as appropriate to prevent tooth decay ❖ Regular taking of medicines, like asthma medications, can decrease salivary flow ❖ Remind parents/caregivers that medicines contain sweeteners that can cause tooth decay and to brush the child's teeth after giving medicines

Figure 14.13 Dental anticipatory guidance for children of three to five years old, recommended by Texas Department of State Health Services (Source: Dental Anticipatory Guidance [E08–12876]; Used with permission from Texas Department of State Health Service).

tooth is within a year, a small lesion can be monitored, while the tooth with an extensive lesion should be extracted.

Diagnosis of pulp status in primary teeth is discussed in Table 14.11. A primary tooth with diagnosis of normal pulp or reversible pulpitis is a candidate for vital pulp therapy. The most commonly used vital pulp therapy techniques in primary teeth include a protective base, indirect pulp treatment and vital pulpotomy. Direct pulp capping is contraindicated in caries exposure of primary teeth due to its low success rate and can only be used when the involved tooth with limited lifespan. Vital pulpotomy has been the most used therapeutic method to treat vital pulp exposure while/after removing

Risk Category	Diagnostics	Interventions			Restorative
		Fluoride	Dietary Counseling	Sealants	
Low risk	– Recall every six to 12 months – Radiographs every 12 to 24 months	– Drink optimally fluoridated water – Twice daily brushing with fluoridated toothpaste	Yes	Yes	– Surveillance
Moderate risk	– Recall every six months – Radiographs every six to 12 months	– Drink optimally fluoridated water – Twice daily brushing with fluoridated toothpaste – Fluoride supplements – Professional topical treatment every six months	Yes	Yes	– Active surveillance of non-cavitated (white spot) caries lesions – Restore of cavitated or enlarging caries lesions
High risk	– Recall every three months – Radiographs every six months	– Drink optimally fluoridated water – Twice daily brushing with fluoridated toothpaste – Professional topical treatment every three months – Silver diamine fluoride on cavitated lesions	Yes	Yes	– Active surveillance of non-cavitated (white spot) caries lesions – Restore of cavitated or enlarging caries lesions

Notes for caries management pathways tables:

Twice daily brushing: Parental supervision of a "smear" amount of fluoridated toothpaste twice daily for children under age 3, pea-size amount for children ages 3-6.

Optimize dietary fluoride levels: Ideally by consuming optimally-fluoridated water; alternatively by dietary fluoride supplements, in a non-fluoridated area, for children at high caries risk.

Surveillance and active surveillance: Periodic monitoring for signs of caries progression and active measures by parents and oral health professionals to reduce cariogenic environment and monitor possible caries progression.

Silver diamine fluoride: Use of 38 percent silver diamine fluoride to assist in arresting caries lesions. Informed consent, particularly highlighting expected staining of treated lesions.

Interim therapeutic restorations: also may be called protective restorations.[20]

Sealants: Although studies report unfavorable cost/benefit ratio for sealant placement in low caries risk children, expert opinion favors sealants in permanent teeth of low risk children based on possible changes in risk over time and differences in tooth anatomy. The decision to seal primary and permanent molars should account for both the individual level and tooth level risk.

Figure 14.14 Example of a caries management pathways for ≥6 years old (Source: © 2020 American Academy of Pediatric Dentistry and reprinted with their permission. The Reference Manual of Pediatric Dentistry 2020:243–247. Available at: https://www.aapd.org/research/oral-healthpolicies-recommendations/caries-risk-assessment-and-management-forinfants-children-and-adolescents/).

deep caries. Multiple pulp medicaments have been used on pulpotomy with variable success rates reported. Formocresol pulpotomy is the most taught and studied technique and considered as the gold standard. However, increased concerns over the possible carcinogenic effect of formaldehyde after systemic absorption, decreased success rates over time in long-term observational studies, and the possible effect of early exfoliation have made formocresol less desirable nowadays (Coll 2008). Among all the other pulptomy agents used, ferric sulfate and MTA have emerged as promising alternatives to formocresol pulpotomy due to comparable clinical and radiographic success (Loh et al. 2004; Ng and Messer 2008). The superior biocompatibility and high success rate of MTA has made it a preferred pulpotomy agent, while high cost has inhibited its popularity right now. Indirect pulp treatment is another procedure performed in teeth with deep caries, but without signs or symptoms of pulp degeneration. Research has shown that indirect pulp treatment has a higher success rate than formocresol pulpotomy in long-term studies (Vij et al. 2004; Coll 2008) with normal exfoliation time. Therefore, indirect pulp treatment is a valid treatment choice when the pulp is normal or has reversible pulpitis. In the primary tooth, indirect pulp treatment can be done in one to visit; the need for reentering the tooth to remove residual caries is inconclusive according to current literature (Ricketts et al. 2006). As long as the tooth is sealed from bacterial contamination, the chance is good for the caries to arrest, and tertiary dentin to form to protect pulp and ensure pulp tissue healing (Ricketts et al. 2006; Coll 2008). Although indirect pulp treatment showed excellent results in treating normal pulp and reversible pulpitis, it has not been taught or used as much as pulpotomy due to difficulty in diagnosing pulp status in primary teeth, inability to assess pulp status visually and practitioners' long-term confidence in pulpotomy. In any type of vital pulp therapy, the keys for success include accurate diagnosis, careful technique, optimal oral health environment and complete biological seal. The most successful long-term restoration providing an effective seal is a stainless steel crown, especially when multisurface restoration is needed. However, amalgam and composite can also be used if there is sufficient supporting enamel remaining (Holan et al. 2002; Guelmann et al. 2005). The details in all above-mentioned techniques have been discussed in many textbooks and are not in the scope of this chapter.

Pulpectomy is indicated for a tooth with irreversible pulpitis or necrotic pulp. It is a relatively complex procedure which requires prolonged patient cooperation and can be quite challenging for the young patient in this age group. Even though pulpectomy can be successful if performed in teeth with minimal root resorption, most dentists are reluctant to perform pulpectomy and choose extraction and space maintenance over pulpectomy. However this radical treatment may be justified in certain clinical situations even when guarded prognosis is expected. One example is when a primary second molar has irreversible pulpitis before the eruption of the first permanent molar. Pulpectomy is preferred and should be attempted under this circumstance to maintain the tooth in the arch to avoid space loss at least until the adequate eruption of permanent first molar, since a natural tooth is the best space maintainer. When persistent hemorrhage is observed during a pulpotomy after complete removal of coronal pulp, indicating advanced pulp inflammation in radicular pulp, a pulpectomy or extraction should be considered. Extraction is suggested for a primary tooth which is non-restorable, or with signs of severe pulp degeneration such as progressive internal resorption, excessive root resorption, excessive loss of bone support or alveolar abscess. A space maintainer should be considered when a primary molar is extracted. Some orthodontic problems can be observed and treated for children in this age group. The details regarding space maintenance and early orthodontic treatment during primary dentition are discussed in Chapter 15.

Most children in this age group who need minor operative treatment can be managed using basic behavior management technique and nitrous oxide. Unfortunately, when a child needs extensive operative treatment or is not able to cooperate with the dental treatment, use of advanced behavior management techniques, such as sedation and general anesthesia, are not uncommon for this age group. A child older than three years don't usually need a parent to accompany them to the dental chair, however, parental presence/absence should be discussed prior to treatment appointment.

III. 6–12 years old

Many changes happen in this age group. Cognitively, these children become literate, mature, and able to grasp abstract information. Emotionally and socially, they become more aware of their body appearance and peer pressure. Dentally, these children are in mixed or transitional dentition, exfoliation of primary teeth and eruption of permanent teeth are an ongoing process. Close supervision by the dentist ensures a successful transition from primary dentition to permanent dentition. Developing malocclusion is becoming more of a concern of both parent and the child. Referral for orthodontic treatment at an appropriate age should be considered.

By this age, most children are enrolled into school, therefore they are most likely have undergone a dental exam as a requirement for school enrollment. Luckily, most children in this age group should be able to cope with the dental examination with a simply tell–show–do approach. However, when a child of this age group with normal intelligence resists the examination, more significant emotional or psychological problems may exist; further inquiry on history from the parent, and sometimes a referral for further evaluation should be considered. Evaluation of periodontal tissue including selective probing of anterior teeth and permanent first molars and assessment of attachment loss is incorporated into the dental examination. Assessment of developing occlusion is critical for these patients, as they are more aware of their appearance and orthodontic treatment at an appropriate age can be indicated. Risk assessment and anticipatory guidance are still essential parts of the examination visit. Caries risk assessment for children of over six years old recommended by AAPD is shown in Figure 14.7. Recommendations for oral health assessment, preventive services, and anticipatory guidance are shown in Figure 14.8. Anticipatory guidance regarding smoking, substance abuse and intraoral-perioral piecing is included. The school-aged child may be actively involved in sports; the focus of injury prevention counseling is shifted from play safety to sports safety. Also, the child's exposure to sugary diet and access to fluoride may change as he/she enters the environment of school. At this age, the child should have developed the skill in maintaining personal oral hygiene; therefore, oral hygiene instruction should be directed towards both the parent and the child patient. Prophylaxis and professionally applied fluoride treatment are still part of periodic examination visit. Rubber cup prophylaxis is usually readily accepted in this age group. In addition to fluoride varnish, topical fluoride in gel or foam formulation delivered by tray is commonly used as well. With the eruption of permanent teeth, as mentioned for the preschooler group, the caries-susceptibility of the deep pits and fissures should be evaluated and the need for sealant placement should be assessed at each periodic visit. Towards the end of this time period, the child is mature enough to participate in decision-making on his/her treatment. It is beneficial for the relationship between the dentist and the patient if the child's opinion and concerns are respected and addressed, in addition, the child is taking a more active role in his/her care.

An example of a caries management protocol for children over six years old is shown in Figure 14.15. It is similar to the protocol proposed for three to five year olds. Use of xylitol is introduced

| Risk Category | Diagnostics | Interventions | | | Restorative |
		Fluoride	Dietary Counseling	Sealants	
Low risk	– Recall every six to 12 months – Radiographs every 12 to 24 months	– Drink optimally fluoridated water – Twice daily brushing with fluoridated toothpaste	Yes	Yes	– Surveillance
Moderate risk	– Recall every six months – Radiographs every six to 12 months	– Drink optimally fluoridated water – Twice daily brushing with fluoridated toothpaste – Fluoride supplements – Professional topical treatment every six months	Yes	Yes	– Active surveillance of non-cavitated (white spot) caries lesions – Restore of cavitated or enlarging caries lesions
High risk	– Recall every three months – Radiographs every six months	– Drink optimally fluoridated water – Brushing with 0.5 percent fluoride gel/paste – Professional topical treatment every three months – Silver diamine fluoride on cavitated lesions	Yes	Yes	– Active surveillance of non-cavitated (white spot) caries lesions – Restore of cavitated or enlarging caries lesions

Notes for caries management pathways tables:

Twice daily brushing: Parental supervision of a "smear" amount of fluoridated toothpaste twice daily for children under age 3, pea-size amount for children ages 3-6.

Optimize dietary fluoride levels: Ideally by consuming optimally-fluoridated water; alternatively by dietary fluoride supplements, in a non-fluoridated area, for children at high caries risk.

Surveillance and active surveillance: Periodic monitoring for signs of caries progression and active measures by parents and oral health professionals to reduce cariogenic environment and monitor possible caries progression.

Silver diamine fluoride: Use of 38 percent silver diamine fluoride to assist in arresting caries lesions. Informed consent, particularly highlighting expected staining of treated lesions.

Interim therapeutic restorations: also may be called protective restorations.[20]

Sealants: Although studies report unfavorable cost/benefit ratio for sealant placement in low caries risk children, expert opinion favors sealants in permanent teeth of low risk children based on possible changes in risk over time and differences in tooth anatomy. The decision to seal primary and permanent molars should account for both the individual level and tooth level risk.

Figure 14.15 Example of a caries management protocol for children of >6 years old (Source: © 2020 American Academy of Pediatric Dentistry and reprinted with their permission. The Reference Manual of Pediatric Dentistry 2020:243–247. Available at: https://www.aapd.org/research/oral-healthpolicies-recommendations/caries-risk-assessment-and-management-forinfants-children-and-adolescents/).

for this group. Xylitol chewing gum has been shown to be effective as a preventive agent (Scheie et al. 1998; Machiulskiene et al. 2001; Soderling et al. 2001), while the effectiveness of other xylitol products, such as toothpastes and mouthwashes, is still under investigation. Many primary teeth exfoliate during this time period; the lifespan of the tooth as well as the need for space maintenance should be kept in mind when managing caries in primary teeth. If exfoliation of the tooth is expected within a year, a small lesion can be monitored, while the tooth with an extensive lesion should be extracted if space maintenance is not indicated post-extraction. If restorative treatment is planned for a tooth, SSC is still the preferred treatment when the caries lesion involves interproximal surfaces or multiple surfaces; however multisurface intracoronal restoration can be considered if the involved tooth has a limited lifespan. The details regarding space maintenance and early orthodontic treatment during mixed dentition are discussed in Chapter 15.

Management of primary caries on young permanent teeth presents unique challenges to the dentist. While nonoperative treatment strategy is similar to that of primary dentition, and the operative treatment on small lesion is relatively straightforward, treating deep caries in immature permanent teeth can be complicated since the pulp vitality is fundamental to complete root formation, thus the longevity of the tooth. The diagnosis of pulp status is similar to that of primary teeth. Electric pulp test and thermal tests may be helpful in assessing pulpal status of permanent teeth. The commonly used vital pulp therapy techniques are protective liner, indirect pulp treatment, direct pulp cap, partial pulpotomy and cervical pulpotomy. Every effort should be made to maintain healthy pulp tissue and promote apexogenesis. However, when the pulp tissue deems to be irreversibly damaged or necrotic, apexification using calcium hydroxide or MTA, or pulp regeneration/revascularization should be considered. The details of the above-mentioned technique is discussed in detail in many pediatric and endodontic textbooks. SSC should be considered as a temporary full coverage restoration when significant tooth structure loss is noted after caries removal until the patient is old enough for definitive permanent restoration. A challenge a dentist sometimes faces is to treat severely decayed permanent first molars in this age group. When the tooth is unrestorable, extraction is necessary and the choice is clear and easy. However, the dilemma occurs when the tooth is borderline restorable, needs extensive treatment (endodontic, periodontic, etc.) and the treatment prognosis is questionable. Ideally, when the possibility of extracting a permanent first molar is raised, the decision should be made with input from a general dentist/pediatric dentist and orthodontist.

A panoramic radiography should always be taken to assess the patient's overall dental development, including the existence of the third molars, prior to the decision-making. Other than the patient's need for future orthodontic treatment, his/her behavior, the family's financial status and compliance should be also considered during treatment planning. The extraction of a first permanent molar can lead to mesial and lingual tipping of the second permanent molar, distal drifting of the premolars and overeruption of the surviving antagonist first molar. However, if extracted at an ideal time, favorable spontaneous space closure can be expected. As a general rule for the lower arch to achieve a good occlusion, the lower first molar should be extracted when there is radiographic evidence of early dentin calcification within the second molar root bifurcation, which usually occurs within a chronological age range of 8–10 years. In the upper arch, the developmental position of an unerupted second permanent molar generally ensures a good occlusion post-extraction (Thunold 1970; Penchas et al. 1994). When presenting the extraction as a treatment option for the parent and child, risks and benefits of extraction versus restoration should be discussed in detail and possible needs for future orthodontic treatment should be included in the discussion as well.

Common dental anomalies, such as supernumerary mesiodens, which may be diagnosed earlier and under supervision during primary dentition, are usually managed during mixed dentition. Extraction of unerupted mesiodens is usually done when the adjacent incisors have at least two-thirds root development to avoid damaging the developing incisors and allow their spontaneous eruption. Surgical exposure and orthodontic treatment may be required if adjacent incisors do not erupt within 6–12 months (Giancotti et al. 2002).

Early orthodontic treatment and occlusion guidance usually starts at this age group and is discussed in detail in Chapter 15. The dentist should remember that the orthodontic treatment should only be done when the patient is mature and

motivated enough to maintain good oral health.

Luckily, by this age, behavior management become less a problem. The majority of the patients can be managed successfully with basic behavior management techniques and nitrous oxide.

Recommended Textbooks and Additional Reading

AAPD (2011). American Academy of Pediatric Dentistry Reference Manual (2011–2012). *Pediatr. Dent.* 33 (6).

McDonald, R.E., Dean, J.A., and Avery, D.R. (2011). *Dentistry for the Child and Adolescent*, 9e. Mosby Elsevier.

Pinkham, J.R., Casamassimo, P.S., McTigue, D.J. et al. (2005). *Pediatric Dentistry: Infancy Through Adolescence*, 4e. Elsevier Saunders.

References

Coll, J.A. (2008). Indirect pulp capping and primary teeth: is the primary tooth pulpotomy out of date? *Pediatr. Dent.* 30 (3): 230–236.

Curzon, M.E.J., Roberts, J.F., and Kennedy, D.B. (1996). *Kennedy's Paediatric Operative Dentistry*, 4e. London: John Wright.

Deery, C. (2005). Atraumatic restorative techniques could reduce discomfort in children receiving dental treatment. *Evid. Based Dent.* 6 (1): 9.

Dell'Aringa, A.R., Juares, A.J., Melo, C.D. et al. (2005). Histological analysis of tonsillectomy and adenoidectomy specimens – January 2001 to May 2003. *Braz. J. Otorhinolaryngol.* 71 (1): 18–22.

Drury, T.F., Horowitz, A.M., Ismail, A.I. et al. (1999). Diagnosis and reporting early childhood caries for research purposes. *J. Public Health Dent.* 59 (3): 192–197.

Ersin, N.K., Candan, U., Aykut, A. et al. (2006). A clinical evaluation of resin-based composite and glass ionomer cement restorations placed in primary teeth using the ART approach: results at 24 months. *J. Am. Dent. Assoc.* 137 (11): 1529–1536.

Featherston, J.D. (2004). The caries balance: the basis for caries management by risk assessment. *Oral Health Prev. Dent.* 2 (suppl. 1): 259–264.

Giancotti, A., Crazzini, F., De Dominicis, F. et al. (2002). Multidisciplinary evaluation and clinical management of mesiodens. *J. Clin. Pediatr. Dent.* 26 (3): 233–237.

Guelmann, M., McIlwain, M.F., and Primosch, R.E. (2005). Radiographic assessment of primary molar pulpotomies restored with resin-based materials. *Pediatr. Dent.* 27 (1): 24–27.

Holan, G., Fuks, A.B., and Keltz, N. (2002). Success rate of formocresol pulpotomy in primary molars restored with stainless steel crown vs amalgam. *Pediatr. Dent.* 24 (3): 212–216.

Holland, I.S., Walls, A.W., Wallwork, M.A. et al. (1986). The longevity of amalgam restorations in deciduous molars. *Br. Dent. J.* 161 (7): 255–258.

Loh, A., O'Hoy, P., Tran, X. et al. (2004). Evidence-based assessment: evaluation of the formocresol versus ferric sulfate primary molar pulpotomy. *Pediatr. Dent.* 26 (5): 401–409.

Machiulskiene, V., Nyvad, B., and Baelum, V. (2001). Caries preventive effect of sugar-substituted chewing gum. *Community Dent. Oral Epidemiol.* 29 (4): 278–288.

Mallampati, S., Gatt, S., Gugino, L. et al. (1985). A clinical sign to predict difficult tracheal intubation: a prospective study. *Can. Anaesth. Soc. J.* 32 (4): 429–434.

Mandari, G.J., Frencken, J.E., and van't Hof, M.A. (2003). Six year success rates of occlusal amalgam and glass ionomer restorations placed using three minimal intervention approaches. *Caries Res.* 37 (4): 246–253.

Ng, F.K. and Messer, L.B. (2008). Mineral trioxide aggregate as a pulpotomy medicament: a narrative review. *Eur. Arch. Paediatr. Dent.* 9 (1): 4–11.

Nixon, G.M. and Brouillette, R.T. (2005). Sleep. 8: paediatric obstructive sleep apnea. *Thorax* 60 (6): 511–516.

Nuckton, T.J., Glidden, D.V., Browner, W.S. et al. (2006). Physical examination: Mallampati score as an independent predictor of obstructive sleep apnea. *Sleep* 29 (7): 903–908.

Nunn, M.E., Dietrich, T., Singh, H.K. et al. (2009). Prevalence of early childhood caries among very young urban Boston children compared with US children. *J. Public Health Dent.* 69 (3): 156–162.

Penchas, J., Peretz, B., and Becker, A. (1994). The dilemma of treating severely decayed first permanent molars in children: to restore or to extract. *ASDC J. Dent. Child.* 16 (3): 199–205.

Pinkham, J.R., Casamassimo, P.S., McTigue, D.J. et al. (2005). *Pediatric Dentistry: Infancy Through Adolescence*, 4e. Elsevier Saunders.

Randall, R.C. (2002). Preformed metal crowns for primary and permanent molar teeth: review of the literature. *Pediatr. Dent.* 24 (5): 489–500.

Reich, E., Lussi, A., and Newbrun, E. (1999). Caries-risk assessment. *Int. Dent. J.* 49 (1): 15–26.

Ricketts, D.N.J., Kidd, E.A.M., Innes, N. et al. (2006). Complete or ultraconservative removal of decayed tissue in unfilled teeth. *Cochrane Database Syst. Rev.* (3) https://doi.org/10.1002/14651858.

Scheie, A.A., Fejerskov, O., and Danielsen, B. (1998). The effects of xylitol-containing chewing gum on dental plaque and acidogenic potential. *J. Dent. Res.* 77 (7): 547–552.

Seale, N.S. (2002). The use of stainless steel crowns. *Pediatr. Dent.* 24 (5): 501–505.

Soderling, E., Isokangas, P., Pienihakkinen, K. et al. (2001). Influence of maternal xylitol consumption on mother-child transmission of mutans streptococci: 6 year follow-up. *Caries Res.* 35 (3): 173–177.

Thunold, K. (1970). Early loss of the first molars 25 years after. *Rep. Congr. Eur. Orthod. Soc.*: 349–365.

Vargas, C.M., Crall, J.J., and Schneider, D.A. (1998). Sociodemographic distribution of pediatric dental caries: NHANES III, 1988–95. *J. Am. Dent. Assoc.* 129 (9): 1229–1138.

Vij, R., Coll, J.A., Shelton, P. et al. (2004). Caries control and other variables associated with success of primary molar vital pulp therapy. *Pediatr. Dent.* 26 (2): 214–220.

Wambier, D.S., dos Santos, F.A., Guedes-Pinto, A.C. et al. (2007). Ultrastructural and microbiological analysis of the dentin layers affected by caries lesions in primary molars treated by minimal intervention. *Pediatr. Dent.* 29 (3): 228–234.

Welbury, R.R. (2001). *Pediatric Dentistry*, 2e. London: Oxford University Press.

15

Orthodontics for the General Practitioner

15.1 Introduction to Orthodontics

The word orthodontics is derived from the Greek *orthos* = straight and *odon* = teeth. Dr. Edward Angle, considered the father of modern orthodontics, developed the first dental classification of malocclusion in 1890 and designed several different appliances, the "E" arch being his signature one. Since then many trends and technological advances have transformed the paradigms of orthodontics dramatically. This chapter will focus on presenting those trends with particular emphasis on diagnosis and treatment planning.

Objectives of Orthodontic Therapy

The principal objective of orthodontic therapy is to provide patients a balanced and stable functional occlusion and improved facial esthetics. Indications for orthodontic treatment include the need or desire to correct or alleviate an unacceptable dental or facial appearance, maintain a normal growth and development process, improve function, prevent trauma to the occlusion; and to facilitate treatment as an adjunct to restorative, periodontal, or prosthodontics therapy in the child, adolescent, and adult population.

The determination to either provide orthodontic care in the general practice setting

Physical Evaluation and Treatment Planning in Dental Practice, Second Edition.
Géza T. Terézhalmy, Michaell A. Huber, Lily T. García and Ronald L. Occhionero.
© 2021 John Wiley & Sons, Inc. Published 2021 by John Wiley & Sons, Inc.
Companion Website: www.wiley.com/go/terezhalmy/physical

or refer to the orthodontic specialist will depend largely on the personal experience and training of the general practitioner. It is important to remember that when a general practitioner provided orthodontic care, he or she is expected to follow the same guidelines and standard of care as the specialist.

What is a Malocclusion?

Malocclusion is a multifactorial developmental process and may be defined as a disharmony or misalignment of the skeletal or dental components, influenced by cranial base bones, maxilla and mandible, dento-alveolar processes, teeth, growth patterns and muscular forces. Although genetics certainly plays an important role, environmental factors are also important determinants. All of these factors should be evaluated during a comprehensive orthodontic examination. It is important for the practitioner to recognize normal occlusion and normal facial morphology in order to differentiate normal from the abnormal in all the stages of the dentition and provide appropriate therapy or referral as necessary (Figure 15.1).

15.2 Diagnosis and Malocclusion Classification

Medical and Dental Histories

The orthodontic diagnostic process should start with a determination of the patient's chief complaint and whether treatment is sought for functional or esthetic reasons or both. This should be followed by a thorough review of the patient's medical and dental histories. Of particular interest is the patient's drug history. The use of prostaglandin-inhibitors and bisphosphonates may interfere with bone resorption and bone deposition (Zahrowski 2009), while phenytoin, calcium channel blockers and some immunosuppressants such as cyclosporine may trigger gingival overgrowth (Doufexi et al. 2005). Allergies, especially to nickel and latex, are important findings.

Dental factors to consider include the patient's oral hygiene, caries risk, the presence of active carious lesions, history of trauma to the dentition, and periodontal status. Orthodontic treatment of teeth with a history of trauma is best delayed from three months to up to one to two years after the incident depending on the nature and

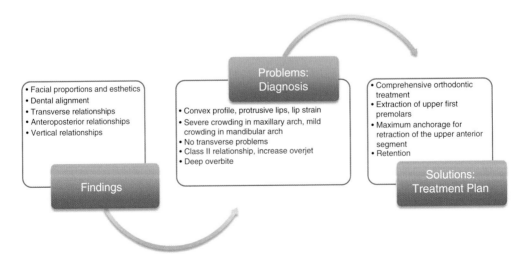

- Facial proportions and esthetics
- Dental alignment
- Transverse relationships
- Anteroposterior relationships
- Vertical relationships

Findings

Problems: Diagnosis

- Convex profile, protrusive lips, lip strain
- Severe crowding in maxillary arch, mild crowding in mandibular arch
- No transverse problems
- Class II relationship, increase overjet
- Deep overbite

- Comprehensive orthodontic treatment
- Extraction of upper first premolars
- Maximum anchorage for retraction of the upper anterior segment
- Retention

Solutions: Treatment Plan

Figure 15.1 Example of the problem-oriented approach to diagnosis and treatment planning.

severity of the trauma (Kindelan et al. 2008). Periodontal considerations include the health of the supporting structures, in particular bone height and crown-root ratio. Possible familial patterns of malocclusion should be investigated.

Current Functional Assessment

It is widely accepted that "function determines form." Deleterious habits (e.g. lip biting, thumb sucking, pacifier use, and mouth-breathing) and muscular forces can influence the growth and occlusion of a patient. A thorough temporomandibular joint (TMJ) assessment should be accomplished to identify any potential underlying discrepancies such as tenderness or pain of the TMJ and/or masticatory muscles.

A determination of the patient's range of motion (ROM) (i.e. maximal mouth opening, left and right excursion and protrusive movements) should be accomplished. Functional shifts between centric occlusion (CO) and centric relation (CR) must be identified because a CO-CR discrepancy may result in a forward or lateral positioning of the mandible and a "false bite" (Figures 15.2 and 15.3).

Comprehensive Orthodontic Examination

This section briefly describes the numerous elements and assessments necessary to accomplish a complete orthodontic examination. Not

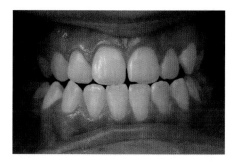

Figure 15.2 CO-CR discrepancy. Patient shows first occlusal contact.

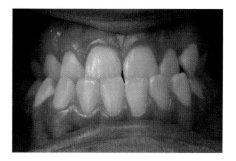

Figure 15.3 Patient shifts mandible forward into occlusion.

every patient will require a full set of records, especially if only limited treatment will be provided, but every comprehensive exam should include a clinical occlusal evaluation.

Extraoral Evaluation

Extraoral balance and facial harmony are considered critical determinants of treatment planning to correct skeletal and dental malocclusions. The extraoral examination should focus on a determination of facial symmetry and profile, vertical and transverse proportions, lip protrusion and smile esthetics. This evaluation should be complemented with extraoral photographs. At least three extraoral views should be taken: frontal, smiling, and profile views. Other photographs such as a ¾ view, a smile close-up view, and a smiling profile view are helpful. Based on the recommendations of the American Board of Orthodontics, the criteria for quality extraoral photographs (Figures 15.4–15.6) include:

- Orientation of the patient in the natural head position.
- One (1) lateral view, facing to the right.
- Two (2) anterior views – one with lips relaxed and one smiling.
- Teeth in occlusion.
- White, or light, background free of shadows and distractions.
- Ears exposed, eyes open and looking straight ahead – glasses and other distractors removed.

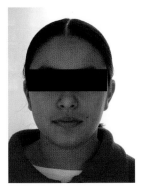

Figure 15.4 Frontal – extraoral view.

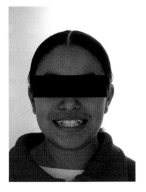

Figure 15.5 Frontal – smiling, extraoral view.

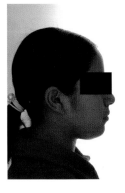

Figure 15.6 Profile – extraoral view.

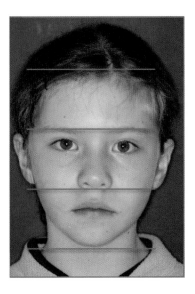

Figure 15.7 Vertical proportions.

Facial proportion is determined by dividing the face into vertical thirds (rule of thirds) measured from the trichion to the glabella, from the glabella to the subnasale, and from the subnasale to the menton (Figure 15.7).

Evaluation of the lower third is particularly important because it is most likely to be affected by treatment. The lower third can be further divided into thirds: one third from subnasale to stomion and two-thirds from stomion to soft-tissue menton.

The rule of fifths, describes the ideal transverse proportions of the face. Application of the concept consists of tracing vertical lines through the inner canthi of the right and left eye, which ideally should be coincident with the alar base of the nose. The medial fifths reflect the widths of the eyes and coincide with the gonial angles of the mandible and the outer fifths are measured from the outer canthus to the ear (Figure 15.8).

In evaluating the profile, facial convexity and the antero-posterior position of the jaws are assessed (Figures 15.9–15.11). Lip position, lip strain, and nasiolabial angle are evaluated since incisal position has great influence on lips position. Lip strain and bi-maxillary protrusion may indicate the need for dental extractions (Figures 15.12 and 15.13). Conversely, if the patient has retrusive lips and an obtuse nasiolabial angle, dental extractions are best avoided.

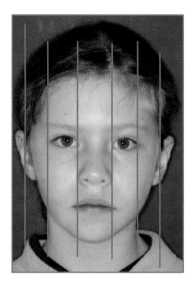

Figure 15.8 Transverse proportions.

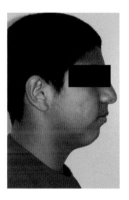

Figure 15.9 Convex profile.

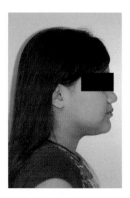

Figure 15.10 Straight profile.

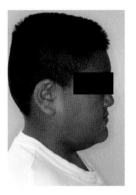

Figure 15.11 Concave profile.

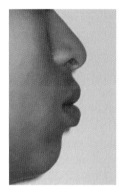

Figure 15.12 Bimaxillary protrusion with acute nasiolabial angle.

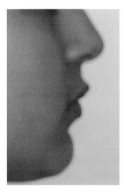

Figure 15.13 Straight profile with normal nasiolabial angle.

Intraoral Evaluation

Data collected during the intraoral examination related to the patient's dental occlusion should include a determination of the angle molar relationship, canine relationship, arch form, overbite, overjet, cross bites, open bites, teeth present or absent, rotation or dental malposition, crowding, spacing, dental–facial midline deviation, and oral health assessment (caries activity and periodontal screening (adult patient).

Clinical data should be complemented with intraoral photographs. At least five intraoral views should be taken: upper and lower occlusal views, right and left lateral views, and a frontal view. This can be complemented with overjet or overbite shots and any other views the clinician deems necessary. Based on the recommendations of the American Board of Orthodontics, the criteria for quality intraoral photographs (Figures 15.14–15.18) include:

- Teeth should be in occlusion.
- Occlusal plane should be parallel to the picture frame.
- Frontal view: there should be equal display of the posterior teeth.
- Lateral views: Anteriorly it should display the entire ipsilateral central incisor. Posteriorly it should display at least the entire first

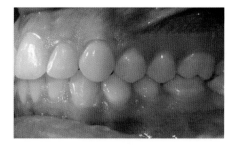

Figure 15.16 Left lateral intraoral view.

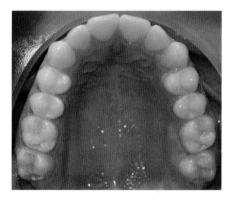

Figure 15.17 Maxillary occlusal view.

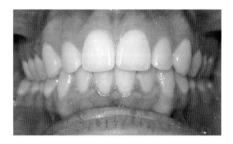

Figure 15.14 Frontal intraoral view.

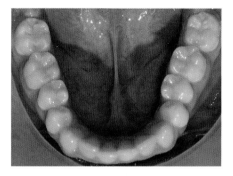

Figure 15.18 Mandibular occlusal view.

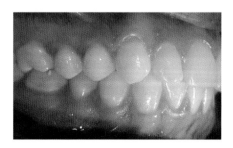

Figure 15.15 Right lateral intraoral view during orthodontic records.

permanent molar. If the image was taken with a lateral mirror be sure to correctly flip the image horizontally.
- Occlusal views: The entire arch should be in the frame and the mid palatal raphe/midline should be centered to the frame; the labial surface of the central incisors should be parallel to the bottom of the frame in the lower arch view.

Predicated on the data collected during the extraoral and intraoral examination, and an assessment of other diagnostic information including:

- Study models.
- Lateral cephalogram and cephalometric analysis.
- Panoramic film.
- Others: selected radiographs such as periapical films, bitewings, occlusal films, posterior–anterior films, cone beam CT, hand wrist films, full mouth radiographic series or other diagnostic records that the clinician deemed necessary.

Study Models

Study models provide a three-dimensional view of the maxillary and mandibular dental arches and their occlusal relationship. Either plaster of Paris study models or Digital (OrthoCAD™, emodel®) models may be used. Data such a metric measurement of arch length, width, symmetry, and shape; as well as tooth size, a determination of the Curve of Spee, and space analysis are more easily obtained from study models. Digital models facilitate Bolton analysis.

When making impressions (alginate or PVC), maximum displacement of soft tissues will facilitate visualization of teeth, supporting bone and soft tissue anatomy. Trimming and finishing of the study models should be according to the specifications of the American Board of Orthodontics (Figure 15.19).

In evaluating the potential orthodontic patient a variety of occlusal assessments or measurements are usually accomplished (see Box 15.1).

Box 15.1 Common Orthodontic Assessments

Arch-length discrepancy
Mixed dentition analysis
Bolton analysis

Anterior–posterior relationships
Angle molar relationship
Transverse relationship
Vertical relationship
Radiographic analysis

Arch-Length Discrepancy (Adult Patient)

Crowding and misalignment of teeth is the most common chief complaint of patients interested in orthodontic treatment. A malposed tooth may be described as: inclined, centrically or eccentrically malpositioned, displaced, rotated, transposed, or a combination of all these characteristics.

Arch-length discrepancy is defined as the difference between the available arch-length and the required arch-length. Available arch-length is determined by measuring the space available from the mesial surface of the first permanent molar to the mesial surface of the first permanent molar on the other side. To determine the arch length required, it is necessary to add the mesiodistal width of all the permanent teeth present. When only one tooth is missing, the clinician may substitute the width of the

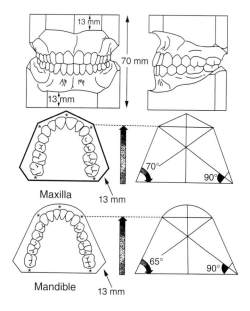

Figure 15.19 Dental cast guide from the American Board of Orthodontics.

missing tooth with the measurement of the contralateral tooth.

Mixed Dentition Analysis

The difference between the tooth size arch-length analysis of the permanent dentition and the mixed dentition is the need to predict the size of the unerupted permanent canines and premolars. Following the eruption of the four mandibular incisors and the permanent molars, arch-length and width dimensions are established and will be very similar to the adult dimensions.

The most accurate method for predicting unerupted tooth size is the Hixon and Old-father Analysis refined by Staley and Kerber (Irwin et al. 1995). It requires study models and periapical radiographs of the lower molars and a prediction graph. The great advantage of non-radiographic methods, like the Tanaka Johnston and Moyers analysis, is that they only require the measurement of the erupted incisors (and in some cases the use of tables); the disadvantage is that they are less accurate.

Bolton Analysis

The Bolton discrepancy, also known as tooth size discrepancy, evaluates the ratio between the widths of maxillary and mandibular teeth. The Bolton analysis consists of a determination of the anterior ratio and an overall ratio. The anterior ratio is calculated by dividing the sum of the mesio-distal widths of the mandibular anterior teeth (from canine to canine) by the sum of the mesio-distal widths of the maxillary anterior teeth multiplied by 100. The mean anterior ratio is 77.2. The mean overall ratio is 91.3, which follows the same methodology but adds the widths of all the teeth from first molar to first molar (Bolton 1958).

The value obtained is compared to the standardized tables to determine the existence of interarch tooth size incompatibilities that could affect the overbite or overjet of the finished case. If the value is reduced, the discrepancy is typically due to disproportionally large maxillary teeth.

Anterior–Posterior Relationships

Overjet is determined by the measurement between two antagonistic anterior teeth comprising the greatest overjet. It is measured from the facial surface of the most lingual tooth (usually mandibular) to the middle of the incisal edge of the more facially positioned tooth (usually maxillary). It is measured in millimeters and can be a positive or negative number like in an anterior crossbite.

Angle Molar Relationship

As mentioned before, Edward H. Angle published the first classification of malocclusion in 1890. The Angle classification system describes the anterior–posterior relationship of the first permanent molars; although it may also be used to describe the anterior–posterior relation of canines and premolars.

An Angle *Class I* occlusion is characterized by the mesiobuccal cusp of the upper first permanent molar occluding with the buccal groove of the lower first molar. Class I occlusion is further divided into normal occlusion and malocclusion. In both instances the relationship between the upper first permanent molar and the lower first molar is the same; however, the latter is characterized by crowding, rotations, or other irregularities.

When the mesiobuccal cusp of the upper first permanent molar occludes anterior to the buccal groove of the lower first molar, the patient is said to have *Class II* malocclusion. Class II malocclusion may be further divided into two subtypes: division 1 and division 2 malocclusion. Both subtypes exhibit the same molar relationship, but differ in the position of the upper incisors:

- Class II division 1 malocclusion – the upper incisors are proclined labially creating a significant overjet.
- Class II division 2 malocclusion – the upper central incisors are tipped lingually and the upper lateral incisors are proclined labially.

In *Class III* malocclusion the mesiobuccal cusp of the upper first permanent molar occludes posterior to the buccal groove of the lower first molar.

Terminal plane: This term refers exclusively to the primary dentition. It describes the anterior–posterior relationship of the second primary molars, and is determined by how the distal surface of the lower primary second molar relates to the upper primary second molar (e.g. flush terminal plane, mesial step, or distal step [Figures 15.20–15.22]). Terminal plane is predictive of the position in which the permanent molars first erupt, the differential growth of the maxilla and the mandible, as well as the late forward drift of the permanent molars (use of leeway space) in the final molar relationship.

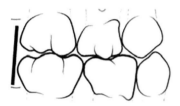

Figure 15.20 Primary dentition molar classification: Flush terminal plane.

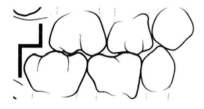

Figure 15.21 Distal step.

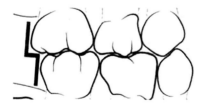

Figure 15.22 Mesial step.

Transverse Relationship

Asymmetric occlusal relationships can result from discrepancies within the occlusion and/or the maxillary-mandibular relationship. Condylar and mandibular trauma may contribute to the development of skeletal asymmetries.

Posterior crossbite describes a malocclusion that involves one or more teeth in which the maxillary teeth occlude lingual to the mandibular antagonist. It is important to distinguish between a dental crossbite and a skeletal crossbite or a combination of both. They can also be classified as unilateral or bilateral. Most unilateral crossbites are bilateral in nature but are hidden by a compensatory functional shift.

Vertical Relationship

Overbite is scored as the amount of overlap of the maxillary and mandibular incisors. It can be measured in millimeters or percentage of overlap of the lower incisor and reported as a positive number.

Anterior open-bite or lateral-open bite describes a space between antagonistic teeth and its location in the arch or teeth involved. It should be reported as a negative value in millimeters.

Radiographic Analysis

Panoramic Radiograph Evaluation Panoramic radiographs offer a broad view of the entire maxillary and mandibular dentition. The clinician should assess all the elements of the radiograph including presence or absence of teeth, root development, root position and parallelism, crown- root ratio, osseous pathology and bone height among others.

Lateral Radiographs and Cephalometric Analysis Broadbent developed the first cephalostat in 1931; it serves as a positioning device that assures the reproducibility of relations between an X-ray beam, the patient's head, and an X-ray film. The principal objectives of the cephalometric analysis are (Jacobson and Caufield 1985):

- Evaluate the underlying anatomical basis of a malocclusion.
- To relate the position of the upper and lower jaws with the cranium, teeth and among each other.
- Identify growth patterns and direction of growth.
- Evaluate soft tissues.
- To evaluate changes during and after treatment.

Anatomical Landmarks The first step and key to an accurate cephalometric diagnosis is to precisely locate the appropriate anatomical landmarks (Figure 15.23).

- **Sella** (S): Center of the pituitary fossa.
- **Nasion** (N): Most anterior point of the frontonasal suture.

- **Orbitale** (Or): Most inferior point of the orbital rim.
- **Porion** (Po): Most superior point of the external auditory meatus, anatomical, or mechanical.
- **Point A** (A): Most posterior point in the anterior concavity of the maxilla.
- **Punto B** (B): Most posterior point in the anterior concavity of the mandible.
- **Anterior nasal spine** (ANS): Anterior tip of the nasal spine.
- **Posterior nasal spine** (PNS): Most posterior aspect of the palatine bone.
- **Pogonion** (Pog): Most anterior point of the mandible symphysis.
- **Gnathion** (Gn): Most anterior and inferior point of the symphysis.
- **Menton** (Me): Most inferior point of the mandible symphysis.
- **Articulare** (Ar): A point in the intersection of the mandibular ramus and the basilar portion of the occipital bone.

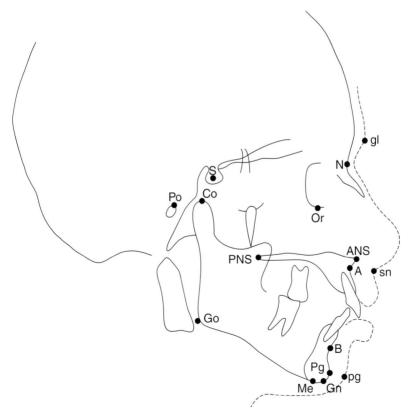

Figure 15.23 Cephalometric anatomical landmarks.

- **Condylion** (Co): Most superior point of the mandibular condyle.
- **Gonion** (Go): Most posterior and inferior point of the mandible, mandibular angle.
- **Glabella** (Gla'): Most prominent anterior point in the midsagittal plane of the forehead.
- **Pronasale** (Pr): Nose tip.
- **Subnasale** (Sn): The point at which the nasal septum merges, in the midsagittal plane, with the upper lip.
- **Stomion** (St): Junction of the upper and lower lip.
- **Labrales superius** (Ls): The median point in the upper margin of the upper membranous lip.
- **Labrales inferius** (Li): The median point in the lower margin of the lower membranous lip.
- **Soft tissue Pogonion** (Pog'): The most prominent point of the chin in the midsagittal plane.

Cephalometric Planes The second step is to score or draw the cephalometric planes described in Figure 15.24 by connecting the defining anatomical landmarks. They will represent a structure or a reference line that will be used to evaluate the spatial relation between structures (Figures 15.24 and 15.25).

- **Sella-nasion** (SN): formed by connecting point S and point N. Represents the anterior cranial base, it is a relative stable structure and is used as a reference point to measure positional changes of the maxilla and mandible.
- **Frankfort horizontal** (FH): formed by connecting Po and Or it is also used as a horizontal reference line to the face.
- **Facial plane** (N-Pog): formed by connecting nasion and pogonion.
- **Palatal plane** (PP): formed by connecting ANS and PNS.

Figure 15.24
Cephalometric planes.

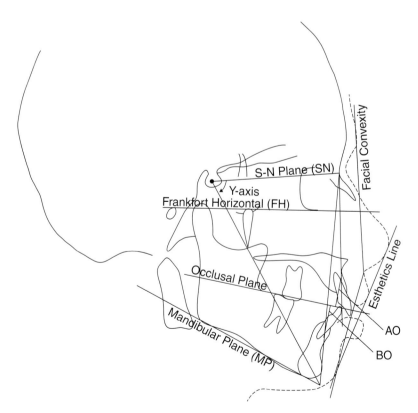

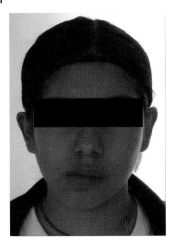

Figure 15.25 Frontal view of patient with laterognathia.

- **Occlusal plane**: formed by connecting the occlusal surfaces of the occluding posterior teeth.
- **Mandibular plane** (MP): formed by connecting Me and Go, it follows the inferior border of the mandible.
- **Y-Axis** (S-Gn): formed by connecting S and Gn, it is used to determine the growth pattern of the patient.
- **E plane (esthetic line)**: Line that goes from the tip of the nose to the tip of the chin.

Cephalometric Measurements and Interpretation

The use of diagnostic software such as like QuickCeph© or Dolphin© will aid the practitioner in tracing planes and measuring angles but remains dependent on accurate landmark identification. Common cephalometric determinants and interpretations include:

Anteroposterior Measurements

SNA angle (82°±2°): Indicates the anteroposterior position of the maxilla relative to the cranial base. High values: prognathism, Lower values: retrognathism, may be affected by the inclination of the craneal base.

SNB angle (80°±2°): Indicates the anteroposterior position of the mandible relative to the cranial base. High values: prognathism, Lower values: retrognathism.

ANB (2°±2°): It represents the anteroposterior relationship of the maxilla and mandible. If within the norm: Class I skeletal pattern. Positive high values 4° or more: Class II skeletal pattern. Negative values: Class III skeletal pattern.

Wit's analysis (female – 0 mm, male – 1 mm): A perpendicular line traced from A-point to the occlusal plane and from B-point to the occlusal plane, relates the position of the maxilla and the mandible, it is measured in millimeters.

Vertical Measurements

SN-MP (32°±4.5°): Angle formed by the MP and cranial base. Measures growth direction. Higher values: Vertical growth. Lower values: Horizontal growth.

FMA (25°±5°): Angle formed by the MP and Frankfort horizontal. Measures growth direction. Higher values: Vertical growth. Lower values: Horizontal growth.

Y axis (SGn)-FH (59.4°±3.6°): Anteroinferior angle that determines the overall growth pattern of the face. High values: Vertical growth. Low values: Horizontal growth.

Y axis (SGn)-SN (67°±4°): Angle formed between Y axis and the cranial base. Will help determine the facial type/growth pattern of the patient

Dental Measurements

U1-SN (104°±6°): Angle formed by the long axis of the upper incisor and SN. Measures the inclination of the upper incisor. Increased value: proclination. Lower value: retroclination.

U1-NA (22°/4 mm±6°/3 mm): Determines the inclination and anteroposterior position of the upper incisor.

L1-NB (25°/4 mm±6°/3 mm): Determines the inclination and anteroposterior position of the lower incisor.

L1-MP (IMPA) (90°±5°): Indicates the inclination of the most prominent lower incisor to the MP, High values: proclination, it value is influenced by the growth direction, forms the Tweed triangle in conjunction with FMA and FMIA.

U1-L1 (130°±6°): Interincisal angle, provides information of the incisors inclination.

Soft Tissue Measurements

Pog-NB (3 mm±2 mm): Millimetric value measured from pogonion perpendicular to NB line.

Facial convexity Gl-Sn-Pog (169±4°): Determines the convexity of the patient's profile. High values: Concave profile. Low values: Convex profile.

E-plane: (LS-E line – 4 mm±2 mm) Indicates soft tissue balance with the lips.
(LI-E line – 2 mm±2 mm).

The analysis of these values will aid the clinician to identify and understand the anatomical basis of the malocclusion in all three planes of space and will also give insight on the patient's skeletal relationship, dental position and inclination; and provide quantitative data on the relationship between soft and hard tissues. The evaluation of vertebral maturation can help assess the growth potential of the patient (Baccetti 2001). This information should be integrated with the rest of the information derived from the other records to reach a final diagnosis.

15.3 Orthodontic Interventions Commonly Accomplished by the General Practitioner

During the primary and mixed dentition the general practitioner should be able to diagnose and offer preventive and interceptive orthodontic treatment. The objective for the practitioner is to lessen the severity or future effects of a malformation and to eliminate its cause. Proposed preventive measures may include localized tooth movement, redirection of ectopically erupting teeth, correction of isolated dental crossbite, space maintenance or recovery of recent minor space loss where overall space is adequate. The key to successful interception is intervention in the incipient stages of a developing problem to lessen the severity of the malformation and eliminate its cause.

Non-nutritive Sucking Habits

Current understanding of child development suggests that sucking behaviors arise from psychological needs. Normally developed infants have an inherent, biological drive to suckle. About 70–90 % of children have some history of a non-nutritive sucking habit. When this habit persists beyond the age of 24–36 months the patient may present with an anterior open bite, posterior crossbite and/or increased overjet (Bishara et al. 2006).

The diagnosis of a sucking habit is established through the medical–dental history and clinical evaluation. Treatment planning should be done with the parent and the patient, since patient compliance is critical for treatment success. Treatment recommendations according to patient's age:

- <36 m. – Assure parent that behavior is acceptable for age.
- 3–4 y.o. – Reminder or reward therapy.
- >4 y.o. – Consider fixed appliance in agreement with parents and patient.

The Crib appliance and Bluegrass appliance are some of the more common appliances used to stop digit sucking habits and can be modified to accommodate a palatal expander in case a posterior crossbite is present. Due to potential relapse, the appliance is usually left in place for at least the same amount or double the time it took to stop the habit.

Space Maintenance

The principal objective for space maintenance therapy is to maintain the mesiodistal relationship of the arch following the premature loss of a primary tooth or teeth and to prevent or reduce the severity of developing malocclusion during the transition from a mixed to adult dentition (Figures 15.26 and 15.27).

Predisposing factors to premature loss of primary teeth include caries, trauma, ankyloses, and ectopic eruption. Special considerations during treatment planning include but are not limited to:

- Time elapsed since tooth loss.
- Status of dental development:
  - Dental age;
  - Predicted eruption–root development of the permanent successor (more than ½ will accelerate eruption, less than ½ will delay it);
  - Amount of bone over successor.

- Congenital absence of the permanent successor.
- Oral hygiene and cooperation.

While the premature loss of anterior teeth does not warrant space maintenance, some appliances have been proposed for esthetics purposes like the Groper appliance. The following tables (Terlaje and Donly 2001) summarize the indications for space maintenance appliances depending on the patient's dentition status (Tables 15.1 and 15.2):

It is imperative that all four mandibular incisors and first permanent molars be present before a LLHA (Lower Lingual Holding Arch) is delivered due to the high potential for obstruction of the eruption path of the lower incisors (Figures 15.28 and 15.29).

Posterior Crossbites

The presence of a posterior crossbite is one of the most prevalent malocclusions observed

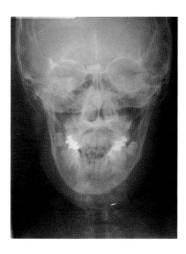

Figure 15.26 Postero-anterior (PA) radiograph of a patient with laterognathia.

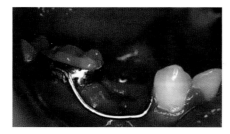

Figure 15.27 Band and loop to prevent mesial drift of second primary molar after early loss of first primary molar.

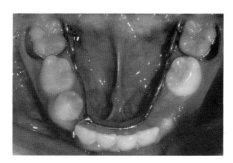

Figure 15.28 Lower lingual holding arch with spur to prevent midline shift.

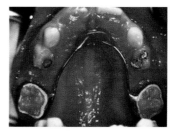

Figure 15.29 Nance appliance after bilateral loss of upper second primary molars.

Table 15.1 ** "Distal shoe and saddle" appliance should be used until the permanent molars are fully erupted; the appliance can be changed to accommodate the one indicated during the mixed dentition.

PRIMARY DENTITION	Unilateral	Bilateral
1st primary molar	Band/crown and loop	Band/crown and loop x2
2nd primary molar	Upper arch = No tx until 6's erupt → Distal band and loop **→ Transpalatal Arch	Upper arch = No tx until 6's erupt → Distal band and loop x2 **→ Nance appliance
	Lower arch = Distal shoe ** →LLHA	Lower arch = Distal shoe x2 **→LLHA
Multiple missing teeth	Saddle appliance **	

Source: Modified from Terlaje and Donly (2001).

Table 15.2 Space maintainers indicated for mixed dentition.

MIXED DENTITION	Unilateral	Bilateral
1st primary molar	No treatment, unless leeway space is to be preserved	
2nd primary molar	Maxilla: Transpalatal Arch	Nance appliance
	Mandible: Lower Lingual Holding Arch	
Multiple missing teeth	Maxilla: Nance appliance	
	Mandible: Lower Lingual Holding Arch (LLHA)	

Source: Modified from Terlaje, Donly (2001).

in the primary and early mixed dentition. It is diagnosed when one or more maxillary teeth occlude lingual in relation to its antagonistic teeth. It is classified according to its etiology and clinical presentation (AAPD Handbook, Nowak and Casamassimo 2011).

- Anterior or posterior.
- With functional shift: about 90 % of the unilateral posterior crossbites will present a functional shift, is also common to have a midline discrepancy.
- Unilateral or bilateral.
- Dental or Skeletal.

Common etiological factors are:

- Constricted maxilla.
- Reduced intercanine width (vertical canine interference, incisal interference).
- Digit habit.
- Mouth breathing habits.
- Dental lingual malposition, crowding.

For a simple posterior crossbite the appropriate treatment is dependent on the age of the patient and the primary etiology:

- W-arch/Quad-helix: (Slow palatal expansion) are recommended during the primary and mixed dentition for dental and skeletal crossbites. Require little to no compliance from patient.
- Hyrax or Hass appliance: (Rapid palatal expansion) recommended for mixed and permanent dentition for skeletal crossbites. It will require moderate compliance from the patient or parents since activation is usually performed at home.
- Removable Schwarz plate: It is more dependent on compliance and has been reported not to be as successful as fixed appliances, indicated for dental expansion.

Early treatment is indicated when a functional shift is present to promote symmetric growth of the mandible and condyles (Kecik et al. 2007). The total treatment length will normally vary from four to six months. The active phase usually ends with the overcorrection of the posterior crossbite; which has been recommended due to the high relapse tendency demonstrated in these cases. The retention phase will follow to allow all the structures to reorganize to their new position and maintain the correction.

Anterior Crossbites

The presence of an anterior crossbite should be identified during the clinical evaluation and it is important to determine if the etiology is of dental or skeletal origin. A general practitioner can treat a simple anterior crossbite due to dental malposition. Complex cases like pseudo Class III or skeletal Class III should be referred to the specialist for further evaluation and treatment planning (Ngan et al. 1997).

If the extraoral and intraoral exam reveal no significant findings other than the anterior crossbite with no arch-length discrepancy the treatment options are:

- Fixed appliance (Bell's appliance) consists of a palatal arch with a finger spring. It is not compliance dependent but intraoral activation might be more challenging to the inexperienced practitioner (Figures 15.30 and 15.31).
- Quad helix with anterior extensions can address both a posterior and anterior crossbite. The appliance has a continuation of the wire pass the midline on both sides. It is a fixed appliance; activation can be done intra or extraorally by removing the appliance followed by re-cementation.
- Removable Hawley appliance with finger spring, is compliance dependent but has little difficulty for extraoral activation.

As with the posterior crossbites (reverse occlusion), it is recommended that therapy be continued for a few months for retention

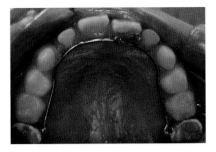

Figure 15.30 Bell's appliance (occlusal view); please note composite stop placed on the lingual of #8 to prevent finger spring from sliding to the incisal edge.

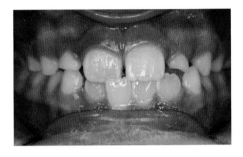

Figure 15.31 Frontal view of the same patient, as shown in Figure 15.30.

after the desired alignment has been achieved. In many cases having a positive overbite and overjet will act as natural retention.

15.4 Management of the Mixed Dentition

The arch width dimensions are typically established in the mixed dentition by about eight years of age, with some minimal increase noted until 13 years of age, followed by progressive but minimal decrease through early and mid-adulthood (Bishara et al. 1997 and 1998). A referral to an orthodontic specialist is recommended when moderate to severe arch-length discrepancies are identified.

Ectopic Eruption of the First Permanent Molar

Ectopic eruption occurs when the tooth erupts away from its normal position. The first permanent molar is the most commonly affected (4% prevalence), followed by maxillary canines and second premolars. The diagnosis is established during the clinical exam due to asymmetry in the eruption of the first permanent molars or during routine radiographic examination. No pain is associated with the undermining resorption of the second primary molar roots.

The cause is often unknown but may be related to an abnormal initial position of the tooth bud, increased mesio-distal width of the second molar or an increase mesial inclination of the permanent molars.

About 66 % of the ectopic eruptions will self-correct and observation and follow-ups are recommended in the six to seven-year-old patient. If the patient is older, severe root resorption is present, or the condition has not improved, intervention is recommended to aid the eruption of the permanent molar in the right position and prevent further loss of arch length and crowding.

Treatment options are:

Orthodontic separator or Brass wire (Figures 15.32–15.34).

Fixed distalizing appliances: Halterman or Humphrey appliance.

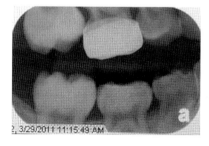

Figure 15.32 Radiographs of an 8 y.o. patient who had ectopic eruption of #3.

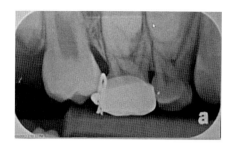

Figure 15.33 Patient was treated initially with a brass wire.

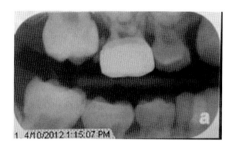

Figure 15.34 Two weeks later the brass wire was replaced with an orthodontic separator which was removed eight days later after correction of ectopic pattern of eruption.

Maxillary Canine Eruption Displacement

The second most commonly impacted tooth is the maxillary canine, with an incidence of 1–2.5 %. Girls are affected more frequently than boys and the canine is usually positioned palatal to its normal location. Some clinical clues that should alert the clinician of the presence of an ectopic erupting canine are:

- Asymmetry between the eruption of the right and left canines.
- Canine not palpable at age 9–10.
- Peg shaped or missing maxillary lateral incisor.

Panoramic film or periapical radiographs should be taken to assess position of the permanent canine in relation to the root of the lateral incisor and its inclination.

Primary canine extraction is the treatment indicated for 10–13 year-old patients, as studies have shown that correction of the canine positioni happens in more than 90 % of cases. If the canine is not overlapping more than half of the root of the lateral, before the age of 10, extraction is normally not indicated (Ericson and Kurol 1988). The presence of root resorption, a complete overlapping of the lateral incisor or central incisor root, or no change in the impacted canine position after initial extraction, should alert the clinician to refer the patient to an orthodontic specialist for evaluation and management to prevent permanent damage to the lateral incisors.

Recommended Resources and Textbooks

Proffit, W., Fields, H., and Sarver, D. (2012). *Contemporary Orthodontics*, 5ee. Mosby Elsevier.

Bishara, S. (2001). *Textbook of Orthodontics*. WB Saunders Company.

McDonald, R., Avery, D., and Dean, J. (2004). *Dentistry for the Child and Adolescence*. Mosby.

Jacobson, A. and Caufield, P.W. (1985). *Introduction to Radiographic Cephalometry*, 8ee. Philadelphia.

Andrews, L.F. (1972). The six keys to normal occlusion. *Am. J. Orthod.* 62 (3): 296–309.

Ngan, P., Alkire, R., and Fields, H. (1999). Management of space problems in the primary and mixed dentition. *JADA* 130: 1330–1339.

Staley, R.N. and Kerber, P.E. (1980). A revision of the Hixon and Oldfather mixed-dentition prediction method. *Am. J. Orthod.* 78 (3): 296–302.

References

Baccetti, T., Franchi, L., and McNamara, J.A. (2001). An improved version of the cervical vertebral maturation (CVM) method for the assessment of mandibular growth. *Angle Orthod.* 72 (4): 316–323.

Bishara, S.E., Jakobsen, J.R. et al. (1997). Arch width changes from 6 weeks to 45 years of age. *Am. J. Orthod. Dentofacial Orthop.* 111: 401–409.

Bishara, S.E., Jakobsen, J.R., Treder, J., and Nowak, A. (1998). Arch length changes from 6 weeks to 45 years. *Angle Orthod.* 68: 69–74.

Bishara, S., Warren, J., Broffitt, B., and Levy, S. (2006). Changes in the prevalence of nonnutritive sucking patterns in the first 8 years of life. *Am. J. Orthod. Dentofacial Orthop.* 130: 31–36.

Bolton, W. (1958). Disharmony in tooth size and its relation to the analysis and treatment of malocclusion. *Am. J. Orthod.* 28: 113–130.

Doufexi, A., Mina, M., and Ioannidou, E. (2005). Gingival overgrowth in children: epidemiology, pathogenesis, and complications. A literature review. *J. Periodontol.* 76 (1): 3–10.

Ericson, S. and Kurol, J. (1988). Early treatment of palatally erupting maxillary canines by extraction of the primary canines. *Eur. J. Orthod.* 10: 283–295.

Irwin, R., Herold, J., and Richardson, A. (1995). Mixed dentition analysis: a review of methods and their accuracy. *Int. J. Paediatr. Dent.* 5: 137–142.

Jacobson, A. and Caufield, P.W. (1985). *Introduction to Radiographic Cephalometry*. Philadelphia, PA: Lee & Febiger.

Kecik, D., Kocadereli, I., and Saatcic, I. (2007). Evaluation of the treatment changes of functional posterior crossbite in the mixed dentition. *Am. J. Orthod. Dentofacial Orthop.* 131: 202–215.

Kindelan, S., Day, P., Kindelan, J. et al. (2008). Dental trauma: an overview of its influence on the management of orthodontic treatment. Part 1. *J. Orthod.* 35 (2): 68–78.

Ngan, P., Hu, A., and Fields, H.W. (1997). Treatment of class III problems begins with differential diagnosis of anterior crossbites. *Pediatr. Dent.* 19: 386–395.

Nowak, A. and Casamassimo, P. (2011). *American Academy of Pediatric Dentistry – The Handbook of Pediatric Dentistry*, Chapter 10, 4e. American Academy of Pediatric Dentistry.

Terlaje, R.D. and Donly, K.J. (2001). Treatment planning for space maintenance in the primary and mixed dentition. *J. Dent. Child.* 68 (2): 109–114.

Zahrowski, J. (2009). Optimizing orthodontic treatment in patients taking bisphosphonates for osteoporosis. *Am. J. Orthod. Dentofacial Orthop.* 135 (3): 361–374.

16

Putting It All Together

Introduction to Treatment Planning

As discussed in Chapter 1, the clinical process is sequentially divided into five main components: (i) data collection; (ii) establishment of the problem (problem list or diagnoses); (iii) development of the treatment plan; (iv) presentation of the treatment plan; and (v) implementation of the treatment plan (Figure 16.1). The intention of this chapter is to provide the fabric for the treatment planning process.

Data collection is the indispensable first step in initiating the clinical process. Interpreting and correlating the database in the light of principles gained from basic biomedical and clinical sciences will lead to the establishment of coherent, defendable, relevant, and timely diagnoses (Table 16.1), which provide the basis for the development of preventive and therapeutic strategies.

16.1 Rational Approach to Treatment Planning

Within the concept of total quality management (TQM), as a treatment plan deviates from optimal design and implementation, its quality (value, outcome) decreases at an accelerated rate. Consequently, in considering preventive and therapeutic options the clinician must consider not only disease-related variables, but such other factors as the availability of material resources (e.g. facilities and equipment); human resources (e.g. the clinician's own

Physical Evaluation and Treatment Planning in Dental Practice, Second Edition.
Géza T. Terézhalmy, Michaell A. Huber, Lily T. García and Ronald L. Occhionero.
© 2021 John Wiley & Sons, Inc. Published 2021 by John Wiley & Sons, Inc.
Companion Website: www.wiley.com/go/terezhalmy/physical

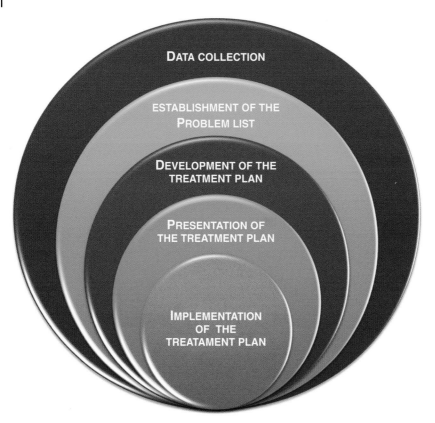

Figure 16.1
The clinical process.

knowledge and technical skills, the availability of an adequate number of qualified support personnel, and a cooperative patient [a patient physically and/or psychologically able to undergo and respond to dental care]); and organizational resources (access to consultants).

The above variables clearly affect outcome and mandate different solutions for identical problems and, at times, may even preclude satisfactory resolution of a specific problem in a given setting. Furthermore, both the clinician and the patient must take into consideration that the treatment of most diseases is predicated on the premise that healing is promoted by modifying the environment of tissues. This, however, requires time. Even if all preventive and treatment procedures were to be implemented on the same day, it would not provide for an immediate optimal healing environment. An effective approach to deal with this problem is to manage disease/illness in phases (Figure 16.2).

Phase I: Priority Treatment

The goal in Phase I is to deal with problems such as pain, infection, trauma, or other issues of immediate concern requiring priority management. The treatment of acute periodontal and endodontic problems, extraction of a symptomatic tooth with hopeless prognosis, biopsy of a suspicious lesion, excavation of caries approaching the pulp and the placement of a temporary restoration, the management of acute mucosal lesions and repairing a fractured prosthesis are all procedures that may be performed in this phase.

Phase II: Disease Control

The goal in Phase II is to arrest or manage disease processes. Procedures for controlling rampant caries, chronic periodontal problems, chronic pulpal problems, elective surgical procedures, preliminary elimination

Table 16.1 Examples of problems/diagnoses requiring consideration.

Systemic problems	Endodontic problems
Restorative problems	Irreversible pulpitis
Reversible pulpitis	Necrotic pulp
Primary or recurrent caries	Acute apical periodontitis
Lost restoration	Acute apical abscess
High restoration	Periodontal problems
Improper proximal contact	Gingival abscess
Tight contact	Periodontal abscess
Open contact	Necrotizing ulcerative gingivitis
Overhang	Postoperative problems
Cracked tooth syndrome	Pain
Trauma	Root surface sensitivity
Injuries affecting hard tissues	Bleeding
Infraction	Injection
Uncomplicated crown fracture	Swelling
Complicated crown fracture	Lost dressing and/or sutures
Crown-root fracture	Increased tooth mobility
Root fracture	Sequestra
Injuries affecting attachment apparatus	Oral surgical problems
Concussion	Nonrestorable tooth
Subluxation	Pericoronitis
Extrusion	Postoperative problems
Lateral displacement	Pain
Intrusion	Bleeding
Avulsion	Alveolar osteitis
Prosthodontic problems	Nerve injury
Missing teeth	Infection
Complete dentures	Air emphysema
Fractured artificial teeth	Soft tissue injury
Fractured denture base	Jaw fracture
Deficient posterior palatal seal	
Removable partial dentures	Oral medicine problems
Fractured artificial teeth	Traumatic ulcers
Fractured base or flange	Recurrent aphthous stomatitis
Fractured metallic connector	Herpes simplex virus infection
Loss of abutment or other teeth	Oral candidiasis
Implant failure	Lichen planus
Fixture fracture	Erythema multiforme
Fastener failure	Xerostomia
	Burning mouth syndrome
	Suspected malignancy
	Temporomandibular disorders
	Socio-economic problems

of occlusal disharmonies, and management of the patient's chief complaint (if not addressed in Phase I) are the activities that are appropriate for this phase.

Phase III: Restoration of Function and Esthetics

The goal in Phase III is to restore function and improve esthetics. Procedures may include restoration of the remaining carious teeth, replacement of defective restorations, and replacing missing teeth.

Phase IV: Reassessment

The goal in Phase IV is to confirm that all problems have been addressed and that no new problems emerged, and to establish an appropriate recall interval for continued

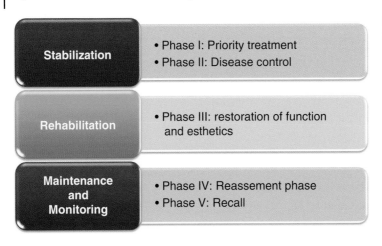

Figure 16.2 Phases of managing disease/illness.

monitoring and maintenance of patients' oral health. A patient satisfaction questionnaire concerning patients' experiences and impressions of treatment and of the treatment environment can provide a mechanism for continued improvement in patient care.

Phase V: Recall

The goal in Phase V is to monitor patients for new or recurrent problems and to implement appropriate corrective and preventive care. Within the concept of TQM, the recall visit also provides an opportunity to evaluate outcomes: (i) the success or failure of preventive and therapeutic strategies; (ii) the success or failure of behavior modification characterized by enhanced oral health–related knowledge; and ultimately, (iii) improved oral health of the patient.

16.2   Putting It All Together

It is important to develop a deliberate pattern of obtaining and reviewing patient information. Similar to a detailed checklist performed repeatedly helps ensure a thorough understanding of all patient factors one must consider in developing a treatment plan and avoid omission of pertinent and relevant mitigating factors.

SUBJECTIVE DATA: CHIEF COMPLAINT (REASON FOR THE VISIT), DENTAL HISTORY, MEDICAL HISTORY

Demographic data –

Age, gender

Chief complaint –

The reason for the visit, a statement of the problem, (character, duration, progression, domain, relationship to function) qualitative description of the symptoms as described by the patient.

Dental history –

Frequency of visits to the dentist
Date of most recent radiographic examination
Types of care received
History of oro-facial injury (date, cause, type)
Difficulties with treatment
Adverse reactions (local anesthetics, latex products, and dental material)

Medical history

Drug allergies or other adverse drug effects
Medications (prescribed Rx, OTC, vitamins, dietary supplements, special diets)
Past or present illness
Last time examined by a physician
Family history
Social history
Review of organ systems

OBJECTIVE DATA: "MEASUREMENTS" TAKEN BY THE CLINICIAN (VITAL SIGNS, CLINICAL EXAMINATION, RADIOGRAPHIC EXAMINATION, LABORATORY DATA)

Physical examination

Vital signs
Head and neck examination (head, face, facial bones, ears, nose, hair, neck lymph nodes, TMJ, salivary glands, neurological deficit)
Intraoral examination (lips/commissures, mucosa, hard palate, soft palate/tonsillar area, tongue, floor of mouth, gingivae, breath, teeth/occlusion/periodontal status

Consultations

Medical
Dental

ASSESSMENT: DIAGNOSIS DERIVED FROM SUBJECTIVE AND OBJECTIVE DATA (PROBLEM LIST, REASON FOR THERAPEUTIC INTERVENTION)

Problem list
Treatment plan

Phase I
Phase II
Phase III
Phase IV
Phase V

16.3 Presentation of the Treatment Plan

Once a treatment plan (with alternative treatment options) has been developed, it must be communicated to the patient or guardian in a clear and concise manner. The purpose of the case presentation is to provide clinicians with the opportunity to discharge their "duty of disclosure" and for patients to obtain the necessary information essential to exercise their right of "self-determination."

Informed Consent

In order to make informed choices, patients need to know their rights as patients. Those rights include the doctrine of informed consent. Before undergoing any oral healthcare–related procedure, patients are legally entitled to an explanation (in terms and phrases that they understand) of the plan so that they can give what is called "informed consent." In those cases in which the patient is unconscious or in some emergency situations, informed consent is implied.

Obtaining informed consent means that patients are given an opportunity to take an active role in the decision-making process that will affect their oral health. It provides an opportunity for patients to become informed oral healthcare consumers.

Step 1

The problem list or diagnostic summary is to be presented to patients and/or guardians in understandable terms. This will set the stage for a discussion of the patient's health status (both systemic and oral) and provide an opportunity to educate patients about the etiology, severity, and prognosis associated with each problem.

Step 2

Discuss with patients various treatment options (including the availability of additional diagnostic tests and procedures), potential benefits of the treatment recommended, possible negative outcomes of the proposed treatment, the probability of success (good outcome), and the consequences of not treating a problem.

Step 3

Inform patients of the time required to complete treatment, the cost for the services recommended, as well as the costs of alternative options. Patients have the right not only to ask questions about the costs of recommended services, but to make choices about their oral healthcare. Articulate clearly that exercising these rights also means that patients assume some responsibility for the success of the clinical process.

Step 4

To maximize the effectiveness of proposed preventive and therapeutic interventions, ensure that patients have an unequivocal understanding of their responsibility to follow the recommendations they have agreed to. It is also the patients' responsibility to provide feedback to the clinician about any problems or concerns that may arise while under treatment. In this context, the principle of "due care," patients performing their role in the clinical process, applies. Patients' failure to participate in the process, to the best of their physical and cognitive ability, constitutes negligence on their part.

Step 5

Educate patients about the dynamic nature of treatment plans. They should understand that as the sequential phases of the treatment plan are implemented, initial therapeutic interventions may provide additional data relevant to the true nature and extent of the problem, occult disease may become overt, and patient response to treatment and the effectiveness of preventive care may all mandate modification of the initial treatment plan.

Step 6

At the end of the case presentation patients should be provided an informed consent form for their signature. This is to certify that they understand the reason for the treatment; that they had an opportunity to discuss the treatment plan, including costs, and alternative treatment options, with the clinician; and that they understand that there may be variations in treatment and costs if new findings are made.

16.4 Consultations and Referrals

Once a patient–doctor relationship has been established and the clinician has agreed to treat a patient, the practitioner is obligated to conduct the management of that patient's illness with "due care." Failure to render due care constitutes negligence. Negligence is the legal term for omission of care either by failure to diagnose or to adequately treat. This clearly implies that clinicians also have an obligation to seek consultation with or initiate referral to other healthcare providers whenever the welfare of the patient might be safeguarded or advanced by having recourse to those who have special skills, knowledge, and experience. Table 16.2 summarizes the various reasons why the primary clinician may initiate the consultation or referral process.

Consultation is an act of deliberation between healthcare providers related to a diagnosis or its treatment. A consultant may either be asked to give professional advice (opinion) or to provide a service. Consequently, consultation provides access to expert knowledge, sophisticated procedures, quality patient management, and patient reassurance.

Role of a Consultant in the Consultation Process

If the request is for professional advice (opinion), the authority for the patient's

Table 16.2 Reasons for consultations or referrals.

1. The diagnosis is uncertain.

2. There is doubt as to the physical and/or emotional ability of the patient to undergo and respond to dental care.

3. Managing the condition of the patient is not within the field of training of the primary clinician.

4. The primary clinician is knowledgeable about the patient's condition and its treatment but believes that a specialist is better prepared to manage the problem.

5. The patient's condition is not responding to treatment.

6. The patient or his or her agent requests a second opinion.

management is retained by the primary clinician. He or she retains full responsibility, including legal, for the welfare of the patient. The consultant assumes no direct authority in the management of the patient and is not required to write orders.

Role of the Consultant in the Referral Process

If the consultant is asked to provide a service, authority for the patient's management is transferred to the consultant with a mutually clear understanding of the purpose and duration of the referral. The consultant assumes full responsibility, including legal, for the patient's welfare. If the consultant believes that additional consultations are warranted, it must be communicated to the primary clinician before further action is taken.

Role of the Patient in the Consultation/Referral Process

The patient is an interested party in the consultation or referral process, but the choice of the consultant should not be left entirely up to the patient. Inform the patient of the reason for the consultation. Brief the patient regarding events that may occur while the patient is in the care of the consultant. Provide the patient insight into the mannerisms and personality of the consultant. Establish uniform definitions that are understood by all (the primary clinician, the consultant, and the patient).

Role of the Primary Clinician in the Consultation and Referral Process

Initiating the Consultation or Referral Process

The office of the primary clinician must coordinate the appointment with the consultant and ensure that the patient has an appointment and that it is scheduled in an appropriate time frame. In routine situations there is no particular immediacy. The appointment may be scheduled at the convenience of both the consultant and the patient.

In urgent situations, a diagnosis should be established and/or treatment initiated fairly rapidly. The patient should be seen in a matter of days. In emergency situations, the gravity of the problem must be clearly explained to the patient and the consultant. The patient should be seen within a matter of hours.

Monitoring the Consultation and Referral Process

The primary clinician has an obligation to monitor the status of the consultation and referral process. A patient may not show up for the scheduled appointment. Likewise, the consultant may be slow in rendering an opinion or in providing a summary of services rendered. When there is a difference of opinion between the primary clinician and the consultant, the problem should be resolved out of earshot of the patient. If there is strong disagreement concerning the diagnosis or the proposed treatment, the patient must be given both opinions and an option for further consultation.

Documenting the Consultation and Referral Process

In the consultation and referral process, the request from the primary clinician and the opinion rendered or a summary of services provided by the consultant should be in writing. The consultation document is an official permanent record. While written as a confidential doctor-to-doctor communication, the consultation document is also available to the patient and others (e.g. peers and insurance companies) for review. Proper utilization and preservation of information in the consultation process are ensured by appropriate documentation methods, which, as in all aspects of the clinical process, should follow the problem-oriented method of record keeping.

16.5 Conclusion

Privileges given to clinicians by society and by patients are quite remarkable. Clinicians are permitted to ask searching personal questions, listen to personal secrets, and touch, manipulate, and explore another individual's body. It is evident that a clinician with proper credentials from society, and consent from a patient, is permitted actions accorded no other individual. With these privileges comes the responsibility to think clearly (professionalism, clinical judgment), act decisively (timely diagnosis and treatment), and care tenderly (sensitive to and considerate of patients' feelings).

The combination of privilege and responsibility mandates the establishment of a patient-doctor relationship that is to clearly benefit the patient and not one that is disguised as a means of rewarding a clinician's own need for approval or advantage. The characteristic that distinguishes, promotes, and maintains a healthy patient–doctor relationship is adherence to the principles of (i) "duty of disclosure" by the clinician; (ii) "self-determination" by the patient; and (iii) "due care" in the clinical process, both by the clinician and the patient.

Suggested Reading

American Dental Association (2007). ADA Council on Dental Practice, Division of Legal Affairs. Dental records. www.ada.org (accessed 17 December 2020).

Appelbaum, P.S. (2007). Assessment of patients' competence to consent to treatment. *N. Engl. J. Med.* 357 (18): 1834–1840.

Sfikas, P.M. (2006). Informed consent. How performing a less invasive procedure led to a claim of battery. *JADA* 137: 101–103.

Index

Physical Evaluation and Treatment Planning in Dental Practice, Second Edition.
Géza T. Terézhalmy, Michaell A. Huber, Lily T. García and Ronald L. Occhionero.
© 2021 John Wiley & Sons, Inc. Published 2021 by John Wiley & Sons, Inc.
Companion Website: www.wiley.com/go/terezhalmy/physical